NIH: An Account of Research in Its Laboratories and Clinics

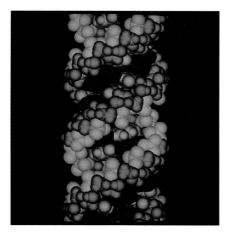

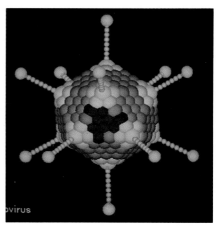

1. RNA helix modeled from fiber diffraction data, with base pairs in red and pink, backbone in gray and white.

2. ADENOVIRUS from electron micrograph data showing typical plate of nine proteins in red.

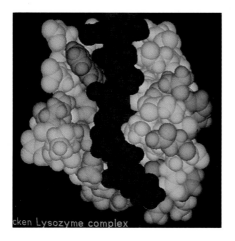

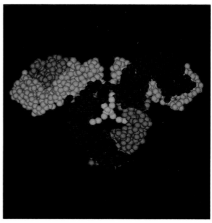

3. LYSOZYME section from crystallographic data, showing active site with sugar substrate in place (red).

4. IMMUNOGLOBULIN-G from crystallographic data, with heavy chains in red and blue, light chains in green.

MACROMOLECULES OF (1) a nucleic acid, (2) a virus, (3) an enzyme, and (4) an antibody as illustrated by means of a computer. On instruction by RICHARD J. FELDMAN of the NIH Division of Computer Research and Technology, a DEC PDP-11/70 computer, using Evans and Sutherland displays, converts data obtained by X-ray crystallography and other means into images in which atoms (or larger aggregates: amino acids in image 4) are simulated in perspective and color coded. Structures containing up to 10,000 atoms can be depicted and manipulated. See Pratt chapter, "Computers in Research."

NIH: An Account of Research in Its Laboratories and Clinics

Editor

DeWitt Stetten, Jr.

Office of the Director
National Institutes of Health
Bethesda, Maryland

Associate Editor

W. T. Carrigan

Office of the Director
National Institutes of Health
Bethesda, Maryland

1984

ACADEMIC PRESS, INC.
(Harcourt Brace Jovanovich, Publishers)
Orlando   San Diego   New York   London
Toronto   Montreal   Sydney   Tokyo

Academic Press Rapid Manuscript Reproduction

The National Institutes of Health does not necessarily endorse any opinions or judgments expressed in this book.

ACADEMIC PRESS, INC.
Orlando, Florida 32887

United Kingdom Edition published by
ACADEMIC PRESS, INC. (LONDON) LTD.
24/28 Oval Road, London NW1 7DX

Library of Congress Cataloging in Publication Data

Main entry under title:

NIH: An account of research in its laboratories and clinics.

Includes index.
1. Medicine--Addresses, essays, lectures. 2. Medicine
--Research--United States--Addresses, essays, lectures.
3. National Institutes of Health (U.S.)--Addresses, essays,
lectures. I. Stetten, DeWitt, Date   . II. Carrigan,
W. T. [DNLM: 1. National Institutes of Health (U.S.)
2. Laboratories. 3. Research--United States. W 20.5 L123]
RA11.D6L33   1984   610   83-45576
ISBN 0-12-667980-0 (alk. paper)   **117267**

PRINTED IN THE UNITED STATES OF AMERICA

85 86 87 88   9 8 7 6 5 4 3 2

To Marney

(Marjorie Roloff Stetten, Ph.D.)

1915–1983

For many years an intramural research scientist at NIH,
she gave stalwart support to the ideas and ideals
expressed in this work.

Contents

Contributors

Numbers in parentheses indicate the pages on which the authors' contributions begin.

Robert S. Adelstein (277), National Heart, Lung, and Blood Institute, National Institutes of Health, Bethesda, Maryland 20205

W. French Anderson (297), National Heart, Lung, and Blood Institute, National Institutes of Health, Bethesda, Maryland 20205

C. B. Anfinsen (257), Department of Biology, The Johns Hopkins University, Baltimore, Maryland 21218

Edwin D. Becker (443), Office of the Director, National Institutes of Health, Bethesda, Maryland 20205

John G. Bieri (71), National Institute of Arthritis, Diabetes, and Digestive and Kidney Diseases, National Institutes of Health, Bethesda, Maryland 20205

Roscoe O. Brady (324), National Institute of Neurological and Communicative Disorders and Stroke, National Institutes of Health, Bethesda, Maryland 20205

Bryan Brewer (271), National Heart, Lung, and Blood Institute, National Institutes of Health, Bethesda, Maryland 20205

Irwin M. Chaiken (266), National Institute of Arthritis, Diabetes, and Digestive and Kidney Diseases, National Institutes of Health, Bethesda, Maryland 20205

Robert A. Cohen (12), Chestnut Lodge, 500 W. Montgomery Avenue, Rockville, Maryland 20850

Roger M. Cole (113), 6200 Maiden Lane, Bethesda, Maryland 20817

Vincent DeVita, Jr. (499), National Cancer Institute, National Institutes of Health, Bethesda, Maryland 20205

Harry Eagle (99), Albert Einstein College of Medicine, Bronx, New York 10461

William A. Eaton (337), National Institute of Arthritis, Diabetes, and Digestive and Kidney Diseases, National Institutes of Health, Bethesda, Maryland 20205

Virginia J. Evans (86), 5824 Bradley Boulevard, Bethesda, Maryland 20814

D. Carleton Gajdusek (395), National Institute of Neurological and Communicative Disorders and Stroke, National Institutes of Health, Bethesda, Maryland 20205

Clarence J. Gibbs, Jr. (395), National Institute of Neurological and Communicative Disorders and Stroke, National Institutes of Health, Bethesda, Maryland 20205

Abraham Goldin (499), National Cancer Institute, National Institutes of Health, Bethesda, Maryland 20205

Jay H. Hoofnagle (141), National Institute of Arthritis, Diabetes, and Digestive and Kidney Diseases, National Institutes of Health, Bethesda, Maryland 20205

Bernard L. Horecker (230), Laboratory of Molecular Enzymology, Roche Institute of Molecular Biology, Nutley, New Jersey 07110

Herman M. Kalckar (305), 16 Channing Street, Cambridge, Massachusetts 02138

Ruth L. Kirschstein (379), National Institute of General Medical Sciences, National Institutes of Health, Bethesda, Maryland 20205

I. J. Kopin (35), National Institute of Neurological and Communicative Disorders and Stroke, National Institutes of Health, Bethesda, Maryland 20205

Mortimer B. Lipsett (416), National Institute of Child Health and Human Development, National Institutes of Health, Bethesda, Maryland 20205

Robert G. Martin (281), National Institute of Arthritis, Diabetes, and Digestive and Kidney Diseases, National Institutes of Health, Bethesda, Maryland 20205

Charles L. McIntosh (481), National Heart, Lung, and Blood Institute, National Institutes of Health, Bethesda, Maryland 20205

Alton Meister (234), Biochemistry Department, Cornell University Medical College, New York, New York 10021

Phillip G. Nelson (108), National Institute of Child Health and Human Development, National Institutes of Health, Bethesda, Maryland 20205

Elizabeth F. Neufeld (330), Department of Biological Chemistry, School of Medicine, University of California, Los Angeles, California 90024

William E. Paul (154, 167, 176), National Institute of Allergy and Infectious Diseases, National Institutes of Health, Bethesda, Maryland 20205

Karl A. Piez (274), Collagen Corporation, Palo Alto, California 94303

Arnold W. Pratt (456), Division of Computer Research and Technology, National Institutes of Health, Bethesda, Maryland 20205

J. E. Rall (527), Office of the Director, National Institutes of Health, Bethesda, Maryland 20205

Frank J. Rauscher, Jr. (349), American Cancer Society, New York, New York 10017

Jacob Robbins (416), National Institute of Arthritis, Diabetes, and Digestive and Kidney Diseases, National Institutes of Health, Bethesda, Maryland 20205

Sanford M. Rosenthal (6), National Institute of Arthritis, Diabetes, and Digestive and Kidney Diseases, National Institutes of Health, Bethesda, Maryland 20205

Norman P. Salzman (387), National Institute of Allergy and Infectious Diseases, National Institutes of Health, Bethesda, Maryland 20205

Katherine K. Sanford (86), National Cancer Institute, National Institutes of Health, Bethesda, Maryland 20205

Alan N. Schechter (262, 337), National Institute of Arthritis, Diabetes, and Digestive and Kidney Diseases, National Institutes of Health, Bethesda, Maryland 20205

Edward M. Scolnick (368), Merck Sharp & Dohme Research Laboratories, West Point, Pennsylvania 19486

J. Edwin Seegmiller (314), Department of Medicine, School of Medicine, University of California, San Diego, La Jolla, California 92093

Norman E. Sharpless (443), National Institute of Arthritis, Diabetes, and Digestive and Kidney Diseases, National Institutes of Health, Bethesda, Maryland 20205

Michael B. Shimkin (349), Department of Community and Family Medicine, School of Medicine, University of California, San Diego, La Jolla, California 92093

DeWitt Stetten, Jr. (1), Office of the Director, National Institutes of Health, Bethesda, Maryland 20205

Herbert Tabor (220), National Institute of Arthritis, Diabetes, and Digestive and Kidney Diseases, National Institutes of Health, Bethesda, Maryland 20205

Donald B. Tower (46), 7105 Brennon Lane, Chevy Chase, Maryland 20815

Thomas A. Waldmann (154, 158, 181), National Cancer Institute, National Institutes of Health, Bethesda, Maryland 20205

Bernhard Witkop (193), National Institute of Arthritis, Diabetes, and Digestive and Kidney Diseases, National Institutes of Health, Bethesda, Maryland 20205

Notes and Acknowledgments

Several NIH Institutes have undergone name changes through the years. These changes are chronicled in the Prologue (Chapter 1). In the text the Institutes are designated as named at the time alluded to.

The names of persons who have worked at NIH or its antecedent, the Hygienic Laboratory, are in capital letters the first time mentioned by each author. Thus Associates, Fellows, Guest Workers, Visiting Scientists, etc., are indicated as NIH personnel. Occasionally, however, the work cited was done before or after the investigator's NIH experience.

The Index of Names lists all scientists whose work is treated in the text, without reference to affiliation.

From the start of this undertaking, I have been fortunate in having the support, advice, and active participation of several assistants, all experts in their fields. One is my indispensable secretary and aide, Nancy Yellin. Another is Storm Whaley, Associate Director for Communications, NIH, who steered us through the bureaucratic minefields. Editing began in late 1981 when Bill Carrigan and his staff in the Office of Program Planning and Evaluation responded to my request for assistance. Bill's group included Gertrude Kelly, who shared importantly in the editing and compiled the name index, and Carole Cone, who rendered expert assistance in the preparation of camera-ready copy. Diagrams were drawn by Bill Stancliff of the Division of Research Grants. The staff of Academic Press has lent valuable advice. Certainly the work could not have materialized in this form without the conscientious, enthusiastic cooperation of these collaborators. I am deeply grateful.

DeWitt Stetten, Jr.

Foreword

We seem to be living through a period (transient, I hope) of public disillusion and discouragement over government and all its works. At all levels, bureaucracy in general is mistrusted, here and abroad. The word is out that government doesn't really work, can't get things right, wastes public money, fumbles along, stalls, gets in the way.

At such a time, it lifts the heart to look closely at one institution created by the United States Government which has been achieving, since its outset, one spectacular, stunning success after another. The National Institutes of Health is not only the largest institution for biomedical science on earth, it is one of this nation's great treasures. As social inventions for human betterment go, this one is a standing proof that, at least once in a while, government possesses the capacity to do something unique, imaginative, useful, and altogether right.

My own first contact with the institution was during the summer of 1944, working as a junior naval officer in the typhus fever laboratories directed by Dr. Norman Topping. I was being coached in the methods then in use for research on scrub typhus, and I was swept off my feet by the quality of the scientists working in those crowded laboratories. NIH was a small affair at that time, with infectious disease and cancer as its principal concerns. After World War II the institution began to expand, taking on one broad area of human disease after another, but the institutional commitment to quality has remained solid as a rock. Under Dr. James Shannon's direction, biomedical research began to flourish within the country's major universities and medical schools, and despite current anxieties over a shrinking budget, the extramural programs flourish still.

But at the center of the NIH scientific effort, driving the whole vast enterprise along, is the research conducted on the Bethesda campus itself—the so-called Intramural Research Program. Although this represents only a minor portion of the total NIH budget—around 10 percent—for sheer excellence and abundant productivity the institution cannot be matched by any other scientific enterprise anywhere.

This book contains the personal accounts of some of the leading figures in the intramural program, describing their own experiences in the laboratories and clinics. In this sense, the book is a historical document. But the reader will note that the science being discussed is not part of the past; it is today's science as well, and much of it can be taken as signposts to the future.

I shall not detain the reader with any attempt at a summary of the work. The list of Nobel laureates whose careers were molded within the walls of NIH speaks for itself, and the record of scientific discovery contained in the bibliography of intramural NIH simply staggers the mind.

But one aspect of the intramural program deserves special mention and emphasis. It is as a training ground for young investigators, who have come to Bethesda for their postdoctoral education in research, that the institution has achieved its most singular influence on the progress of American science. For three decades the youngest and brightest candidates for careers in biomedical research have competed for the opportunity to learn how to do science in this place. Most of them worked here for two or three years and then deployed out to the universities to continue in research, and a high percentage of these alumni then turned into the country's leaders of academic science.

It has, in short, been a success story from start to finish, although the "finish" is, I trust, nowhere near. The NIH laboratories are something for the Government to boast about, to dine out on, and to be immensely proud of. It is my hope that the same intelligence and scientific good taste will be displayed for the institution's future as were used to build the magnificent instrument now at hand.

LEWIS THOMAS, M.D.
President Emeritus
Memorial Sloan–Kettering
Cancer Center
New York, New York

1

PROLOGUE

DeWitt Stetten, Jr.

Bethesda, Maryland, a suburb northwest of Washington, D.C., contains two major Federal centers of biomedical research. One, on the east side of the Rockville Pike, is the National Naval Medical Center and its related Uniformed Services University of the Health Sciences. The other, on the west side, is the main campus of the National Institutes of Health. NIH is the principal research arm of the Public Health Service, U.S. Department of Health and Human Services.

This work describes the scientific efforts and achievements of NIH, not only on the Bethesda campus but also at installations in Baltimore, in Research Triangle Park of North Carolina, in the Bitterroot Valley of Montana, and at a few smaller sites. We shall focus on the laboratories and clinical facilities, on the people who do research there, and on the studies they have completed or are presently conducting.

At the outset it may be well to state what this book is not. Most of the funds appropriated to NIH are distributed in the form of awards, including research grants and contracts to non-Federal institutions, awards to institutions and individuals for research training, and grants to provide research centers and resources. The supported activities conducted outside NIH will not be included here; nor will the political and fiscal history of NIH be detailed. Rather, we shall be concerned primarily with events that have occurred in the intramural clinics and laboratories since NIH moved to Bethesda in 1938.

At present NIH comprises 11 Institutes:

- National Institute on Aging (NIA).

- National Institute of Allergy and Infectious Diseases (NIAID). [Formed from older laboratories as the National Microbiological Institute. Renamed NIAID in 1955.]

DeWITT STETTEN, Jr., M.D., Ph.D., Senior Scientific Advisor, National Institutes of Health.

NIH: AN ACCOUNT OF RESEARCH
IN ITS LABORATORIES AND CLINICS

ISBN 0-12-667980-0

- National Institute of Arthritis, Diabetes, and Digestive and Kidney Diseases (NIADDK). [Formed from older laboratories as the Experimental Biology and Medicine Institute. Superseded by the National Institute of Arthritis and Metabolic Diseases in 1950. Renamed National Institute of Arthritis, Metabolism and Digestive Diseases in 1972. Renamed NIADDK in 1980.]

- National Cancer Institute (NCI).

- National Institute of Child Health and Human Development (NICHD).

- National Institute of Dental Research (NIDR).

- National Institute of Environmental Health Sciences (NIEHS).

- National Eye Institute (NEI).

- National Institute of General Medical Sciences (NIGMS).

- National Heart, Lung, and Blood Institute (NHLBI). [Established as the National Heart Institute. Renamed National Heart and Lung Institute in 1969. Renamed NHLBI in 1976.]

- National Institute of Neurological and Communicative Disorders and Stroke (NINCDS). [Established as the National Institute of Neurological Diseases and Blindness. Renamed National Institute of Neurological Diseases and Stroke in 1968. Renamed NINCDS in 1975.]

Each of the above Institutes except NIGMS houses an intramural program. Two of them, NIEHS and NIA, conduct all their intramural activities away from the Bethesda campus. NIEHS has laboratory buildings at Research Triangle Park, North Carolina, while NIA scientists work entirely in the Gerontology Research Center in Baltimore, Maryland. NCI, in addition to its laboratory and clinical programs in Bethesda, has extensive laboratory activities at the Frederick Cancer Research Center in Frederick, Maryland, and clinical investigations in Baltimore and at the National Naval Medical Center. NIAID operates a major research laboratory in Hamilton, Montana. Other Institutes conduct smaller projects at Poolesville, Maryland; Phoenix, Arizona; Woods Hole and Framingham, Massachusetts; and Guam.

The intramural studies of NCI, because of its size and complexity, come under three Divisions: Cancer Treatment, Cancer Biology and Diagnosis, and Cancer Cause and Prevention.

Three other NIH Divisions conduct research: the Clinical Center, the Division of Computer Research and Technology, and the Division of Research Services. These also provide services to the Institutes. For the present purposes, it is clearly appropriate to include their investigations among intramural activities.

The history of the relationship between the National Institute of Mental Health and the other components of NIH is complex. NIMH was a member of the NIH family of Institutes from 1949 to 1967, when it became a separate bureau. It is now a part of the Alcohol, Drug Abuse, and Mental Health Administration, Public Health Service. The intramural programs of NIMH and NIH, however, are closely associated in a happy and productive relationship. NIMH scientists still share laboratory and clinical facilities with NIH scientists; the scientific director of NIMH meets regularly with his counterparts from the NIH Institutes; and matters of space allocation and personnel are in the domain of the NIH Deputy Director for Intramural Research. Two of the following chapters, concerned mainly with NIMH studies from 1953 to 1973, are quite appropriate to a history of NIH intramural science.

Yet another component of NIH, administratively introduced through a reorganization of PHS in 1968, is the National Library of Medicine. This is predominantly a service institution, but intramural studies are addressed to problems of biomedical communications. One example is a continuing development of electronic methods for scanning, storing, retrieving, and distributing scientific information.

Two buildings on the Bethesda campus house the Bureau of Biologics of the Food and Drug Administration. The Bureau derives from the Division of Biologics Standards, which was a part of NIH until 1972. Its scientists have continued to interact with their counterparts in the Institutes.

The dimensions of intramural NIH—the size of a research venture—can be measured in terms of numbers of people, areas of laboratory and clinical space, and amounts of money dedicated to the program. About half of the nearly 14,000 persons on the NIH staff devote most of their time and effort to intramural activities, and many others divide their time between intra- and extramural. The intramural staff includes about 2200 with doctoral degrees, of whom about half are M.D.'s. Approximately half of the intramural doctoral scientists hold full-time tenured positions in the Civil Service or the PHS Commissioned Corps, and the remainder are mainly nontenured fellows, associates, and visiting scientists. In addition to

the 14,000, there are about 1000 visiting fellows and guest
workers.   All NIH scientists tenured and nontenured, when
first named in each of the following chapters, are indicated
by capital letters.

The total NIH campus including the satellites covers about
1400 acres and contains laboratory, clinical, and administrative buildings comprising 5.3 million square feet.

The current annual appropriations for NIH total approximately $4 billion.   About 10 percent of this is budgeted
for intramural science.   Most of the remainder is distributed in research grants, training grants, and research contracts.   Thus, the intramural programs engage the majority
of the personnel and a distinct minority of the appropriated
funds.

Comparison of the foregoing numbers with others describing
institutions in this country and abroad will reveal that the
intramural NIH, considered in its entirety, is by far the
largest biomedical research program in the world.   Its investigators enjoy a high degree of intellectual freedom, as in
the choice of scientific pursuits. It should be stressed that
autonomy in selection of research subjects is not merely tol-
erated but encouraged.

The resources, equipment, and clinical opportunities are
unparalleled.   The investigators' administrative duties are
kept at a minimum.   They have no teaching responsibilities
unless they choose to create them.   They are not required—
indeed, not allowed—to compose grant applications as their
academic colleagues must do.   They have access to a wealth of
services: veterinary, bibliographic, shop and engineering,
art, photography, etc.   In sum, they have at their command
all the advantages of a comprehensive modern medical center,
with expert consultation available at both the main campus and
the associated animal farm in Poolesville.

For all these reasons, the quality of research and of
those who have been assembled to conduct it has waxed steadily
over the years.   NIH ranks high among the world's biomedical
research institutions. This has been confirmed, for instance,
by recent studies on citation of articles as a measure of
their value to other scientists.   Over a 15-year period the
300 articles most frequently cited in the biomedical sciences
included no less than 45 by members of our intramural staff.
Many NIH scientists have held distinguished outside posts and
won notable national and international awards.   Six have received the Nobel Prize.

The following chapters frequently address ways in which
the science has been prosecuted.   How have scientists been
attracted and retained?   How are fruitful collaborations

fostered across laboratory and Institute lines? What major
themes of research activity have predominated during the past
four decades?

Probably these questions have no definitive answers. In
the seeking, however, we may be able to respond to a fundamental question often posed in one form or another: Why does
NIH need an intramural program?

The program must, and does, speak for itself. The extramural activities of NIH—our grant and contract programs—have
numerous and vocal advocates. Every medical school, every
biomedical research institution acclaims them. Our intramural
activities, on the other hand, have no such constituency. Indeed, many of our supporters would prefer to see the entire
appropriation distributed to the non-Federal sector. But
there is, in the last analysis, a most persuasive argument for
the intramural research program. It lies in the abundance and
excellence of the results.

Those results are the substance of this work.

2

THE EARLY DAYS

Sanford M. Rosenthal

The Hygienic Laboratory when I arrived in 1928 consisted of two modest two-story buildings at 25th and E Streets N.W., Washington, D.C. Heurich's brewery was on one side of E Street and the Naval Hospital on the other. Our residential neighbors were the poor, living in rundown row houses. My salary of $4000 a year was to prove munificent in the Depression years ahead, when a neighboring gasoline station would advertise eight gallons for a dollar.

The staff included about 40 research workers and a scattering of helpers. Trained technicians were nonexistent, and anyhow, there was no complicated instrumentation.

The laboratory operated on two professional levels, Commissioned Officers on the upper and Civil Service appointees on the lower. The upper level was a fire brigade for investigating outbreaks of new or unusual diseases. The lower level consisted of divisions of chemistry and pharmacology, but had no concerted function. It was headed by men from universities who followed their own interests, though at times some were pressed into service by an outbreak of poisoning of unknown origin.

The director of the Hygienic Laboratory (1915-1937) was GEORGE W. McCOY. He was a gaunt, restless man with an intense, penetrating glance that took in everything about you. He had served as a Commissioned Officer since 1900, working on leprosy and plague. A self-taught bacteriologist, he discovered in ground squirrels an organism (Pasteurella tularensis) that later proved to be the cause of tularemia. He was aptly dubbed "the director who did not direct."

McCoy was possessed with Scotch thrift. He had a Model A Ford at his disposal, but I often saw him get into the delivery truck for a visit to the Surgeon General's office. When I needed a Warburg apparatus ($500), he agreed, but said he

SANFORD M. ROSENTHAL, M.D., Scientist Emeritus, Laboratory of Biochemical Pharmacology, National Institute of Arthritis, Diabetes, and Digestive and Kidney Diseases.

NIH: AN ACCOUNT OF RESEARCH
IN ITS LABORATORIES AND CLINICS

ISBN 0-12-667980-0

would need the S.G.'s approval. I really suspect that he
retired early because he couldn't tolerate the wave of expansion that overtook Government activities in the late 1930s.

I have often pondered McCoy's genius for choosing productive research people. He sought dedication and industry in
young researchers and rarely imposed his decisions on them.
Between the lack of laboratory training and the rather primitive conditions for handling infectious materials, there is
little wonder at the frequency of serious disease among the
workers.

To compare the achievements of this small group of scientists with the output of today's mammoth institutions, with
their highly trained specialists and technical support, is
to pose an interesting question of which approach to research
is more successful. I do not ignore the giant steps made by
the moderns who with great skills and advanced technology have
extended the horizons of their fields. I only regret the loss
of creative talents in today's world because the laboratory
door is closed to those without proper qualifications. Few of
the scientists described below could have obtained a research
appointment today had they applied at the beginning of their
careers.

Since the story of the Hygienic Laboratory is really the
story of its workers, I shall set down my impression of some
of them and their accomplishments.

JOSEPH GOLDBERGER was still puttering around the laboratory in 1928, though he died the following year. Before coming
to the Hygienic Laboratory, he had done field work in typhus
and yellow fever (which he contracted). In 1914 he was placed
in charge of a team of 41' to study pellagra, thought at the
time to be an infectious disease. He proved in human studies
(including self-inoculation of blood from a patient) that
pellagra was of dietary origin. Then he returned to the laboratory to reproduce the disease in dogs ("black tongue") by
dietary restriction. He discovered that brewer's yeast was
preventive, and in 1924 it was introduced clinically.

EDWARD FRANCIS was a colorful character, always cheerful
and ready with quaint and humorous phrases—except when he was
battling for his life with some terrible disease he had contracted. He had worked with McCoy in isolating *P. tularensis*.
When a human epidemic of "deer fly fever" occurred in Utah,
Francis was sent to investigate. He recognized and later established the organism as that recovered from ground squirrels
and, by a beautiful piece of detective work, showed that the
disease—tularemia—was endemic in rabbits and was transmitted
to humans through the bite of the deer fly.

I recall visiting Francis's laboratory when he was working on the transmission of Rocky Mountain spotted fever by bedbugs. When I asked how he kept his bedbugs, he heated the pan of a guinea pig cage with a bunsen burner. Several plump bedbugs crawled forth.

RALPH LILLIE was the laboratory pathologist. Everybody dumped their autopsy material on him, but I never knew him to grumble or refuse collaboration. He was a superb pathologist and mastered the task of evaluating histologic changes in the confusion presented by different animal species. Few of us knew that he was making fundamental contributions in histochemistry, an emerging technique by which he first demonstrated the virus of psittacosis in tissues. His descriptions of the pathology of such diseases as tularemia, typhus, and psittacosis are classics in the field. A meticulous worker, Lillie escaped the infections that downed so many colleagues. He was a fine teacher, and there are many distinguished pathologists who served in his laboratory.

CHARLES ARMSTRONG was a big, quiet man who showed his Nordic ancestry. When Goodpasture succeeded in growing poliovirus in hens' eggs, Armstrong tackled the problem of producing poliomyelitis in small animals. He succeeded with intracerebral inoculation of mice, greatly advancing the study of the disease. Fortunately, he did not contract it, though he nearly died from psittacosis and epidemic choriomeningitis. Having isolated the choriomeningitis virus from humans, he later reproduced the disease in mice by intracerebral inoculation.

On one occasion an epidemic struck the Hygienic Laboratory. Because of an outbreak of psittacosis in nearby Maryland, infected parrots were brought to the laboratory for Armstrong to study. In a short time the disease spread through the north building, attacking Armstrong and 10 other workers. Armstrong's assistant HARRY ANDERSON died. McCoy drove everybody out of the building and alone took over the work and cared for the parrots. Out of this came Lillie's demonstration of a virus in tissues of the infected birds.

The "Dental Institute" consisted of one scientist, TRENDLEY DEAN. He was assigned to study a local endemic of mottled enamel in Arkansas. The condition was known to be related to fluoride intake, so a survey of the teeth of the inhabitants was made, along with analyses of drinking water for fluoride content. The analyses were carried out by ELIAS ELVOVE of the Laboratory of Chemistry. Elvove, a chemist of the old school, distrusted the fuzzy thinking of the less precise biologists. He also distrusted the primitive colorimeters of the time and made his color comparisons by looking down into long test tubes. When the data from the survey were assembled, he pointed out that the teeth with mottled enamel had few or no cavities. Thus was born the epoch of fluoride prevention of dental caries.

ROLLA DYER was another soldier in the fight against epidemics. His special interest was rickettsial diseases: murine typhus, spotted fever, and Q fever. After becoming immune to Q fever by contracting it, he established that the rat flea was the transmitting agent of murine typhus, while the similar Q fever was caused by a different organism *(Coxiella burnetii)* and transmitted by ticks.

HENRY SEBRELL began his research with Goldberger and continued in the field of nutrition. He produced riboflavin deficiency in animals and pioneered in the recognition of this condition in man. In other studies he showed that onions could produce a severe anemia in dogs (because of the sulfhydryl-containing oil). When newspaper publicity brought down the onion producers in a storm, he pacified them by stating that the amounts required were beyond those normally ingested. So far as I know, he and I are the only surviving workers of this period of the Hygienic Laboratory.

ROSCOE SPENCER worked on Rocky Mountain spotted fever at the laboratory in Montana and the Hygienic Laboratory. He produced an effective vaccine from infected ticks, and later from virus grown in hens' eggs. In the 1940s, after serving as director of the National Cancer Institute, he studied cell survival and adaptation, using paramecia and bacteria.

MANSFIELD CLARK, a quiet, retiring man who spoke a different language from the rest of us, was preparing to leave for Johns Hopkins Medical School to head the Department of Biochemistry. His studies on oxidation-reduction potentials were a major accomplishment of the Hygienic Laboratory. To protect Clark's instruments from cockroaches, the table legs were placed in cans of kerosene. This did not present the hazard one might think, for evaporation of the kerosene was slow, and someone showed that a lighted match quickly submerged in it would not ignite.

The head of pharmacology, CARL VOEGTLIN, was interested in arsenicals and sulfhydryl compounds and had asked me to work with him. Inspired by Clark's oxidation-reduction findings, he started an ambitious program of applying them to living tissues. It gradually became apparent after innumerable readings with a platinum electrode inserted into isolated tissues that a multiplicity of extraneous factors made valid interpretations impossible. Voegtlin turned to cancer research and left me to my own devices.

One moment proved unforgettable in light of a subsequent tragedy. We saw the Hindenburg dirigible on its way to the landing field in New Jersey. This was before the days of large

transport planes, and the huge balloon with its delicate gon-
dola passed silently and majestically only a few hundred feet
over our heads. It had a silvery sheen in the morning sunlight, and we could make out faces pressed against four or
five windows. Who would have suspected that in a few hours
it would be consumed in flames? If only it had been inflated
with helium instead of hydrogen, aviation might have taken a
different course.

When McCoy retired, we all had the feeling that it foreshadowed the end of a pioneer era. Indeed, the offer of the
Luke Wilson estate in Bethesda for the National Institute of
Health soon followed. Bethesda was a quiet suburban community
of a few thousand people, and the Chamber of Commerce feared
that NIH with its diseases and animals might be harmful to
business and development. Rolla Dyer, our new director, was
able to convince them of its material benefits, and the Hygienic Laboratory passed into history.

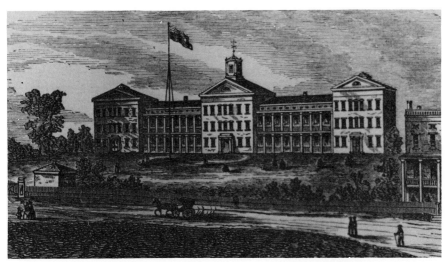

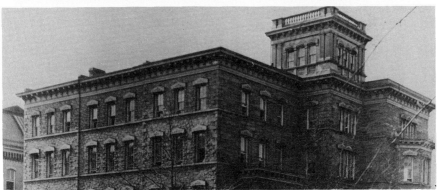

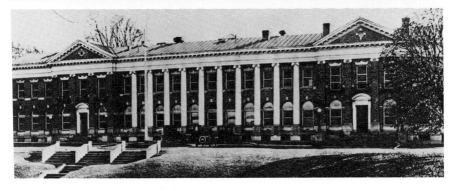

THE HYGIENIC LABORATORY, predecessor of NIH, at its three locations (reading down): Marine Hospital, Stapleton, Staten Island, New York, 1887-1891; top floor of four-story Butler Building, Capitol Hill, Washington, D.C., 1891-1903; 25th and E Streets, N.W., Washington, D.C., 1903-1938.

STUDIES ON THE
ETIOLOGY OF SCHIZOPHRENIA

The early creation of the National Institute of Mental Health filled an important gap in the research assault on health problems. Mental disorders were particularly inaccessible because of difficulties in diagnosis and uncertainties in the behavioral and analytic approaches. Many scientists schooled in the disciplines of chemistry, physics, and traditional biology were skeptical of the "softer" approaches of the psychologist and the psychiatrist. This chapter will be of particular interest in that it describes a multidisciplinary approach to a major mental health problem, schizophrenia.

NIMH scientists have explored many possible contributing factors to this common and costly disease, from underlying genetic defects to failure of parental communication. They have studied the disease in the light of recent important advances in biochemistry, neurology, and molecular biology—notably, the discoveries concerning neurotransmitters. Over the period covered here—mainly 1953 to 1973—schizophrenia has come to be viewed as a relatively specific syndrome that can often be solidly diagnosed and rationally treated.

D. S.

3

STUDIES ON THE
ETIOLOGY OF SCHIZOPHRENIA

Robert A. Cohen

Some Predecessors

Of all the Institutes brought together to constitute the National Institutes of Health, the National Institute of Mental Health was the least firmly based on an accepted foundation of rigorous scientific research. This was inconsonant with the seriousness of the problem of mental illness. At midcentury over half of the country's hospital beds were occupied by mental patients. Suicide, though underreported, was recognized as a major problem, as were alcohol and drug abuse. The human and economic costs of mental illness far outweighed the tragic burdens imposed by cancer, cardiovascular disease, or arthritis.

There were several reasons for the relative dearth of psychiatric research. One was the complexity of determining the cause or causes of an individual's abnormal behavior as displayed in his personal relations with others in his culture. Compared with this, the pathophysiology of a disease with clearly definable lesions affecting a single organ or entire system appeared simple indeed.

Not that distinguished scientists had ignored mental disease, but many of their findings failed the test of replication. For example, Virchow, in the late nineteenth century, described a specific brain lesion in dementia praecox, but like others before and after, he had discovered an artifact. Moreover, professors of medicine often had little interest or experience in the study and treatment of the mentally ill. Their contributions were largely in the realm of pathological anatomy or neurology or whatever science was advancing at the time. It was hoped that a Meynert or a Hitzig or a Flechsig

ROBERT A. COHEN, M.D., Ph.D., Director of Psychotherapy, Chestnut Lodge, Rockville, Maryland. Formerly Deputy Director, Mental Health Intramural Research Program, National Institute of Mental Health.

would discover a specific defect and at long last bring
order to this amorphous and frustrating field.

Investigators looked for single causes, as in the infectious diseases. Indeed, such advances as were made encouraged that approach. The development of the Wassermann test,
Ehrlich's salvarsan treatment for syphilis, Noguchi's identification of *Treponema pallidum*, Wagner von Jauregg's malarial
treatment for dementia paralytica, and GOLDBERGER'S discovery
of the cause, cure, and prevention of pellagra removed large
populations from the mental hospital. These patients were
brought into the orbit of general medicine, where they could
be diagnosed and treated with the same respect and concern
that physicians showed others who sought their help and whose
disorders they understood.

Aside from the bewildering complexity of mental disease
and the slow pace of scientific discovery in the field, a
diagnosis of manic-depressive illness or schizophrenia may
have been more harmful, through its stigmatizing effect, than
useful. Any serious mental disorder was popularly considered
a reflection of a weakness, less respectable in kind and quite
different in character from sarcoma, myocardial infarction, or
multiple sclerosis. Mental patients were alienated from society, and doctors who treated them (called "alienists," from
the French *aliéné*—insane) often led professional lives out
of the mainstream of medicine. Few medical schools even had
departments of psychiatry, and the lectures offered were sporadic and cursory. All this, added to other factors, accounted for the small number of specialists and the paltry
sums available for research.

In 1928 Adolf Meyer, the first Henry Phipps Professor of
Psychiatry at Johns Hopkins, could look back on the preceding
35 years and say:

> Psychiatry was then, as it still is in many places,
> largely an institutional and legal task. Under the
> rise of state care, it had . . . been gathering from
> almshouses and detention houses persons who proved to
> be impossible in the community, but who nevertheless
> were in need of more promising treatment than that of
> retaliation or mere exclusion. Psychiatry could deal
> with individuals only to a slight extent. . . . Real
> science in medicine was identified with the dead house
> and the use of the microscope. . . . As an example of
> the diversity of expectations from a laboratory worker
> of those days, a task waiting for him on the shelves
> [was] a collection of dessicated feces to be analyzed
> —the aim being to find the disease in pure culture.

When Meyer first came to the United States in 1892 to work as one of six assistant physicians at the Kankakee (Illinois) State Hospital, one of his colleagues acting as superintendent boasted that he alone could do all the medical work for the 2200 patients. Such was the setting to which the average mentally disturbed patient at the turn of the century was confined for safekeeping—though there were, of course, significant exceptions.

The interest of the Public Health Service in the problems of mental illness derived from its responsibility for medical inspection of the thousands of immigrants who were pouring into the country. In 1904 Thomas W. Salmon was sent to Ellis Island to assist in mental examination and to develop tests for serious disorders or mental defects.

Increasing numbers of the foreign-born were admitted to the already overburdened state hospitals. WALTER TREADWAY was assigned to study the problem. Beginning in 1914, he carried out a series of surveys, at first related to immigration and mental illness and later extended to the physical and mental health of school children, including a survey of state and local community policies related to the broad field of mental disease and deficiency. Eventually the surveys encompassed drug addiction, which, with its associated crime, had given rise to much public alarm.

In 1929 a Narcotics Division was authorized, with Treadway as Director. In the following year its responsibilities were broadened and it was renamed the Division of Mental Hygiene. It was led in turn by three remarkably able Directors: Treadway, LAWRENCE KOLB, and ROBERT FELIX. In 1939 Kolb, with the strong support of Surgeon General Thomas Parran, first proposed the establishment of a National Neuropsychiatric Institute modeled on the pattern of the National Cancer Institute, which had been created two years earlier. Although the idea was endorsed by the professional specialty societies, it was vigorously opposed by the House of Delegates of the American Medical Association through fear that it might lead to state medicine. The proposal then lay dormant for several years.

Experiences during World War II shocked both the profession and the public. Of the 4.8 million men called up for military duty, 1.8 million were rejected because of neuropsychiatric disorders and mental and educational deficiencies. Forty percent of those later given medical discharges were dismissed for psychiatric disorder, and 60 percent of all hospitalized patients of the Veterans Administration were within that category.

Meanwhile, the fraction of the country's 3000 psychiatrists who served with the armed forces made convincing contributions to the maintenance of morale and to crisis management of acute breakdowns under stress. Thus reinforced, Kolb's successor, Felix, with the continued support of Parran, gained congressional approval for the National Mental Health Act, signed into law by President Truman on July 3, 1946. Under its authority the National Institute of Mental Health was established on April 15, 1949.

With a charter broader than those of the other NIH Institutes, NIMH set forth four goals: to conduct research and demonstrations relating to the cause, diagnosis, and treatment of psychiatric disorders; to foster such research by public and private agencies and to coordinate their studies and the useful application of their results; to train personnel in matters relating to mental health; and to assist the states in the use of the most effective methods of prevention, diagnosis, and treatment.

Even before the establishment of the Division of Mental Hygiene, the Public Health Service had carried out intramural psychiatric research. Treadway's studies have been mentioned. Kolb, as Medical Director of the Addiction Research Center at Lexington, Kentucky, the first hospital for drug addicts, had reported in 1935 an impressive series of investigations with HIMMELSBACH, ISBELL, WIKLER, and others. In Bethesda, JOHN CLAUSEN, a sociologist, was carrying out a program of community studies, and WADE MARSHALL had developed a productive neurophysiology laboratory. In 1951 SEYMOUR KETY came to set up basic research programs for both NIMH and the National Institute of Neurological Diseases and Blindness. In 1952 the writer arrived to develop the clinical research program of NIMH, and a few months later MILTON SHY came to establish the clinical research program of NINDB. The Clinical Center was formally opened to patients on July 6, 1953.

The directors of the research programs were given extraordinary freedom, both in the choice of areas for study and the recruitment of professional staff. The NIH Institutes fostered multidisciplinary research, and all the fields clearly relevant to the problems selected for study were strongly represented. But NIMH, unlike the other Institutes, had few models to follow. At the time the National Mental Health Act was passed, only $2.5 million from all sources was being spent annually in the United States on research in psychiatry and related fields.

Looking back over the years, one saw the examples set by the discovery of the cause and treatment of the behavioral disorders stemming from central nervous system lues and pellagra. Psychiatric clinics associated with leading medical schools and hospitals, while predominantly staffed with clinical psychiatrists, usually included also a psychologist and an internist, occasionally even a geneticist, an experimental psychologist, a physiologist, a pharmacologist, a biometrist, and more rarely an anthropologist or sociologist.

Back still further, there were such prophetic statements as that of Sir Henry Maudsley a century ago:

> It is deserving of remark that the different nervous centers of the body manifest elective affinities for particular poisons. . . . That medicinal substances do display these elective affinities is a proof, at any rate, that there are important though delicate differences in the constitution or composition of the different nervous centers, notwithstanding that we are unable to detect the nature of them. It may be also that there is shadowed out in these different effects of poisons on the nervous system a means which may ultimately be of use in the investigation of the constitution of the latter.

It was Maudsley, too, who said:

> Sorrows which find no vent in tears may make other organs weep.

In the 1880s Thudichum had undertaken a 20-year program designed to determine the chemical constitution of the brain. And in 1905 Van Gieson in New York had proposed a Correlation of the Sciences:

> The aim being to provide for an exhaustive study of the causes and conditions that underlie mental disease from the standpoint of cellular biology, which is now elevated to the dignity of a special science.

Of this proposal Adolf Meyer observed that it was remarkably comprehensive, but had a fatal flaw. There was no place for man as we know him—as an integrated whole.

Two research programs were particularly relevant to the NIH setting. In the 1920s Mrs. Stanley McCormick became disheartened by her schizophrenic husband's lack of progress during several years of psychoanalysis. She consulted Walter Cannon about establishing a research center devoted to the development of an organic, preferably endocrine treatment. Roy Hoskins, a former student of Cannon's, left his post as Professor of Physiology at Ohio State University School of Medicine to head a new research institute at the Worcester (Massachusetts) State Hospital. In its 20 years (1927-1946), this institute made notable contributions both to the study of schizophrenia and to the disciplines represented on its staff.

And in London, the Institute of Psychiatry at Maudsley Hospital and at the University of London, then under the direction of Professor Aubrey Lewis, had conducted—and still conducts—impressive and critical studies in the field. As Sir Aubrey said, the roll call of psychiatry's fundamental sciences is absurdly long. Since it is concerned with disorders of behavior, its investigation must rest on psychology and the social sciences. And since it is also concerned with the pathology of mental disease and the bodily changes that can affect behavior, it must incorporate the biological and physical sciences that provide the basis for medical research.

It was with these examples in mind that we in the Mental Health Institute undertook an ambitious multidisciplinary program. The early focus was on the establishment of laboratories or clinical branches in the relevant disciplines, because we felt that this would help us keep abreast of advances in the respective fields. Unique opportunities afforded by the Clinical Center were that it could bring to the clinician normal persons who would not otherwise consult him in his practice, and that it introduced to those studying normals the situations encountered in the clinic.

It was felt that truly interdisciplinary studies would not be undertaken unless the theories that guided research in each of the disciplines were considerably modified. Moreover, it was expected that in so heterodox a congregation a parochial point of view would be difficult to maintain unless the facts supporting it were substantial and impressive to those with a different body of data at hand.

The Institutes sharing the NIH Clinical Center concur in regarding disease as an experiment of nature. Hence, the focus of NIMH research is not solely on treatment, but includes the study of experiences and biological processes that underlie adaptive behavior. To describe in detail the diverse investigations that the Institute has conducted would of course exceed the scope of this chapter. Some of the contributions from the study of schizophrenia, however, will give an impression of the range, character, and quality of the work undertaken.

Nosology

Schizophrenia is a serious affliction that strikes in the prime of life. Most cases start between the ages of 15 and 24, fewer between 25 and 34, and still fewer in succeeding decades. Incidence is lowest in childhood and old age. It is estimated that 1 percent of the population is schizophrenic and that 2 percent will have an episode at some time in their lives. Even with the recent deployment of community mental health centers designed to provide treatment and social support in outpatient settings, one-quarter of all hospital beds in the United States and one-half of all the mental hospital beds are occupied by schizophrenic patients.

Despite the fact that descriptions of behavior viewed today as schizophrenic date back at least 3500 years, there is still only modest agreement in establishing the diagnosis. Some advocate classification by symptoms, others by putative cause. Some are convinced that life experiences underlie the disorder, others that genetic or nongenetic biological factors are paramount.

Modern classification of mental illnesses is patterned after the system proposed in 1896 by Kraepelin, who attempted to bring order out of the chaotic disagreements of the time. Heinroth, for example, had described 48 separate and distinct diseases. Neumann declared that there was only one disease process, which manifested itself in a progression of symptoms from melancholia to mania to confusion to dementia—a progression that might be arrested at any stage by mechanisms yet unknown. Kraepelin reviewed the life histories and detailed medical records of patients whose illness had reached a terminal stage. He grouped cases with similar outcomes, each group including many with symptom complexes previously regarded as different diseases. He designated as "dementia praecox" a clinical picture characterized by early onset, hallucinations, delusions, stereotypies, inappropriate affect, and stupor, usually progressing to irreversible deterioration.

Several years later Bleuler published an equally classic study. He agreed in principle that Kraepelin's patients had related illnesses, but viewed the pattern as more loosely organized. He designated one group of symptoms as primary, caused directly by an unknown etiologic agent, and other symptoms as psychological reactions secondary to the primary changes. The disease process, he believed, might be arrested but was in no instance completely reversible. He emphasized the split between thought and affect, suggesting the term *schizophrenia* (Greek, divided + mind). He felt that Kraepelin had described not one disorder but several related ones, and considered it more accurate to place them in the "group of schizophrenias."

Kraepelin and Bleuler made a major advance in classification, setting a pattern still followed in efforts to increase nosologic precision. But diagnosis in psychiatry remains highly subjective. It depends on the patient's history, on signs and symptoms elicited in interaction with the observer, and to a large extent, on individual judgment. Investigators

are currently searching for biological markers. Among the
candidates are levels of platelet monoamine oxidase, urinary
excretion of catecholamine metabolites, the dexamethasone
suppression test, and the effect of methylphenidate and
amphetamine on symptoms. But such aids have not yet proved
definitive.

Nor is diagnosis made easier by the fact that normal persons under certain conditions employ most schizophrenic mechanisms.

In recent years a number of descriptive nosologic systems
have been introduced. Agreement among raters in each system
is usually high, while agreement among systems is only moderate. Patients are now described in terms of one or more of
these systems and according to standardized diagnostic interviews. This approach has improved the quality and validity of
comparative studies.

The variety of symptoms now diagnosed as schizophrenic is
narrowing. Long-term outcome is no longer a diagnostic criterion. The statement that schizophrenia is "a relatively
specific syndrome and neither a disease entity nor an arbi-
trary figment nor an epithet" (Gottesman and Shields) ex-
presses a prevalent view.

The NIH Intramural Program: Four Early Studies

The remainder of this chapter will be devoted to four of
the many studies of schizophrenia carried out in the NIMH
intramural research program. One of these is concerned with
relationships and thought disorder in families with a schizophrenic member; another addresses genetic aspects; another
takes as its starting point the relationship between social
isolation and schizophrenia; and the last arises in an attempt
to test a biological theory advanced to explain certain
symptoms.

Schizophrenics and Their Families:
Research on Parental Communication

One encounters the nature/nurture controversy in the earliest publications on psychiatry. It has been noted for centuries that mental illness seems to run in families, and
every resident in training soon observes that some of his
schizophrenic patients become more disturbed when visited by
anxious parents. In keeping with the usual medical practice
of treating the person who has the illness, it had been the

custom to discourage visits for a time, devoting major efforts
to the patient while giving the parents a degree of support.
In the decade preceding the opening of the Clinical Center,
however, investigators had begun to examine these family relationships instead of manipulating them for the patient's
presumed benefit.

- Fromm-Reichmann described an unusually intense and
  prolonged attachment between the mother and her adult
  schizophrenic child. She suggested that in such instances the mother might be considered "schizophreno-
  genic," in the sense that normal growth toward independence had been obstructed.

- Jackson and Bateson observed a "double bind" phenomenon
  in the relationship between some schizophrenics and
  their parents. The parents conveyed insistent, diamet-
  rically opposed expectations, with the result that
  whatever the child did was wrong.

- Lidz and Fleck reported that the homes of schizophrenics
  were marked by serious parental strife or eccentricity.
  Hence, the illness might be regarded as an alteration in
  the patient's sense of reality that served as an escape
  from insoluble domestic conflicts.

- Johnson and Szurek conducted simultaneous but separate
  psychotherapy with antisocial, hyperaggressive children
  and their parents. They found instances in which the
  child seemed to be acting out a parent's ambivalent
  repressed wish. The parent, consequently, could not
  give effective guidance in that area.

The program selected for this section was one of several
family studies undertaken soon after the Clinical Center
opened. LYMAN WYNNE headed the research team from the beginning. MARGARET THALER SINGER joined the group later and became a full partner. The program was based on clinical
observations made during family therapy sessions in which
patient, parents, and siblings participated.

The investigators noted differences between families with
a schizophrenic member and those with a member having another
mental disorder. Relationships were marked by a high degree
of *pseudomutuality*. Personality theory assumes that normal
development requires (1) continuing relationships with significant others (beginning with a nurturing one with the
mother) and (2) a sense of identity, evolving in the context
of those relationships, that gives continuity and coherence

to experience. The progression from dependent infancy to independent and interdependent maturity is fostered by a mutual relatedness, which accepts, survives, and benefits from the stresses of growth and the divergences inevitably occurring during the life course. In pseudomutual relationships, divergence is experienced as a threat that will lead to total disruption of the family group. Change is not perceived accurately, acknowledged, or accepted, and efforts are made to preserve the feeling that all remains the same. Thus the relationship is built upon a denial of reality and becomes progressively more fragile.

The investigators found that in families with a schizophrenic member, communications were obscure and resulted in entanglements that seemed to sustain the patient's symptomatology. The family members had difficulty in maintaining foci of attention, in arriving at a closure of issues under discussion, and in establishing consensually understood meanings. It was as if a smoke screen had enveloped the field of family interaction—a screen that made it impossible for the members to see, feel, or experience what was actually going on or to take any action leading to useful change. The investigators termed this family tendency *communication deviance*.

A brief example of such behavior in the family of a schizophrenic patient is reported by Wynne and Singer:

> Daughter (the patient), complainingly: Nobody will listen to me. Everybody is trying to still me.
>
> Mother: Nobody wants to kill you.
>
> Father: If you're going to associate with intellectual people, you're going to have to remember that "still" is a noun and not a verb.

Satisfied that the communication deviance they and their co-workers had noted in the course of conjoint family investigation occurred in all of the families treated, Wynne and Singer developed a study designed to quantify the deviance and to determine the extent to which it occurs in mental disorders generally. The data were no longer the interactions that took place during family treatment sessions. In a precisely structured procedure, each family member alone and the family as a group were asked to view Rorschach cards, and their responses were recorded verbatim.

These responses were not interpreted in the usual way. They were looked upon as typical samples of communication that would reveal how the subjects and the examiner interrelated and how they shared or did not share meanings. It was hypothesized that even in this experimental situation, the family members would display the same communication patterns they regularly displayed in the emotionally charged atmosphere of the therapeutic group. The duties involved in administering the test, interpreting the data, and caring for the families during their stay in the Clinical Center were allocated in a manner that kept those concerned with each procedure blind to information gathered in the others.

The investigators analyzed communication deviance in 114 families. In 20 of these, the patients had unremitting schizophrenia; in 24, remitting schizophrenia; and in 25, the patients were considered borderline. In 25 other families the patients were severely neurotic or delinquent. Twenty families served as normal controls. All in all, 228 parents, 114 patients, and 141 patients' siblings took part in the study.

None of the parental pairs with a schizophrenic child scored below the median in communication deviance. Only two of the parents with normal or neurotic children scored above the median, while those with borderline offspring were equally distributed above and below. In other words, schizophrenic patients came from families in which both parents had high deviance scores; normals and neurotics, from parents with low scores. Borderlines tended to come from families in which one parent had a high and the other a low score. The severity of the patient's disorder varied directly with the extent of the communication deviance of the parents. Although the siblings were not clinically disturbed, their deviance scores were directly related to the severity of the patient's disorder.

The study was cross-sectional and could not answer the question whether the parents' communication deviance preceded or followed the development of their child's illness. However, several longitudinal studies of children at high risk for schizophrenia are under way. In one carried out by Goldstein at the University of California (Los Angeles), the adolescents whose problem behavior had brought the families to the clinic were entering adulthood five years after enrollment. Seven out of eight diagnosed at followup as falling within the schizophrenic spectrum had parents who had shown high communication deviance. Of 26 considered normal or neurotic at followup, 19 were from families with low to moderate deviance. While the data strongly suggest that parental communication deviance plays a causal role in schizophrenia, it is at least possible that the high parental scores were a subclinical expression of schizophrenia and that the offspring's disorder might have been inherited.

Genetic Studies in Schizophrenia

The work of Wynne, Singer, and their associates strongly supports the view that parental communication deviance should be considered a possible etiologic factor in the development of schizophrenia. They did not conclude that it was a sole or necessary cause. From the inception of their research program, they assumed that the disorder probably resulted from interaction between experiential and biological variables. Early in their work they began the study of response dispositions that are probably inherited and can be measured by psychophysiological, neurophysiological, and perceptual methods.

The Wynne-Singer investigation was just getting under way when the attention of many members of the staff was forcefully directed to a consideration of genetic factors in schizophrenia. Identical schizophrenic quadruplets and their parents had been admitted to one of the NIMH patient care units. They remained in the hospital almost three years. Investigators from all five of the laboratories in the Clinical Investigations Program participated in a series of studies. The findings are reported in *The Genain Quadruplets*, edited by DAVID ROSENTHAL.

The presence of this unique and very cooperative family stimulated lively discussion and serious review of the nature/nurture literature. Rosenthal designed most of the psychological studies of the family members, but his greatest contribution was his penetrating and critical review of the research advanced in support of the various etiologic theories of schizophrenia. He placed these in three categories: "monogenic-biochemical" theories, which deny significant experiential influences; "life-experience" theories, which deny genetic influences; and what he termed "diathesis-stress" theories—several in number—which advance different hypotheses about the nature of the heredity-environment interaction but accept the idea of dual causality. Most investigators seemed to place themselves in the diathesis-stress group. But there was still ample room for disagreement about the relative importance of each factor and the kinds of genetic, biological, psychological, and sociological influences thought to be involved.

The most persuasive evidence for a powerful genetic factor had come from studies on twins. Among identical twins of schizophrenics, 76 to 86 percent were reported to be concordant for the illness, as compared with 12 to 17 percent of fraternal twins. Rosenthal contended that several of the procedures employed in these studies skewed the findings. He examined the data, made allowances for the errors that might have been inherent in the methodology, and recalculated the concordance rates. While the total values for monozygotic (identical) twins were lower, the rate was still four times that for dizygotic (fraternal) twins.

The analysis of several of the Wynne-Singer clinical studies had just been completed as the report on the Genain quadruplets approached its final form. The entire intramural staff was impressed by Margaret Singer's almost uncanny ability to group family members on the basis of their Rorschach records alone—even records of patients she had never seen, thus ruling out any possibility of contamination. She attributed her success to reliance on similarities in *form* of the responses rather than in *content*.

An obvious criticism of twin studies is the fact that, with few exceptions, the subjects have been reared together. Because monozygotic twins are more apt to be treated alike than dizygotic twins, and more apt to think of themselves as one, the experiential and environmental factors could not be convincingly separated from the hereditary. To address this problem, Rosenthal, Kety, and PAUL WENDER independently proposed a study of children who had been adopted in infancy or early childhood. This would meet the reservations about the twin studies and might serve as a control for the Wynne-Singer project. The three investigators agreed to collaborate and the adoption studies were undertaken.

Denmark was selected as the site because of the excellent adoption and psychiatric registers. The collection of data began in 1965. The first three studies will be described: Schizophrenics' Offspring Reared in Adoptive Homes, the Extended Family Study, and the Adoptive Parents Study.

Schizophrenics' Offspring Reared in Adoptive Homes.

Between 1924 and 1947, 5500 individuals had been adopted. They ranged in age from 17 to 40 at the time the study began. The records named both the biological and adoptive parents. A search of the psychiatric register then disclosed the biological parents who had been admitted to a psychiatric facility. The records were reviewed by Fini Schulsinger and Joseph Welner, Danish psychiatrists, who prepared abstracts that were independently rated by our three investigators. When there was unanimous agreement on the diagnosis of schizophrenia, the child was selected as an index case. Controls were selected from the same adoption register. Except that their biological parents had not received any recorded psychiatric treatment, they matched the index cases in age, sex, age at adoption, and socioeconomic status of their adoptive and biological parents.

The first report from this study was made after the Danish psychiatrists had blindly interviewed 39 index cases and 47 controls. Three of the index cases were diagnosed as schizophrenic and 10 others as falling within a "schizophrenic spectrum," which included chronic and acute schizophrenia of early or late onset, uncertain schizophrenia, and schizoid and inadequate personality. None of the controls had developed a frank psychosis, and only six were placed in the spectrum.

As more cases were accumulated, the differences became less spectacular. In fact, it was necessary to add to the diagnostic interview the requirement of a divergent profile (Minnesota Multiphasic Personality Inventory) and to include biological parents who had an affective disorder. While the difference between index and control cases was maintained, the controls had more disorders than would be expected in the normal population. This raised a question that could not be definitely answered: Do parents who give up their children for adoption have a higher rate of mental disturbance than the general population (even though they have not sought institutional treatment)?

By an unusual coincidence, another study of schizophrenics' offspring was under way in Oregon. Neither investigating group was aware of the other's work. Leonard Heston studied 47 persons born to schizophrenic mothers confined to the Oregon State Psychiatric Hospital between 1915 and 1945. A control group comprising 50 children of mothers with no known history of psychiatric disorder had been placed concurrently in the same foundling home as the index subjects. Five of the index subjects had developed schizophrenia and 21 displayed diagnosable sociopathy. In the control group, there were none with psychosis and nine with sociopathy.

The Extended Family Study. The index cases in the extended family study were 33 adoptees who had been admitted to a psychiatric facility. The matched control group had no such history. Through use of the register, histories of admission were sought for the biological and adoptive parents, siblings, and half-siblings. Of the biological relatives of the index cases, 21 percent fell within the schizophrenic spectrum, in contrast to 5 percent of the adoptive relatives. Of the biological relatives of the controls, 11 percent were so diagnosed, in contrast to 7.7 percent of the adoptive relatives.

The Adoptive Parents Study. Here the adoptive parents of schizophrenic patients were compared with biological parents who had reared their own schizophrenic children and with adoptive parents of normal young adults. According to a scale that rated the global severity of psychopathology, the biological parents presented moderate to severe neuroses. The adoptive relatives of the schizophrenics displayed milder forms of character disorder, while the adoptive relatives of the normals were found to be normal.

Rorschach responses collected from the three groups of parents were sent to Singer for analysis. She was able to differentiate the biological and adoptive parents of schizophrenics from the adoptive parents of normals with a high degree of accuracy.

The adoption studies of Rosenthal, Kety, and Wender, the earliest of which have just been described, together with Heston's study, are generally regarded as the most compelling evidence available for a genetic factor in the development of schizophrenia. They do, however, pose some questions.

It was clearly established that the mothers of all of Heston's index cases had been diagnosed and treated for the disorder. While it was true that the 5 cases of schizophrenia in the offspring were found only in the index series, 21 of the 42 remaining in that group displayed criminality, mental deficiency, neurosis, and/or sociopathy—conditions not usually associated with schizophrenia.

The first Rosenthal, Kety, and Wender studies were skewed by the fact that the psychiatric register had unavoidably been used in selecting the control adoptees. Absence of the parents from the register did not necessarily preclude mental illness. Since not every mentally ill person seeks or receives treatment, it is probable that the findings represent an underestimate of the incidence of the illness among biological relatives of control (and index) cases.

As the adoption studies progressed, the category "schizophrenic spectrum disorders," with its broad range of conditions, came to include 32 percent of the index group and 25 percent of the controls. Nevertheless, this tended to support a general consensus that nuclear and extended biological families of schizophrenics evince significantly high levels of mental illness. It would seem, however, that what is inherited is not susceptibility to schizophrenia alone, but rather to a whole set of mental disorders, which may or may not be interrelated.

Social Isolation and Schizophrenia

The next study to be described is concerned with the relation of social isolation to schizophrenia. Modern sociological interest in the epidemiology and etiology of the disorder dates to the work of Faris in 1934 and Faris and Dunham in 1939. Faris proposed that schizophrenia results from social isolation. He and Dunham had found that the highest rates of first hospital admissions for schizophrenia came from

central-city areas where residential mobility was high and
socioeconomic status low, from ethnic groups living in non-
ethnic areas, and from foreign-born populations living in
slums—all circumstances in which social isolation might
occur. He suggested that the isolated individual, through
lack of intimate personal contacts, is deficient in his understanding of the reactions of others and may respond to them
unconventionally and inappropriately.

MELVIN KOHN and Clausen of the Laboratory of Socioenviron-
mental Studies proposed an investigation to test this hypothesis. Hagerstown, Maryland, was selected as the site of the
study because the Public Health Service's Division of Public
Health Methods had long conducted carefully documented mor-
bidity studies there. Kohn and Clausen interviewed 45 schizophrenic patients who had been admitted in their first illness
to Maryland state mental hospitals during 1940-1952. Controls
were matched on the basis of age, sex, and occupation or
father's occupation. By virtue of the extensive PHS files,
it was possible to select controls for a period averaging 16
years before hospitalization of the index patients. In half
the cases, index patients and controls had actually been in
the same public school class. Families were included in a
detailed interview schedule.

Patients and controls were categorized as follows: isolates—those whose activities were primarily sedentary with
little or no social interaction; partial isolates—those who
engaged in both social and solitary activities; and nonisolates—those whose activities were primarily social. It was
found that 7 of the patients were isolates and 8 partial isolates, as compared with only 1 in each category among the
controls; that 9 of the patients played only with siblings,
as compared with 6 of the controls; and that 19 of the patients were nonisolates, as compared with 36 of the controls.
(Two of the patients and one of the controls were not classified.)

Investigation of the observed isolation could not establish conclusively that it was self-determined. But neither
could external causes for the isolation be demonstrated. The
isolates had had no more illnesses, no greater degree of
residential mobility or parental restriction, and no more
remote housing. Isolates and partial isolates did not fall
ill earlier than the nonisolate patients, did not require
longer periods of hospitalization, and did not respond less
adequately to treatment.

Kohn and Clausen concluded that their data did not support the hypothesis that social isolation is a predisposing
factor in schizophrenia. They went on to point out that the
development of social isolation may be viewed as a sign that

an individual is no longer capable of functioning in interpersonal relationships. They suggested that instead of determining the relation between social isolation and psychosis,
it might be more fruitful to study the conditions that produce alienation, and then proceed to the processes by which
subsequent experiences transform interpersonal difficulty into interpersonal failure.

In another study they confirmed an earlier finding that
family relationships of schizophrenic patients were significantly different from those of presumably normal individuals
with the same social background. But when they controlled
for social class, they found that this observation applied to
the middle class alone. Family relations of middle-class
schizophrenics resembled those of all lower-class families,
schizophrenic and nonschizophrenic alike. This finding was
consistent with the Faris-Dunham study of the social class
distribution. The obvious inference from these studies—
though the incidence of schizophrenia was low, even in the
lowest social class—is that circumstances of lower-class
life, among other things, might increase susceptibility to
schizophrenia.

Studies on class and family were at that time extensive
but inconsistent and did not provide an understanding of the
processes by which social class might influence personality
development and behavior. Kohn turned to this more basic
problem. A series of elegantly designed studies ultimately
grew into a major program of research into the effects of
class and occupation on values and personality and into the
social processes by which parental values are transmitted to
the offspring. In brief, Kohn established that there is a
consistent and meaningful relationship between people's social class positions and their values and orientation; that
the class-values relationship has important implications for
behavior; and that it can be interpreted as resulting from
systematic differences in conditions of life, particularly
occupational life, associated with social class.

The detailed findings grew out of a nationwide survey.
They have been confirmed independently by investigators in
Taiwan, France, Great Britain, Ireland, Canada, Peru, and West
Germany. Kohn's major study has been replicated and confirmed
in cultures as divergent as those of Poland and Japan. His
book Class and Conformity is widely regarded as a model of
sociological craftsmanship.

Metabolic and Pharmacologic Studies

The intramural program has had from its inception a goal of contributing to the understanding of how behavior is shaped by experience and how biological processes mediate its expression. The Laboratory of Psychosomatic Medicine assumed principal responsibility for the biological studies. The disciplines represented on its staff included psychiatry, internal medicine, biochemistry, and physiology.

One of the early projects of EDWARD EVARTS, the Acting Chief, was the study of the effects induced by lysergic acid diethylamide (LSD). It was believed at the time that the effects were both transitory and innocuous and that the psychosis induced by LSD might be considered a model that could throw light on some of the mechanisms involved in schizophrenia. Evarts enlisted the collaboration of several NIMH laboratories and, in addition, sought consultation from the National Heart Institute's Laboratory of Chemical Pharmacology, headed by BERNARD BRODIE.

The most important result of the consultation was the recruitment of JULIUS AXELROD from NHI to head the Section on Pharmacology in the NIMH laboratory. Axelrod had made several important discoveries. His observation that p-acetylaminophenol is the active metabolite of acetanilid and acetophenetidin was cited in textbooks as a classic example of the correlation of the metabolism of drugs with their pharmacologic effects. Of even greater importance was his demonstration that the sympathomimetic amines were metabolized by the microsomes of liver. This was the first demonstration of the liver oxidative microsomal system, which was subsequently found to play a principal role in the metabolism of most drugs.

Axelrod's interest in LSD had been sparked by its antagonism and chemical resemblance to serotonin, which Gaddum had shown to be present in the brain. Several biochemical associations of interest to investigators of mental illness were involved. SHORE and Brodie discovered that reserpine, a tranquilizer, depleted brain serotonin; and Vogt and CARLSSON reported that it also reduced the level of brain norepinephrine. Evarts, Axelrod, BERNHARD WITKOP, and ROSCOE BRADY published a report on the metabolism of LSD.

By the time this study was completed, it had become clear that LSD was capable of producing serious side effects. The project was discontinued, and Axelrod returned to work on the microsomal enzyme systems involved in the metabolism of narcotic drugs.

In 1956 Kety left his position as Director of Basic Research and joined the laboratory as Chief, changing its name to the Laboratory of Clinical Science. LOUIS SOKOLOFF accompanied him as Chief of the Section of Cerebral Metabolism and began the work that led eventually to the deoxyglucose method for measuring local rates of glucose utilization in the brain. Under Kety's direction the laboratory embarked on a critical review of the biological theories of the etiology of schizophrenia and undertook to repeat the experiments that appeared most promising. In one instance after another, the reported finding was not confirmed, most frequently because the controls in the original study had been inadequate. This became so common an occurrence that someone wryly suggested changing the name of the laboratory to Laboratory of Negative Results.

Axelrod's participation in these replication ventures followed an intriguing suggestion of the Canadian investigators Hoffer and Osmond. They had advanced the theory that schizophrenia might be due to the aberrant metabolism of epinephrine* to adrenochrome. At that time epinephrine was believed to be metabolized and inactivated by monoamine oxidase, but little was known about its fate in the body. Axelrod was unable to find evidence to support the adrenochrome theory. The study, however, led to major discoveries about the metabolism of epinephrine and the neurotransmitter norepinephrine.

Axelrod's attention was drawn to a report by Armstrong, McMillan, and Shaw that patients with pheochromocytoma, an epinephrine-secreting tumor, excreted large amounts of 3-methoxy-4-hydroxymandelic acid in the urine. This suggested that the pathway for metabolism of epinephrine might be O-methylation. Axelrod found that epinephrine was rapidly metabolized when incubated in liver homogenates with ATP (adenosine triphosphate) and methionine. It appeared that ATP and methionine were converted to the methyl donor S-adenosylmethionine, a compound first implicated by CANTONI, and that epinephrine was indeed metabolized by an O-methylating enzyme.

In a series of brilliant studies, Axelrod and his coworkers described the enzyme, catechol-O-methyltransferase. They demonstrated that it metabolized all catechols tested. Further, they established that the catecholamines are metabolized by two pathways: O-methylation as described above and deamination by monoamine oxidase. And they found other methylating enzymes—one in rabbit lung that could convert tryptamine into the hallucinogen dimethyltryptamine.

---

*The chief neurohormone of the adrenal medulla, or "marrow" of the adrenal gland. Epinephrine (from Greek *epi* + *nephros*, or near + kidney) is also called adrenaline, Adrenalin (Parke, Davis), or adrenalin (from Latin *ad* + *renes*, or near + kidneys). The third spelling, according to some authorities, is incorrect, as the word without the terminal "e" is a trademark and should be capitalized.

Normally occurring compounds found to be substrates for catechol-O-methyltransferase were norepinephrine, dopamine, dopa, 3,4-dihydroxymandelic acid, 3,4-hydroxyphenylglycol, 3,4-hydroxyphenylglycol acetic acid, and 2-hydroxyestradiol. While the enzyme's activity was highest in liver, it was found in all tissues studied, including the brain.

A paradoxic finding, reported by CROUT, was that the action of norepinephrine was rapidly terminated even when the enzyme and monoamine oxidase were inhibited. Axelrod explained this in demonstrating that the liberated neurotransmitter was taken up and held in physiologically inactive form in the dense core granules of sympathetic nerve terminals. This knowledge made possible the elucidation of sites and modes of action of a variety of drugs that affect norepinephrine's fate. These discoveries had direct application in the study and treatment of cardiovascular, neurologic, and psychiatric disorders.

[See also Kopin chapter, "Neurotransmitters and Neuropsychopharmacology."]

Some Results

The studies described above were among the pioneering explorations in their respective areas of investigation. They were in the forefront of a veritable explosion of interest in schizophrenia research. Questions left unresolved were, of course, recognized by the scientists themselves. Their subsequent work answered some of the questions, raised others, and clarified issues that need consideration.

In a World Health Organization study supported by NIMH, nine teams of psychiatrists from developed and developing countries (JOHN STRAUSS and WILLIAM CARPENTER, then of NIMH, were the United States team) found similar symptom pictures in widely differing cultures. It was noted on followup that in the developing countries, schizophrenia followed a more benign course.

The preponderance of evidence, including greatly expanded adoption studies by Kety, Rosenthal, and Wender, leaves little doubt that genetic factors contribute to the development of the disorder. A wealth of psychophysiological studies and investigations of cognitive processes have defined clear differences between schizophrenics and normal control subjects, pointing to central nervous system structures and processes that must be involved in schizophrenic behavior. The Nobel Prize-winning work of Axelrod and Von Euler led to the discovery of additional neurotransmitters and to their implication in schizophrenia and other disease states. It also increased our understanding of normal physiology.

A range of family studies revealed distorted power relationships, prolonged symbiotic attachments between parent and child, and/or communication deviance, clearly implicating family experience as a contributory factor in the maintenance and possibly development of the disorder. WILLIAM POLLIN and JAMES STABENAU, of the NIMH Adult Psychiatry Branch, for example, studied a series of identical twins who were discordant for schizophrenia. And usually it is only one child in a family who is the "identified patient." No exogenous factor, however, has been established as a sufficient cause.

Kohn pointed out that the observations of the sociologist cannot be explained without invoking concepts of stress and/or genetics. In the nature/nurture controversy, it is tempting but hardly scientific for the advocate of nature to take as proof of his own hypothesis the failure to prove nurture a sufficient cause, and vice versa. Granting the fact that our increased knowledge has not yet established precisely the extent to which either or both are involved, the words of Lucretius seem as apt today as when first expressed centuries ago:

> Though education may apply a similar polish to various individuals, it still leaves fundamental traces of their various temperaments. It must not be supposed that innate vices can be completely eradicated; one man will still incline more readily to outbursts of rage; another will give way a little sooner to fear; a third will accept some contingencies too impassively. And in a host of other ways men must differ one from another in temperament and so also in the resultant behavior. To unfold here the secret causes of these differences is beyond my power. I cannot even find names for the multiplicity of atomic shapes that give rise to this variety of types. But I am clear that there is one relevant fact I can affirm; the lingering traces of inborn temperament that cannot be eliminated by philosophy are so slight that there is nothing to prevent men from leading a life worthy of the Gods.

Commentary

One looks back at the 28 years that have passed since the opening of the Clinical Center with the feeling that it was good to be young in a young institution. Reminiscing about

the early days of the Institute, JOHN C. EBERHART, the first
Director of the NIMH Intramural Research Program, remarked,
"It had early leaders with vision, maturity, limited personal
ambition, but strong organizational ambition."

During the period in which the foregoing studies were
carried out, JAMES SHANNON served as Director, NIH; JOSEPH
SMADEL, G. BURROUGHS MIDER, and ROBERT BERLINER, successively, as Deputy Director for Science; JACK MASUR as Director, Clinical Center; and Robert Felix as Director, NIMH.
Although critical, they gave unstinting support once their
searching questions were satisfactorily answered. They re-
sourcefully adapted a set of general-purpose government regulations and procedures to the specific requirements of a
broad range of disciplines. They provided an environment and
governance that encouraged and supported creativity, and
enlisted the dedication of the staff to their goals for the
institution.

Finally, all of us, directors and investigators alike,
owe much to those officers of the Public Health Service whose
vision of the future of biomedical and behavioral science
found expression in this research institute, designed to
foster interaction and close collaboration between the basic
laboratory and the clinic.

Selected References

Axelrod, J., and R. Weinshilbaum. Catecholamines. N Engl J
    Med 27:237-242, 1972.
Brand, J.L. The National Mental Health Act of 1946: A retro-
    spect. Bull Hist Med 39:231-245, 1965.
Kohn, M.L. Class and Conformity: A Study in Values. Home-
    wood, Ill.: Dorsey Press, 1969.
Rosenthal, D. (ed.). The Genain Quadruplets. New York: Basic
    Books, 1963.
Rosenthal, D., and S.S. Kety (eds.). The Transmission of
    Schizophrenia. Oxford: Pergamon Press, 1968. [Note par-
    ticularly papers by M. Bleuler, M.L. Kohn, P.H. Wender,
    D. Rosenthal and S.S. Kety, and L.C. Wynne.]
World Health Organization. The International Pilot Study of
    Schizophrenia. Geneva: WHO, 1973.
Wynne, L.C., and M.T. Singer. Thought disorder and family re-
    lations of schizophrenics: I. A research strategy. Arch
    Gen Psychiatry 9:191-198, 1963.

Introduction

NEUROTRANSMITTERS AND
NEUROPSYCHOPHARMACOLOGY

This chapter describes investigations in the Laboratory of Clinical Science, National Institute of Mental Health, from 1957 to 1972. It is no exaggeration to say that the results have opened a new era in the understanding and treatment of mental illness and neuropsychiatric disorders.

The classic experiment showing that stimulation of the vagus nerve released a heart-slowing material into the bloodstream had a far-reaching impact. Otto Loewi's "Vagusstoffe" turned out to be one of several chemicals that act specifically to transmit impulses either from one nerve cell to another, as at a synapse, or from a nerve cell to an effector, such as a muscle or gland. The past half-century has seen a flowering of neurochemistry as knowledge of the neurotransmitters and their receptor sites expands.

Moreover, we are in an age of rational creation of new drugs. In earlier times drugs had to be "discovered" through empirical detection of pharmacologic activity, at first in natural substances and later in synthetics. Now, with increasing frequency, drugs are tailor-made. A molecule may be designed, say, to compete with a neurotransmitter for a certain receptor site, interfering with transmission of the message. Or, once it is known that the body produces an enzyme that catalyzes destruction of a specific neurotransmitter, inhibitors of that enzyme may be developed to spare the transmitter and promote its effectiveness.

In these and related ways, a large number of novel drugs have been elaborated. Both agonists and antagonists of neurotransmitters have enriched the pharmacopoeia. The science of pharmacology is now moving rapidly along the path proposed by Paul Ehrlich. Therapeutic advantages are being realized through the rapid-fire molding of well-aimed "magic bullets."

D. S.

4

NEUROTRANSMITTERS AND
NEUROPSYCHOPHARMACOLOGY

I. J. Kopin

Background

The concept that nerve terminals can emit a message-transmitting agent was first proved by Otto Loewi in 1921 when he showed that a substance released into the perfusate of an isolated frog's heart during stimulation of the vagus nerve could slow another frog's heartbeat. The substance was later identified as acetylcholine. Ulf von Euler, in 1948, found that norepinephrine was the active substance in sympathetic nerves innervating bovine spleen, and W. Stanley Peart showed that it was released upon stimulation of the splenic nerves. Subsequently Marthe Vogt demonstrated norepinephrine in brain and suggested that it was a neurotransmitter both there and at peripheral sympathetic nerve endings. By 1950 only acetylcholine and norepinephrine had been identified as potential neurotransmitters, but shortly thereafter serotonin and dopamine were found in the central nervous system. At the close of the decade, these four compounds were considered to be the major neurotransmitters in brain.

The 1950s brought into Western medicine a series of substances that formed the basis for a revolution in the management of psychiatric disorders. Reserpine, a potent hypotensive and tranquilizer, was isolated; the first of the monoamine oxidase inhibitors with antidepressant effect was discovered; chlorpromazine was found to be an effective antipsychotic, and related tricyclic antidepressants were introduced; lithium had been suggested for treatment of mania; the tranquilizer meprobamate was in wide use; and chlordiazepoxide was introduced for treatment of anxiety. This array of relatively specific therapeutic agents replaced sedatives and hypnotics, opened locked mental hospital doors, and provided pharmacologic tools

---

I. J. KOPIN, M.D., Director, Intramural Research Program, National Institute of Neurological and Communicative Disorders and Stroke.

for investigators. It had become possible to examine the "disturbances in brain chemistry" that Freud had envisioned as the basis of many psychiatric disorders.

The emergence of psychopharmacology, largely through technologic advances that afforded precise measurement of biogenic amines* and their metabolites, set the stage for an explosion of research on neurotransmitters and the relation of chemistry to behavior. Subsequent advances in understanding the processes regulating neurotransmitters resulted in the first rational neurotherapy: L-dopa for the management of Parkinson's disease. Other dramatic results were drugs for treatment of hypertension (methyldopa) and arrhythmia (propranolol) as well as a host of new psychotherapeutic agents.

After the opening of the Clinical Center in 1953, investigators throughout the rapidly growing National Institutes of Health made important discoveries at an amazing rate. No one immersed in this milieu could escape being swept up in the enthusiasm of the eager, bright young investigators from all corners of the world who came to learn, make their mark, and return to their institutions to conduct research, teach, and become leaders in the biomedical sciences.

The neurosciences were no exception, and investigators in several Institutes contributed importantly to the unfolding of basic concepts of neurotransmitters and the development of neuropsychopharmacology. It is impossible in a brief account to describe all the major contributions to this large field. However, an illustration of the excitement, the interactions among scientists, and the processes leading to advances may be provided by a somewhat detailed account of one segment of research in a single laboratory. I will attempt to follow the evolution of the concepts of chemical neurotransmitters and neuropsychopharmacology, using as a focal point research on catecholamines in the Laboratory of Clinical Science, National Institute of Mental Health, between 1957 and 1972.

Many of the fundamental discoveries of processes involved in the regulation of chemical neurotransmitters were unfolded in relation to norepinephrine, a biogenic substance of the catecholamine group. The biosynthesis, storage, release, receptor activation, and termination of action were delineated first for norepinephrine at peripheral nerve endings and then extended to the brain. Subsequently these processes were defined for other neurotransmitters.

---

*Biologically generated neurotransmitters containing an amine (from "ammonium" + "ine"). They are small molecules incorporating the amino group, NH_2.

Fate of the Catecholamines

In 1955 SEYMOUR KETY, then Chief of the newly created Laboratory of Clinical Science, called attention to the intriguing suggestion by Hoffer, Osmond, and Smythies in Canada that abnormal metabolism of epinephrine to form excessive amounts of adrenochrome (which they thought to be hallucinogenic) was responsible for the symptoms of schizophrenia. This prompted JULIUS AXELROD, who had recently been appointed Chief of the Laboratory's Section on Pharmacology, to look into catecholamine metabolism.

At that time almost nothing was known about the fate of epinephrine or norepinephrine. Both were known to be substrates for the enzyme monoamine oxidase (MAO).* But even drastic inhibition of MAO did not potentiate the actions of administered epinephrine. It was therefore clear that this enzyme was not required for inactivating the transmitter, a process that would be essential to efficient nerve function.

In March 1957 Marvin D. Armstrong and Armand McMillan published an abstract in *Federation Proceedings* reporting that 3-methoxy-4-hydroxymandelic acid, which they named vanillylmandelic acid (VMA), was the major urinary metabolite of epinephrine and norepinephrine in humans. Axelrod considered the possibility that O-methylation occurred before deamination —before MAO came into play—and was the route of metabolic inactivation of the catecholamines. He showed that epinephrine was rapidly destroyed upon incubation with homogenates of rat liver (source of hormone-metabolizing enzymes), methionine (source of a methyl group), and ATP (adenosine triphosphate, a source of energy). Destruction did not occur, however, if ATP or methionine was omitted from the homogenate. He then obtained some S-adenosylmethionine from GABRIEL de la HABA, who was working with its discoverer, GIULIO CANTONI, and showed that this active methyl donor could substitute for methionine and ATP. Evidently the essential factor in liver was a methylating enzyme.

Since the metabolite VMA was methylated in the 3 position, Axelrod assumed that methylation occurred in this position on the epinephrine molecule. A telephone call to BERNHARD WITKOP initiated the synthesis of a new compound by SIRO SENOH, the first of many Japanese Visiting Scientists at NIH. At Axelrod's suggestion, Senoh synthesized methylated epinephrine, or "metanephrine." This compound proved to be identical to that formed in incubating epinephrine with S-adenosylmethio-

---

*That is, were known to be transformed in reactions catalyzed by MAO.

nine and liver homogenates. The *O*-methylating enzyme in liver was soon purified, found to *O*-methylate other catechols, and named catechol-*O*-methyltransferase (COMT). Metanephrine was found in the urine of rats and humans. It was clear that a new route for the metabolism of epinephrine and norepinephrine had been discovered.

Tracing the Biogenic Amines

Meanwhile Kety had arranged for the synthesis of tritiated epinephrine and norepinephrine* and had introduced into our laboratory a newly available instrument, the liquid scintillation spectrophotometer. The object was to use these labeled compounds to trace the metabolism of catecholamines in normal subjects and schizophrenic patients. Early experiments with radioactive substances were tedious. Each sample vial had to be placed in a refrigerated shielded scintillation spectrometer, the scalar readings recorded, and the sample replaced. Our early version of the spectrophotometer was soon superseded by one with an automatic sample changer, and isotopic tracers were quickly adopted throughout the laboratory. ELWOOD La-BROSSE and JAY MANN, with Seymour Kety, instituted quantitative studies on the separation of catecholamines and their metabolites.

At about this time, interest in biogenic amines and their role in the nervous system was rapidly increasing. Controversies about methodology and a need for current views on the biosynthesis, disposition, and actions of these substances led to the first Symposium on Catecholamines, sponsored by NIH's Division of Research Grants and National Heart Institute. It was held at the Clinical Center in October 1958, and the papers were published in *Pharmacological Reviews*.

At the time of the symposium, I was a Research Associate, with Seymour Kety as my preceptor. The Research Associate program, newly established at NIH, supported young physicians for two years of full-time research in the NIH intramural program, with a view to drawing them into careers in clinical investigation. I was intrigued by the controversy over the roles of MAO and COMT in terminating the actions of catecholamines. Inhibition of MAO was known to elevate tissue levels of norepinephrine, suggesting that the enzyme was instrumental in inactivating the neurotransmitter; and inhibition of COMT was known to potentiate administered catecholamines but not the effects of sympathetic nerve stimulation, suggesting a

---

*Epinephrine and norepinephrine tagged with tritium, ^{3}H, a radioisotope of hydrogen.

role in the inactivation of catecholamines outside nerves.
Kety encouraged me to carry out some double-isotope experiments designed to distinguish alternative metabolic pathways
of epinephrine. This undertaking set the course of my research
career.

With Julius Axelrod, I studied the metabolism of [^{3}H]epinephrine* and [^{14}C]metanephrine** and was able to show that
O-methylation was the predominant pathway of the administered
catecholamine in rats and humans.

Inactivation of Catecholamines in Relation to Nerve Impulse

While metabolic studies on humans proceeded, Julius Axelrod with HANS WEIL-MALHERBE and ROBERT TOMCHICK began to investigate the disposition of [^{3}H]epinephrine in animals. They
found that much of the tritiated catecholamine was retained in
the tissues long after its actions had been dissipated. GORDON WHITBY showed this to be so for norepinephrine as well.
It appeared to Axelrod that the tissues retaining the catecholamines were those well supplied with sympathetic nerves.
GEORG HERTTING, who began working with Axelrod at the time,
suggested an approach to testing this idea: sympathectomy, or
nerve removal. Together with Whitby, we removed the superior
cervical ganglion in cats and found that the [^{3}H]norepinephrine was rapidly depleted, confirming Axelrod's impression.

Hertting and Axelrod showed that the tritiated catecholamine was released during sympathetic nerve stimulation. Together with LINCOLN POTTER (the first of Axelrod's long series
of Research Associates), they found that the rate of spontaneous disappearance of [^{3}H]norepinephrine from tissues depended
on the nerve impulse flow and was retarded by ganglionic
blocking agents or by decentralization.

Hertting with SIDNEY HESS in the Heart Institute showed
that reserpine depleted both tritiated and endogenous norepinephrine at the same rate. This observation confirmed the
validity of using tritiated norepinephrine as a tracer for
measuring turnover.

The Roles of MAO and COMT Distinguished

Certain drugs, such as cocaine, blocked uptake of norepinephrine into nerves and also potentiated the effects of

_____

*Tritiated epinephrine (see previous footnote).
**Metanephrine tagged with the radioisotope carbon-14.

sympathetic nerve stimulation. Thus uptake into nerves was postulated as a major means for terminating the action of released neurotransmitter. Electron microscopy demonstrated that nerve terminals contain vesicles. Potter and Axelrod showed that labeled norepinephrine was taken up into a fraction containing dopamine β-hydroxylase, the enzyme responsible for converting dopamine to norepinephrine. Together with D. G. WOLFE and K. C. RICHARDSON, they demonstrated by radioautography* that the labeled catecholamine was stored in dense core vesicles of sympathetic nerves.

At about this time (1962), EDNA GORDON, Hertting, and I showed that norepinephrine taken up into the tissues followed a different metabolic path from norepinephrine destroyed immediately after intravenous injection or release from nerve endings. O-Methylation (by COMT) was the primary route of metabolism outside the nerve, whereas deamination (by MAO) predominated when norepinephrine escaped from storage sites into the neural cytoplasm (see figure).

Examining the Effects of Drugs

Axelrod and his co-workers, in a series of elegantly simple but crucial animal experiments, showed that psychoactive drugs influence the processes essential to neurotransmitter function. Two postdoctoral fellows from abroad, JACQUES GLOWINSKI and LESLIE IVERSEN, joined Axelrod, and together they demonstrated that [^{3}H]norepinephrine, injected into the cerebral ventricles, would label the brain's norepinephrine stores. Thus the effects of drugs on neurotransmission could be examined. It was shown that the stimulant amphetamine releases the catecholamines, antidepressants inhibit their uptake, and MAO inhibitors slow their metabolism. ROSS BALDESSARINI and I found that brain slices took up [^{3}H]norepinephrine and released it upon stimulation with an electric current or subjection to potassium ion at depolarizing concentrations.

Diversification

In the mid 1960s many budding branches of the field developed. In my laboratory JOSEPH E. FISCHER, JOSE MUSACCHIO, DALE HORST, and I embarked on a series of studies to define the properties and the role in drug action of false adren-

---

*A technique for localizing radioisotope in tissue slices by means of photographic emulsion.

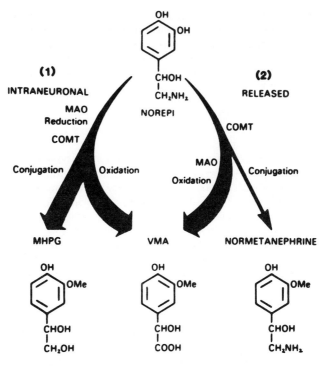

NOREPINEPHRINE, the chief sympathetic neurotransmitter, is metabolized by two major pathways. (1) Within nerves, it is first transformed (deaminated) by the enzyme monoamine oxidase (MAO), then reduced, and further metabolized (O-methylated) by the enzyme catechol-O-methyltransferase (COMT). Subsequent paths differ quantitatively in rats and humans. The main urinary metabolite in the rat is 3-methoxy-4-hydroxyphenylglycol (MHPG); in the human, vanillylmandelic acid (VMA). (2) Norepinephrine released at nerve terminals (but not recaptured) is first O-methylated, then deaminated. The main urinary metabolites of normetanephrine in rats and humans are MHPG and VMA, but some of the O-methylated product escapes deamination and is excreted as normetanephrine.

ergic* transmitters. These are substances chemically related to norepinephrine that are synthesized, stored, and released in the same manner as the authentic transmitter but cannot adequately replace it at the site of action, the receptor. RICHARD WURTMAN, SOLOMON SNYDER, and others in Axelrod's lab-

---

*Adrenergic: pertaining to the adrenal hormones adrenaline (epinephrine) and noradrenaline (norepinephrine).

oratory initiated and developed studies on the circadian
rhythms of pineal gland production of melatonin, a substance
known to suppress gonadal function and reported to have other
effects.   IRA BLACK studied regulation of liver enzymes by
adrenergic mechanisms, and Axelrod further developed the use
of tritiated S-adenosylmethionine as a tool for studying
methylation reactions.   These seminal activities led to the
discovery of new enzymes and metabolic pathways and, years
later, to productive studies on the role of methylation in
membrane function.

The results of fundamental studies on neurotransmitters
and psychopharmacologic agents began to have their impact on
psychiatry, anesthesiology, neurology, and other clinical
areas.   Led by Seymour Kety, psychiatrists such as JOSEPH E.
SCHILDKRAUT, WILLIAM BUNNEY, and Baldessarini began to develop
heuristic hypotheses relating biogenic amines to psychiatric
disorders.   Neurologists such as THOMAS CHASE were interested
in studying these agents in neurological disorders, encouraged
by the success with L-dopa in Parkinson's disease.   Research
on both humans and animals was undertaken to develop methods
for assessing biogenic amine function, in order to test hypotheses concerning neuropsychiatric disorders and psychoactive drugs.   [See also chapter by Robert A. Cohen.]

"The NIH Neuron"

Tyrosine hydroxylase, the rate-limiting enzyme in norepinephrine formation, was discovered in SIDNEY UDENFRIEND's laboratory in the Heart Institute.   GORAN SEDVALL and I showed
that sympathetic nerve stimulation accelerated formation of
norepinephrine by increasing tyrosine hydroxylation.   Regulation of the biosynthetic processes for catecholamines became
a focus of attention.   HANS THOENEN, ROBERT MUELLER, Wurtman,
and Axelrod showed that the enzymes in the adrenal medulla and
sympathetic nerves could be induced by endocrine as well as
neural regulators.   RICHARD KVETNANSKY in my laboratory made
similar observations in stressed animals.

By the end of the decade, the concept of an adrenergic
nerve ending had evolved from that of a simple norepinephrine-
releasing terminal to that of a complex structure in which
norepinephrine was synthesized by a sequence of defined enzymes adaptive to functional requirements, was stored in a
chemical complex contained in dense core vesicles, was released by a calcium-dependent exocytotic (secretory) process,
and was whisked away from the receptor site by uptake into the

presynaptic* nerve ending. The model of the sympathetic nerve
terminal gained the nickname "NIH neuron." Such phenomena as
tachyphylaxis to tyramine,** supersensitivity to catecholamines after chronic denervation or cocaine administration, and
the actions of many psychoactive drugs were related to alterations in the synthesis, storage, release, or inactivation of
norepinephrine.

In 1970 Julius Axelrod was awarded the Nobel Prize for
his many contributions to the development of these concepts
of neurotransmitter function. Since this milestone in his
career, Axelrod's interests have expanded to embrace important related fields, such as membrane biochemistry and regulation of receptors. After 1970, studies on neurotransmitters
accelerated everywhere and came to include a host of new substances—for example, the opiatelike endorphins and enkephalins and other peptides.

Clinical Applications

In Axelrod's laboratory, basic science observations had a
direct influence on clinical investigation. PERRY MOLINOFF developed a sensitive assay for the enzyme dopamine β-hydroxylase, RICHARD WEINSHILBOUM demonstrated its presence in human
plasma and its genetic control, and ROLAND CIARANELLO began
studies of genetic regulation of catecholamine-synthesizing
enzymes. Radioenzymatic methods based on methylating enzymes
previously discovered by Axelrod were developed at NIH and
elsewhere to assay the minute quantities of catecholamines and
their metabolites in human cerebrospinal fluid and plasma.
These methods have been of great value in laboratories concerned with cardiovascular disorders (particularly hypertension), neuropsychiatric states (anxiety, stress, affective
disorders), and clinical pharmacology. Since 1972 these clinical activities, studies on receptors and their regulation,
and the appearance of a host of putative neurotransmitters
have shaped research programs here and elsewhere. We have
seen that the 15 years from 1957 to 1972 were critical to
these developments.

---

*Pertaining to the proximal (axon) side of the synapse,
or point at which a nerve impulse passes from an axon of one
neuron (nerve cell) to the dendrite of another.

**Rapid decrease in response to repeated administration
of the epinephrinelike compound tyramine.

Extensions

Investigators in many laboratories at NIMH and NIH collaborated with those in the Laboratory of Clinical Science and, of course, made independent advances in the field of neurotransmitters. At NIMH FLOYD BLOOM, GIAN SALMOIRAGHI, BARRY HOFFER, GEORGE SIGGINS, ERMINIO COSTA, NORTON NEFF, and a host of others have been prolific contributors to the much expanded disciplines of the neurosciences. In the Heart Institute, investigators in Udenfriend's and BERNARD BRODIE's laboratories contributed importantly to the biochemistry and pharmacology of the nervous system. For the future, there is great promise in the disciplines of molecular genetics, the implications of cellular biology for the study of the nervous system and its disorders, and the strong probability of entirely new approaches. The promise is implicit in the flow of brilliant, innovative young scientists through these laboratories and clinics. Their work continues to be a source of exciting new knowledge and its applications.

Selected References

Axelrod, J. Noradrenaline: Fate and control of its biosynthesis. Science 173:598-606, 1971.

Axelrod, J., and R. Weinshilboum. Catecholamines. N Engl J Med 287:237-242, 1972.

Kety, S.S. The central physiological and pharmacological effects of the biogenic amines and their correlations with behavior, in The Neurosciences, G.D. Quorton, T. Melmechuk, and F.O. Schmitt (eds.). New York: Rockefeller University Press, 1967.

Kopin, I.J. False adrenergic transmitters. Ann Rev Pharmacol 8:377-394, 1968.

Kopin, I.J. Metabolic degradation of catecholamines: The relative importance of different pathways under physiological conditions and after administration of drugs. Hbk of Exp Pharmacol 33:270-282, 1972.

Schildkraut, J.J., and S.S. Kety. Biogenic amines and emotion. Science 156: 21-30, 1967.

Introduction

THE NEUROSCIENCES—BASIC AND CLINICAL

The domain of neurology is truly enormous. With central and peripheral components, with sensory and motor pathways and many complex interrelations and interconnections, with voluntary and autonomic functions employing electrical transmission in the axons and chemical transmission in the synapses, such a complex and refined system would be expected to manifest diseases of virtually every etiology.

Thus we find frank infections, both viral and bacterial; a variety of tumors; vascular diseases; and degenerative diseases of mysterious origin, some of which entail alterations well-defined chemically, such as demyelination. There are diseases that act predominantly upon the motor pathways, such as poliomyelitis, while others attack the sensory centers, such as migraine. And the "slow virus" diseases so far discovered affect the central nervous system.

Through brain extensions via the cranial nerves, neurology embraces all the organs of special sense, such as the retina, the cochlea, the semicircular canals, and the end organs of smell and taste; while peripheral nerves bring us sensations of touch, temperature, and pain.

In order to protect this remarkable structure, nature has encased much of it in a bony box (the skull) and a bony canal (the vertebral column). Nevertheless, trauma to the central nervous system is a common catastrophe and has been the subject of much study. It is this multiplicity of parts, functions, and disorders that makes the activities of what is now called the National Institute of Neurological and Communicative Disorders and Stroke (NINCDS) so diverse.

Clinically, neurology relates in one way or another to all specialties of medicine, but to none more than psychiatry. In the following chapter Dr. TOWER reveals the matrimonial entanglements that have existed between the Neurological Institute and the National Institute of Mental Health. Another closely related specialty is ophthalmology. The National Eye Institute was clearly an offspring of the National Institute of Neurological Diseases and Blindness, an ancestor of NINCDS.

We find that NINCDS is conducting research in many of the

46

areas just mentioned. There are scientists in its labora-
tories who are seeking to learn more about the origin and
transmission of the neural impulse. Simultaneously, scien-
tists in the clinic are concerned with the control of epilepsy
and a better understanding of the several chronic and still
incurable degenerative diseases of the central nervous sys-
tem. By attacking on a broad front, we are making steady
progress in these and other branches of the neurological
sciences.

D. S.

5

THE NEUROSCIENCES—BASIC AND CLINICAL

Donald B. Tower

Origin of the Laboratory of Neurochemistry

The "Neurology Institute" was created as the National Institute of Neurological Diseases and Blindness (NINDB) by act of Congress on August 15, 1950. In that year the Institute acquired a director, PEARCE BAILEY (1902-1976), who came to NIH from the Veterans Administration, where he had served as chief of neurology. The NIH Director, WILLIAM H. SEBRELL, Jr., had decided that NINDB would share with the National Institute of Mental Health (NIMH) an intramural basic science program under the direction of SEYMOUR S. KETY. It was not until 1953 that NINDB received an operating budget of its own and was allocated space (with understandable reluctance) from NIMH in the newly opened Clinical Center. NINDB then launched its own intramural clinical research program. [Bailey has provided a detailed account of the founding and early years of the Institute for the period of his directorship, 1950-1959 (1).]

In the spring of 1953 Bailey recruited two key persons, G. MILTON SHY (1919-1967) and MAITLAND BALDWIN (1918-1970), to head the clinical intramural branches in medical and surgical neurology, respectively. Shy and Baldwin both came from the training programs of the Montreal Neurological Institute (MNI), then directed by Wilder Penfield, via subsequent faculty appointments at the University of Colorado Medical School in Denver. They recruited additional staff: COSIMO AJMONE-MARSAN in electroencephalography, IGOR KLATZO in neuropathology, DONALD B. TOWER in neurochemistry, GIOVANNI DiCHIRO in neuroradiology, and RICHARD L. IRWIN in neuropharmacology. The first three were also "graduates" of MNI and, together with several other recruits (CHOH-LUH LI in neuro-

DONALD B. TOWER, M.D., Ph.D., Director Emeritus, National Institute of Neurological and Communicative Disorders and Stroke.

NIH: AN ACCOUNT OF RESEARCH
IN ITS LABORATORIES AND CLINICS
ISBN 0-12-667980-0

surgery, ANATOLE S. DEKABAN in pediatric neurology, JOHN M. VAN BUREN in neurosurgery, and SHIRLEY LEWIS in neurosurgical nursing), formed the largest "satellite" of MNI at any institution outside Montreal.

Additional recruits for the NINDB intramural clinical research program included BENI M. HORVATH in muscle chemistry, PAUL O. CHATFIELD (1917-1959) in neurophysiology, and LAURENCE L. FROST in psychology. LUDWIG von SALLMANN (1892-1975) was recruited from Columbia in 1954 to head the ophthalmology branch. Von Sallmann added ROBERT A. RESNIK in physical chemistry, SJOERD L. BONTING in biochemistry, THEODOR WANKO (1923-1964) in electron microscopy, FRANK J. MACRI in pharmacology, and PETER GOURAS and MICHELANGELO FUORTES (1917-1977) in physiology.

The staff of the various clinical branches and sections soon achieved effective interfaces with neurologically oriented groups in the NIMH-NINDB basic science program, including those of KENNETH S. COLE in biophysics, WADE H. MARSHALL (1907-1972) in neurophysiology, KARL FRANK in spinal cord physiology, WILLIAM F. WINDLE in neuroanatomy, JAN CAMMERMEYER in neuropathology, and ROSCOE O. BRADY in lipid neurochemistry. The combined basic research programs continued under the direction of Seymour Kety from 1951 to 1956 and of ROBERT B. LIVINGSTON from 1956 to 1960, when it was decided that the two Institutes' basic research laboratories should be separated. By 1961 Milton Shy had been appointed Scientific Director of the NINDB intramural research program, with Maitland Baldwin as Clinical Director.

I joined the NINDB intramural program in July 1953, shortly after its inception, and have been privileged to participate in its growth and development for much of its 30 years. Those early days provided many contrasts with the present. Henry Sebrell, NIH Director from 1950 to 1955, was easily approachable and accessible. In those days NIH was very much a "family" affair. The laboratory chiefs from all Institutes met regularly once a week at Top Cottage (where Building 31 now stands) for lunch and discussion of ongoing research. I was not then a laboratory chief but was often invited to present our neurochemical research or to participate in relevant discussions. This informal atmosphere extended to the research staff. Each winter before the congressional budget hearings, Pearce Bailey would invite the branch and section chiefs to his home for brainstorming sessions in preparation for his testimony. On one such occasion we toasted the success of the hearings with glasses of 105-year-old brandy from the dowry of his wife, Dora, who was descended from French nobility.

There were inevitable growing pains in the new research hospital. Typical questions were how to deal with an ongoing craniotomy when the operation lasted past 5 p.m. and no overtime had been authorized for operating room personnel; how to demonstrate that a research bed at NIH legitimately cost more per patient-day than one in a Veterans Administration hospital so that the Bureau of the Budget* would release operating funds for the NIH intramural programs; how to convince the NIH procurement office that the lowest bidder did not necessarily provide an adequate, timely product; or how to persuade Departmental and Congressional watchdogs that intramural scientists really had legitimate reasons for attending scientific meetings. Most such problems (though not the last) were eventually solved.

The Early Clinical Research Program

Meanwhile research began to flourish. Milton Shy inaugurated an aggressive program of investigations on neuromuscular disorders, including the muscular dystrophies, myasthenia gravis, amyotrophic lateral sclerosis ("Lou Gehrig's disease"), peripheral neuropathies, cerebellar ataxias, and related disorders. He devised techniques for taking muscle biopsies and innovative histochemical methods for examining them. The clinical research program was so successful that Shy established a whole school of investigators in the neuromuscular disorders from the clinical associates who "graduated" from his group. After Shy left NIH in 1962, W. KING ENGEL headed the NINDB Medical Neurology Branch and continued this very active research program.

From it came not only the recognition of new diseases, such as central core disease, nemaline myopathy, mitochondrial (megaconial or pleoconial) myopathies, and variants of the glycogen storage myopathies, but also new or more effective therapies, particularly in myasthenia gravis, dermatomyositis, and polymyositis. In these conditions, long-term, high single-dose, alternate-day prednisone therapy has been dramatically beneficial. More recently, skeletal muscle cells have been successfully cultured in vitro, where biochemical abnormalities can be rigorously manipulated and immunochemical studies evaluated. Such studies at NIH and elsewhere have led to the definite recognition of myasthenia gravis as an autoimmune disorder.

The other clinical branches were equally active. Epilepsy was the central concern of Baldwin and his colleagues in the

---

*Now Office of Management and Budget.

Surgical Neurology Branch. As graduates of the Penfield school in Montreal, they established a comparable program of diagnostic, surgical, and postoperative procedures for the treatment of focal seizures. The work of a well-coordinated team—the electroencephalographer Ajmone-Marsan, the neuroradiologist DiChiro, the psychologists Frost and later HERBERT C. LANSDELL, the neurosurgical operating room staff (nurse Shirley Lewis, neurophysiologist and microelectrode expert Choh-Luh Li), and the followup neurosurgeon John Van Buren—was essential for this complex type of clinical research and therapy.

The program was built on the Montreal experience. At operation, the affected area of cerebral cortex was exposed under scalp anesthesia, the patient being awake in order to respond to questions. The cortical brain areas were mapped for motor and sensory responses to gentle electrical stimulation, and the brain waves (cortical electrical activity) were recorded from an array of electrodes. In this way the focus of epileptic discharge could be localized and, if not impinging on vital areas, excised to rid the patient of seizure attacks.

The NINDB case series was impressively successful, as recent reviews by Ajmone-Marsan and Van Buren have demonstrated. After Mait Baldwin's untimely death in 1970, Van Buren continued this program until his departure for the University of Miami a few years ago. The new neurosurgical team under PAUL L. KORNBLITH has shifted emphasis to brain tumors, with some very exciting studies on the immunochemical characteristics of glial tumor cells and on tissue culture methods for evaluating the responsiveness of such cells to chemotherapeutic agents.

Research on Vision at NINDB

In opthalmology Von Sallmann assembled a very able team at a time when research in that field was less active than today. Studies on the crystalline lens with reference to cataracts, on the fluid dynamics of the anterior chamber with reference to glaucoma, on the treatment of toxoplasmosis infections of the retina, on the use of lasers to treat retinal or pararetinal structures, and on the retinal neuronal network—all represent activities of this group. The last two topics were addressed, respectively, by Peter Gouras and Mike Fuortes, both of whom achieved wide recognition.

Fuortes studied retinal neurophysiology, especially in the eye of the horseshoe crab *Limulus*. This preparation provided an anatomical and functional model that could be transferred to the more complex mammalian visual apparatus. The retina, a photoreceptive area at the rear of the eye, is in fact an extension of the brain. It is the only portion of the central nervous system that is readily accessible to visual, microelectrode, and chemotherapeutic examination and experiment. Hence the broader significance of such studies.

Reorganization in the 1960s

The 1960s brought a number of changes to NINDB. Pearce Bailey was succeeded as Director by RICHARD L. MASLAND, who served from 1960 to 1968. A neurologist with a special interest in epilepsy, Masland came from Bowman-Gray Medical School and had been recruited by Bailey to head the Collaborative Perinatal Study in 1958. It was he who set up the Institute's separate laboratory research program when the combined NIMH-NINDB operation was terminated. An active Collaborative and Field Research (C & FR) program was established, oriented primarily around the perinatal study. While not intramural by the usual definition, some of the C & FR units soon became so in character and, with the demise of the C & FR program in the early 1970s, joined the intramural organization.

Another major change occurred in 1968: the creation of a separate National Eye Institute (NEI). NINDB lost the "B" from its name and became briefly the National Institute of Neurological Diseases before Mary Lasker and Senator Lister Hill joined forces to have its name changed to the National Institute of Neurological Diseases and Stroke. Early in 1975 the name was changed again to the present National Institute of Neurological and Communicative Disorders and Stroke (NINCDS). As a result, the eye research programs, personnel, space, and budget were transferred out of the Neurology Institute to form NEI, though much of the central visual neurophysiology remained. For the period 1968-1973, the Institute was under the direction of EDWARD F. MacNICHOL, Jr. A biophysicist with special interests in visual systems, Ted MacNichol came from The Johns Hopkins University and, as the Institute's first nonclinically trained director, took more than usual interest in its intramural activities.

The need for more space was an inevitable consequence of the growing research program. This need was met in the late 1960s by the opening of Building 36 and the new surgical wing, Building 10-A, whose circular shape evoked the familiar designation "the silo." NINCDS shares Building 36 with NIMH and the surgical wing with the Heart Institute. Both buildings incorporated technological innovations that enhance research capabilities: e.g., for neurophysiology, computer network terminals and circulating artificial sea water (for marine specimens); for neurovirological studies, isolation lab and animal-holding areas (including cages with individual ventilation and sterilization systems); and for neurosurgery, the latest in electronic monitoring and recording apparatus. The increased research space did not spawn much additional staff but ended the collective breath-holding of already crowded investigators.

Collaborative and Field Research

The C & FR program of NINDB comprised some important actual and potential research units. The infectious diseases group under JOHN L. SEVER did outstanding research on rubella (German measles) during the major epidemic of the mid 1960s. Many pregnant mothers were afflicted, resulting in a large number of progeny with post-rubella congenital anomalies of the nervous system. Sever's group succeeded in isolating the rubella virus simultaneously with groups at Harvard and Walter Reed Army Hospital. This work led to an effective rubella vaccine that can completely protect pregnant mothers and their babies. Masland has provided a detailed account of these events (2). Sever and his colleagues went on to study a number of other neuroviral and neuroimmunological problems. Their discovery of the role of the measles virus in a fatal disabling brain disorder, subacute sclerosing panencephalitis (SSPE), is notable. Such investigations seem relevant to several other sclerosing and degenerative disorders of the nervous system, especially multiple sclerosis.

Amyotrophic Lateral Sclerosis and Parkinson's Disease Dementia

Many neurological disorders exhibit peculiarities of incidence, prevalence, and geographic distribution. An important component of the C & FR program was its neuroepidemiology unit under LEONARD T. KURLAND (now at the Mayo Clinic), later JACOB A. BRODY (now in NIA), and more recently BRUCE S. SCHOENBERG. Much effort was expended by these investigators and their associates on the remarkable focus of amyotrophic lateral sclerosis (ALS) and Parkinson's disease dementia (PDD), discovered on the island of Guam in the western Pacific. NINDB established a small clinical research facility at the Guam Memorial Hospital in Agana. Eventually this remote outpost became a special unit within the NINCDS intra-

mural program, and scientists from many countries continue to
face the challenge of these fatal disorders among the Guamanian natives.

What is especially intriguing about ALS and PDD is that
the brains of patients contain neurofibrillary tangles,
plaques, and other pathologic changes characteristic of Alzheimer's disease and similar senile or presenile dementias.
In the 1950s and 1960s Alzheimer's disease was regarded as
something of a neurological curiosity, but today we recognize
that the senile dementias constitute a major public health
problem. Thus the Guamanian and other studies take on a new
and compelling perspective. Although little can be done
for the Guamanians with ALS, some with PDD seem to benefit
from treatment with L-dopa and other medications. In recent
years DONALD B. CALNE and THOMAS N. CHASE in the Experimental
Therapeutics Branch have focused on developing new anti-
Parkinson therapies, such as bromocriptine.

Epilepsy

Another major outgrowth of the C & FR program was the
epilepsy unit, first headed by J. KIFFIN PENRY. This unit
has remained primarily extramural in its orientation, but has
always maintained intramural sections for studies of anticonvulsant drug pharmacodynamics and for specialized, long-
term telemetric monitoring (remote surveillance of brain
activity) of patients with severe seizure problems. Both
these sections have evolved into intramural units now headed,
respectively, by HARVEY J. KUPFERBERG and ROGER J. PORTER.
Kupferberg's studies have revolutionized the clinical management of the epileptic patient, of whom there are some 4 million in the United States. Building on known methods, Kupferberg and colleagues developed definitive techniques for quantifying the common anticonvulsant drugs in blood, urine, and
other body fluids. As a result, idiosyncrasies of drug metabolism, noncompliance of patients, and correlations of drug
blood levels with seizure control could be easily established,
assuring more effective treatment. On a given regimen, for
example, the simple expedient of following drug levels in the
patient's blood to ensure therapeutically optimal doses has
increased the proportion of seizure-free patients from 47 to
74 percent or better.

Slow Virus Diseases

Perhaps the most dramatic achievements to come out of the C & FR program are those from the unit headed by D. CARLETON GAJDUSEK and CLARENCE J. GIBBS [see chapter by these authors]. In 1959 Gajdusek came to NINDB fresh from recent forays into the highlands of New Guinea, where he had begun to study a curious fatal disorder called kuru. It was characterized by shaking, progressive motor disability, dementia, and death and was restricted to a particular native group, the Fore people. Dick Masland took Carleton under his wing, much to the dismay of many who saw resources seemingly frittered away on a rare disorder of a distant primitive tribe at a time when intramural research could have used the funds for pressing domestic problems. How wrong can one be?

Carleton Gajdusek is a most unusual person—pediatrician, neurologist, virologist, linguist, anthropologist, and much more. From those simple beginnings as a young physician trekking through the New Guinea bush and establishing rapport with its natives, he has built a worldwide Laboratory of Central Nervous System Studies, with satellites or connections in France, the U.S.S.R., central Africa, Australia, China, Japan, Papua-New Guinea, and much of Melanesia and Micronesia in the south and western Pacific. He has conducted or collaborated in experiments in most of these places.

When kuru was first recognized and studied, it was thought to be either a toxic or hereditary disorder because of its restriction to a particular native group and its predilection for women and children. However, examination of brain specimens obtained by Gajdusek led several neuropathologists, WILLIAM J. HADLOW and Klatzo in particular, to note similarities to other degenerative disorders of the nervous system, such as scrapie in sheep, Creutzfeldt-Jakob disease, and Alzheimer's disease. Scrapie was already known to be an infectious disorder of unusual type, though the agent had not been isolated. Accordingly, Gajdusek, Gibbs, and colleagues set out in the 1960s to ascertain whether kuru was transmissible. Fortunately they used chimpanzees and concentrated on intracerebral inoculations of samples from kuru brains. The first successful transmissions of the disease to chimpanzees occurred 22 and 30 months after inoculation, and subsequent trials reduced the average incubation time to 11 months. In the rhesus monkey, however, the incubation time is 8.5 years. Much later it became possible to transmit scrapie, kuru, and Creutzfeldt-Jakob disease to mice, hamsters, and other common mammals.

The work of the Gajdusek group has been truly a team effort. With Carleton so often away in the far corners of the

world, Joe Gibbs in Bethesda has carried major responsibilities. It is he who has received and processed brain specimens, supervised the primate holdings and serial passage
experiments, and kept the complex records. The chimpanzees
and other primates must be held for years, so a major aspect
has been the development and oversight of holding-facilities
in Louisiana, New York State, and Frederick, Maryland. It is
now recognized that kuru and Creutzfeldt-Jakob disease, as
well as scrapie, belong to the group of infectious disorders
caused by slow or latent "viruses." The quotation marks de-
note that these agents are unlike other known viruses in their
physical, chemical, and biological properties. The attribu-
tion of these neurological disorders, hitherto thought to be
degenerative in nature, to transmissible agents is an astounding and revolutionary discovery that has occasioned a
rethinking of the whole question of degeneration and aging in
the nervous system.

For these discoveries and investigations, Gajdusek was
awarded the 1976 Nobel Prize in medicine, the fourth such
award to an NIH scientist and the first for NINCDS (3). I
had the privilege of attending the ceremony in Stockholm that
December. It was quite an occasion! One of Carleton's special interests has been to bring boys from the New Guinea-
Melanesia-Micronesia region to his home in the Washington
area to attend high school and college at his expense, with
a view to their returning to be leaders among their people.
When he went to Stockholm, Carleton took a group of his
"adopted" boys with him. The news media were filled with
interviews and stories. One boy visited a museum housing
South Pacific artifacts and apparently knew more about the
collection than the curator. At the sumptuous banquet, we
hardly recognized Carleton in formal attire seated next to
Princess Christina.

The Voltage Clamp

As already noted, the Neurology Institute acquired its
own basic research units in 1960, ending the administrative
uncertainties inherent in the joint NIMH-NINDB program. In
the highly productive Laboratory of Biophysics, Kenneth Cole
("K.C." to his friends) invented and pioneered the use of the
voltage clamp technique for studying the conduction of nerve
impulses.

By way of background, reference should be made to a favorite subject of study among neurophysiologists: the giant
axon of the squid. This relatively huge nerve fiber lends
itself well to electrical stimulation and recording, bio-

chemical and pharmacological manipulations, and biochemical analyses. Such studies by Cole and colleagues at Bethesda (and Woods Hole, Massachusetts) and by Alan Hodgkin and Andrew Huxley at Cambridge (and Plymouth), England, have yielded most of our knowledge about one of the two major processes by which nerve cells communicate with each other and with target organs like muscles.

In axonal conduction the overall events are *electrical*: the propagation of an action potential, or spike, along the surface of the nerve fiber. (The companion process is synaptic transmission, involving specific *chemical* messengers across the junction between neural elements.) Neural electrical events are powered by the differential distribution of sodium and potassium ions across the axonal membrane. When a nerve impulse progresses down the axon, the permeabilities of the membrane temporarily change to admit sodium ions and lose potassium ions, producing the action potential and the swift transit of the electrical impulse.

This process is now well understood after years of research by the Cole group, the Hodgkin-Huxley group, and others, all critically dependent upon Cole's voltage clamping technique. By using the voltage clamp, one can set the axonal membrane at a predetermined resting value—i.e., manipulate the distribution of sodium and potassium ions across the membrane—and thus evaluate or dissect the various components involved in the conduction process. This was the crucial tool that made all subsequent studies possible.

Initially Cole and his team had to do their experiments during the summer at the Marine Biological Laboratory in Woods Hole. Cole soon beat the system by installing a computer in his Bethesda laboratory and programming it with the basic experimental parameters. Simulated experiments could then be done all year around on the computer and the most crucial or complex ones verified on actual squid axons the next summer at Woods Hole. This sophisticated approach has prospered— except for a disastrous occasion in the mid 1960s when, as a result of a thunderstorm, the entire NIH lacked power for many hours. Among the major casualties were the data from several years' work stored in K.C.'s computer. Nearly six months were required for reprogramming, and many appropriate measures were instituted to prevent a recurrence in the lab or at NIH as a whole.

The Cole voltage clamp was the most essential tool in all subsequent studies on axonal conduction. These studies, particularly in the hands of the Cambridge group, led to the awarding of the Nobel Prize in medicine/physiology (1963) to Hodgkin and Huxley. In their Nobel lectures they were em-

phatic in crediting Cole and his voltage clamp technique for
their success. Today more than ever the technique is of fundamental importance in the study of many nerve, muscle, and
even tissue culture problems.

Central Neural Organization

Wade Marshall's Laboratory of Neurophysiology retained
its dual connections to NIMH and NINDB, but the Section on
Spinal Cord Physiology under Karl Frank became very much an
NINDB activity. Here Mike Fuortes began his work, and many
others, such as TERRY HAMBRECHT, ROBERT E. BURKE, and THOMAS
G. SMITH, received their training under the experienced guidance of Frank and Marshall. Burke went on to head the NINCDS
Laboratory of Neural Control, concentrating on the motor organization of the nervous system in studies impinging on a
wide variety of human movement disorders. Smith, with JEFFERY
L. BARKER and others, formed the Laboratory of Neurophysiology
after their mentor Karl Frank turned to administrative challenges. Smith and Barker have been in the forefront of studies
on the functional significance of various neuromodulatory compounds, the neuropeptides and neurohormones. Here, on this
exciting frontier, the neurobiology of behavior is beginning
to be elucidated. And Hambrecht, an engineer as well as a
physician, has made outstanding contributions in the field
of neural prostheses, both as investigator and as program
director for extramurally supported studies.

Spinal Cord Regeneration

Other major investigations flourished under Bill Windle,
chief of the Laboratory of Neuroanatomical Sciences. Originally from the University of Pennsylvania, Windle came with
a special interest in problems of regeneration in the mammalian central nervous system. When he began his research,
neurologists and neuroscientists universally accepted the
dogma that nerve tracts in the mammalian spinal cord and brain
could not regenerate after injury or transection. Thus accident victims with cord or head injuries and patients with
stroke, multiple sclerosis, tumors, and the like faced a bleak
future of permanent motor and sensory loss. Windle and his
colleagues thought they saw evidence for central spinal cord
regeneration, and this tantalizing hint fired their subsequent
research. The problems are not yet solved, but Windle's conviction that central regeneration can occur, given the right
circumstances, has many authoritative adherents.

One of his disciples, LLOYD GUTH, has worked particularly on the trophic factors that ensure the correct connection between a growing nerve fiber and its target muscle, sensory receptor, or gland and the maintenance of such a connection once established. Guth started in Windle's lab, then headed a section in our Laboratory of Neurochemistry, and is now professor of anatomy at the University of Maryland Medical School. As a recognized expert in the field of central regeneration, he recently evaluated for NINCDS a Soviet scientist's claim to have effected spinal cord regeneration by means of enzyme therapy. Guth carefully repeated the experiments, but could not substantiate the claims.

Asphyxia and Edema

Windle also contributed importantly to knowledge of peri- and neonatal asphyxia and its consequences for brain function, matters of direct relevance to cerebral palsy and related disorders. Toward the end of his NIH career, he devoted increasing time to this work as chief of the Laboratory of Perinatal Physiology in San Juan, Puerto Rico, where NINDB established on the islet of Cayo Santiago a free-ranging colony of rhesus (macaque) monkeys (2). Suffice it to say that this experiment in the domestic production and study of primates was premature, for it was terminated by NIH and NINDS before the current shortages of primates from Asian and African sources might have dictated a different decision.

After Windle's move to the perinatal lab, Igor Klatzo took over the Laboratory of Neuroanatomical Sciences. He initiated a series of important comparative studies on the blood-brain barrier, a mechanism that selectively insulates the central nervous system from most circulating metabolites and thus maintains an optimal internal milieu for cerebral activity. Some of the most interesting data came from studies on the shark brain, in which the barrier organization is much different from that of mammals. Klatzo's hobby of underwater photography contributed to specimen collecting. In the course of studies on the modification of the barrier, he investigated the attendant types of brain edema, or fluid collection, and established much of the basis for our present understanding of this clinical problem so common after trauma, vascular accidents, and surgery.

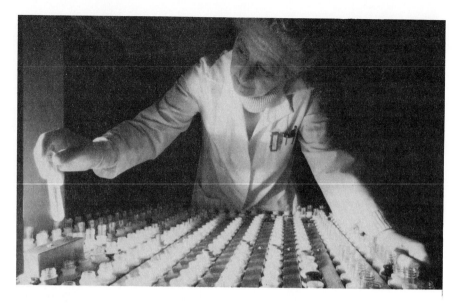

ELIZABETH MINGIOLI, chemist, checks sample in gamma counter, used to measure and analyze immunoglobulins and specific antibodies to viral proteins and human cell antigens.

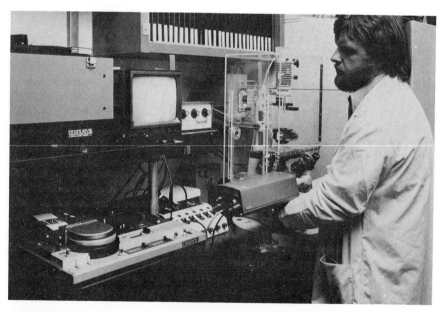

BERNARD RENTIER, virologist, demonstrates equipment for viewing single neuron in a culture infected with mouse hepatitis virus, a mutant of which produces demyelination.

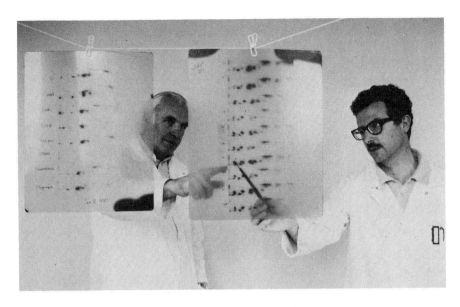

ERNST FREESE AND VINCENT LOPEZ, molecular biologists, discuss electrophoresis film in studying differentiation. The technique employs an electric current to separate compounds.

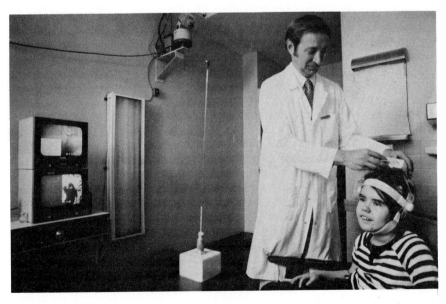

ROGER PORTER, neurologist, adjusts telemetering equipment for broadcasting EEG data. Picked up by the antenna, data are correlated with patient's movements as recorded by TV camera.

Myelin Studies

Klatzo's lab was large and well staffed with such out-standing scientists as MILTON W. BRIGHTMAN, THOMAS S. REESE, and HENRY deF. WEBSTER. Their innovative studies with freeze-fracture electron microscopy and in vivo models of de- and remyelination* are in the forefront of current neuroscience research. Use of the freeze-fracture technique, pioneered by Reese and his colleagues, has revealed many details of how chemical neurotransmitters in the presynaptic nerve ending are stored, released, and renewed in synaptic trans-mission. Webster's studies on optic nerve and on tadpoles subjected to demyelination are particularly relevant to multiple sclerosis, which is characterized by analogous lesions. In collaboration with DALE E. McFARLIN's group in neuroimmu-nology and Roscoe Brady's in lipid neurochemistry, Webster has developed an in vivo system for evaluating factors involved in demyelination and its repair.

Basic Neurobiologic Mechanisms

The newer Laboratories include Molecular Biology under ERNST FREESE, whose interests in mechanisms of differenti-ation** and mutagenesis*** have contributed significantly to the fundamental understanding of these processes. In Mole-cular Genetics, an offspring of Freese's lab, a group under ROBERT A. LAZZARINI is studying the interactions of virus or viral particles with RNA and DNA in neural host cells. Intriguing new information is emerging, such as evidence of entirely different clinical syndromes from the same infec-tive agent, depending upon conditions of infection and prop-agation. Neuro-otolaryngology under T. J. JÖRGEN FEX is ded-icated to understanding processes of neural reception and transduction of auditory signals.

Among the newer Branches are Neuroimmunology under Dale McFarlin, who heads one of the country's pioneering groups in immunologic research on the nervous system, and Experi-mental Therapeutics under Donald Calne and Tom Chase, as already mentioned. Administrative leadership for the intra-mural research is provided by the Laboratory and Clinical Directors. Richard Irwin has ably held the Laboratory direc-

---

*Loss/gain of myelin, a fatty material sheathing and in-sulating nerve fibers and tracts.
**Specialization and ***mutant production in the course of cell development and maturation.

torship through the terms of several Clinical Directors: Van
Buren, Calne, McFarlin, and currently Kornblith (Acting).

Origin of the Laboratory of Neurochemistry

I have been personally involved in the origin and development of the Laboratory of Neurochemistry. When I arrived at
NIH in July 1953 to set up a Section on Clinical Neurochemistry, I was joined by Beni Horvath (a pupil of Szent-Györgyi);
and by 1954, there were three other neurochemistry groups in
NIMH and NINDB: ALEXANDER RICH in physical chemistry, Brady
in lipid chemistry, and R. WAYNE ALBERS in cytochemistry. In
1960, when the combined NIMH-NINDB basic science program was
split, Milton Shy, the NINDB Scientific Director, proposed
that I head a Laboratory of Neurochemistry (LNC) formed from
my unit and those headed by Brady, Albers, and Horvath (succeeded shortly by EBERHARD TRAMS [1926-1982]). Brady formed
his own Branch in 1982, and JANET PASSONNEAU was appointed
Chief when I became Director of NINCDS in 1973.

Hereditary Lipid Storage Diseases

The LNC and its precursors were an exciting and productive
milieu in which to conduct research. I will recount only a
few highlights and relevant comments for the period 1953-1973,
referring for more detail to another report (4). The studies
by Roscoe Brady and his colleagues [see Brady section in the
chapter "Genetic Diseases"] are outstanding and have been
recognized by several significant awards, notably the Lasker
in 1982. What the studies revealed was that certain hereditary lipid storage diseases—Tay-Sachs, Gaucher's, Niemann-
Pick, Fabry's, etc.—are the results of genetic deletion or
attenuation of a specific enzyme. Each such enzyme is responsible for the degradation or disposal of a particular fatty
molecule which, if not metabolized, accumulates in the cells
of brain, liver, spleen, kidney, muscle, etc. Moreover, all
these degradative enzymes were shown to reside in the intracellular organelle called the lysosome and to function as
hydrolases.* This general principle led Brady and others to
uncover biochemical lesions in related diseases, each involving a different enzyme and hence a different lipid.

Once the affected enzymes had been identified, Brady and
his co-workers easily devised simple diagnostic and screening

---

*Enzymes that cleave substrates by hydrolysis, addition
of H_2O.

procedures to permit identification of patients and carriers. A special feature of the tests is their applicability to the amniocentesis technique, so that it is now possible prenatally to identify fetuses at risk and to provide genetic counseling. Before Brady's procedures became generally available, he invited scientists and physicians worldwide to submit specimens to be tested for the presence or absence of key enzyme activities, surely a remarkable public service.

One other feature of this work should be mentioned. To facilitate the research and especially the diagnostic tests, it was necessary to have radioactively labeled substrates— that is, the specific stored lipids on which the affected enzymes normally act. The challenge of synthesizing biologically active substrates comprising such complex lipid molecules was formidable indeed. There was literally one organic chemist in the world, DAVID SHAPIRO at the Weizmann Institute in Israel, who had the necessary expertise. After a preliminary collaborative session at NIH, Shapiro contracted to prepare the needed labeled materials. Funding was provided through the Special Foreign Currency Program, under Public Law 480. To my mind, this was the perfect example of how P.L. 480 was supposed to work. United States funds tied up in Israeli currency at the end of World War II were used to produce needed chemicals for research at NIH and to benefit American patients and their families.

The Sodium/Potassium Ion Pump

In the LNC Wayne Albers has studied in detail the enzyme responsible for transport of sodium and potassium ions across neural membranes. This enzyme is the magnesium-dependent, sodium/potassium-activated ATPase. Minimizing technicality, we may say that this enzyme system catalyzes the conversion (or transduction) of energy generated by nerve cells in the form of adenosine triphosphate (ATP) into an ion transfer process. Excess sodium within the cell is pumped out in return for the inward transfer of potassium ions previously lost from the cell during a period of activity. Albers has contributed significantly to our understanding of this very complex yet absolutely critical process in the functioning of the nervous system. The whole process of nerve conduction and transmission —the ability of nerve cells to communicate with each other— depends ultimately on these ion pumps. It is estimated that their fueling utilizes one-half or more of all the energy expended by the brain, spinal cord, and nerves.

Nerve Membrane Studies

In related studies Eberhard G. Trams concentrated on the intimate details of the physicochemical properties of membranes. This led to his discovery of the ectoenzymes situated on the outer surface of most cells, including neural cells. He was among the first to demonstrate a key role for ecto-ATPases and for at least one of their products, adenosine, which appears to be a crucial intercellular messenger. Trams engaged in an important extracurricular activity. An accomplished airplane pilot, he served for many years as executive officer for a wing of the Maryland Civil Air Patrol, where he was highly regarded by his fellow pilots. His tragic death in a small-plane crash (as a passenger) has deprived us of knowing by what innovative and sometimes unorthodox approaches he would have further probed the ectoenzyme/adenosine phenomenon.

Collaborative Research of LNC

Rather than simply recount my own research, I would prefer to use it to exemplify a significant feature of the NIH intramural research milieu—namely, the important opportunities for collaboration. One of my major interests has been the neurochemical mechanisms of epilepsy. Shortly after starting work at NINDB, we embarked on therapeutic trials of the amino acids asparagine and glutamine in young epileptic patients with relatively intractable seizures. Neither amino acid had ever been administered to human subjects in large amounts, and we wanted to know something about blood and cerebrospinal fluid levels as functions of dose and time after administration. Since our analytic procedures were not entirely appropriate for such studies, we turned to ALTON MEISTER, then a biochemist in the National Cancer Institute, who generously assayed our samples for us.

Later, we evaluated the therapeutic potential of gamma aminobutyric acid (GABA), an amino acid found primarily in nervous tissues as an inhibitory transmitter. Al Meister again helped by determining the GABA content of blood and cerebrospinal fluid samples. His collaboration saved us much time and labor and added greatly to the completeness of the studies. Incidentally, the three amino acids asparagine, glutamine, and GABA did exhibit anticonvulsant activity in some cases, but their costs were not competitive with those of conventional drugs.

In these studies we also needed help in locating sources of amino acids in large amounts. Sam Mann of the Nutritional

Biochemicals Co. in Cleveland, Ohio, was generously helpful in this respect. And in formulating these heat-labile compounds into sterile units for intravenous use, Lewis Sarrett, then with Merck and Co., and Joseph Hawkins, then with the Merck Institute, were able to provide sterile, pyrogen-free preparations. I mention these latter two examples to illustrate that cooperation from industry is often an essential ingredient in the success of a research venture.

Another example comes from my studies in 1958 on 2-deoxy-D-glucose (2-DG), at that time a new-found inhibitor of glucose metabolism. Converted by body cells into 2-DG 6-phosphate, the inhibitor cannot be metabolized further and accumulates intracellularly. When present in sufficient amounts, it restricts the metabolism of glucose 6-phosphate competitively to produce hyperglycemia (excess glucose extracellularly) and cytoglucopenia (severe deprivation intracellularly). In these studies I wanted to analyze incubated brain slices for the various sugar phosphates. Lacking experience with the requisite chromatographic procedures, I turned to an authority, G. GILBERT ASHWELL, in the Laboratory of Biochemistry and Metabolic Diseases, NIAMD. Gil generously taught me the procedures, supplied special reagents, and checked my completed chromatograms. These were the first such studies on brain tissue and were to inspire my colleague LOUIS SOKOLOFF in the Laboratory of Cerebral Metabolism, NIMH, to develop his ingenious and widely applied 2-DG method for examining regional and local cerebral blood flow, glucose uptake, and metabolism in vivo.

In the course of our studies on GABA, GUY M. McKHANN and I wanted to examine the role of this amino acid in the oxidative, or energy, metabolism of the brain, since its position in the pathways of intermediary oxidative metabolism provided a potential shunt around one of the key steps. The metabolism of GABA requires vitamin B_6 as coenzyme. Thus one approach was to study B_6-deficient animals to ascertain whether the deficiency reduced cerebral oxygen consumption and, if so, whether the reduction could be corrected with the vitamin or with GABA. We turned to an expert in nutrition, OLAF MICKELSEN, of the Laboratory of Nutrition and Endocrinology, NIAMD, to help us prepare B_6-deficient kittens. The experiments were eminently successful and corroborated our working hypothesis that GABA can serve as an energy source for brain metabolism.

An analogous study involved measurement of cerebral blood flow and oxygen consumption in a child with the vitamin-B_6-dependency syndrome. McKhann and I collaborated with Wayne Albers, Louis Sokoloff, and NIELS A. LASSEN of Copenhagen, then working in Sokoloff's lab. Comparison of the child's

cerebral metabolism before and after B_6 repletion revealed
that the metabolic rate was significantly reduced in the depleted state, as we had postulated.

Later work with JOHN R. WHERRETT on cerebral proteins
involved the development of a method of enzymatic hydrolysis
that would retain intact the glutamine and asparagine amide
groups that are usually split off by other procedures. Our
studies with Viokase (a pancreatic enzyme concentrate) preceded the later and superior results with Pronase (an enzyme
complex isolated from *Streptomyces griseus*), but were equally
valid and useful. In the course of our studies CHRISTIAN B.
ANFINSEN, then in the Laboratory of Cellular Physiology and
Metabolism, NHI, sought our help in working out the amino
acid sequence of the so-called RNase S-peptide (residues 1-20
of the enzyme RNase, or ribonuclease). Previous analyses
had indicated the presence of one amide group, but it was not
clear whether this was an asparagine or a glutamine residue
and where in the peptide it was located. Our method provided
the answer, unequivocally ruling out asparagine and confirming the presence of a glutamine residue at the 11 position.
Thus the structure of this portion of the enzyme molecule
could be revised to the correct sequence. The studies on
ribonuclease by Anfinsen and colleagues led eventually to
his Nobel Prize in chemistry for 1972.

In other studies on cerebral proteins, Wherrett and I
investigated the metabolism of the amino and amide nitrogen,
using isotope-labeled compounds. This involved analyses of
tissue extracts for the stable isotope ^{15}N in the mass spectrometer. Our instrument was a small model (intended for
oil field analyses) with limited resolution. We repeatedly
compared results with Heinrich Waelsch (1905-1966), who was
conducting parallel studies at the New York Psychiatric Institute. Our protein amide nitrogen seemed to contain a significant excess of ^{15}N, whereas Waelsch's did not; and when
we exchanged samples, he could not confirm our results. So
we turned to WILLIAM COMSTOCK of NIAMD, who applied a large
spectrometer of greater resolution to a portion of the same
preparation. The results agreed with Waelsch's, enabling us
to correct our data before publication.

One final example involved our studies on electrolyte,
or ion, metabolism in the brain. Together with ROBERT S.
BOURKE, we were examining the dynamics of the various fluid
spaces, extracellular and intracellular, in intact brain and
neural tissue slices. In the course of most experimental
manipulations, extra fluid was taken up as edema, or swelling. We wished to learn in which fluid compartment such
accumulations occurred by using indicators of extracellular
space like inulin and sucrose and of total fluid space (in-

cluding intracellular spaces) like chloride and thiocyanate.
Our data seemed consistent and reasonable when compared with
those of other investigators, but we were troubled by electron microscopists' reports that there was no visible extracellular space in sections of mammalian brain tissue.   We
turned to our colleague and electron microscopist, Theodor
Wanko, and together undertook an extensive series of experiments.

We found that the fixation and dehydration techniques then
in use by microscopists for neural tissues caused striking
changes in the fluid dynamics of the specimens, first inducing tremendous swelling by uptake of extra fluid and then
marked shrinkage, so that the specimen might eventually resemble the fresh unprocessed sample but without necessarily
having the same distribution of fluid spaces. Wanko devised
specially buffered fixatives of physiological ionic strength
that minimized such fluid shifts. With his procedures we obtained electron micrographs that clearly showed neural tissues to have ample extracellular spaces, comparable to our
biochemical assays. These studies with Wanko were among the
first to call attention to the artifacts being created, by
the methods of fixation and dehydration then in use.   As a
result Bourke was able to undertake promising studies on brain
edema and its clinical correction.

The Institute's Role in Training

These and many other examples could be cited to illustrate the extraordinary collaborative opportunities in the
NIH intramural programs.   And there is another valuable facet
to such research. As in the clinically oriented neuromuscular
disease program of Milton Shy's group, mentioned above, the
laboratory or basic science programs were important sources
of future research leaders.   Especially during the period
when the Selective Service System obligated young physicians,
the NIH intramural programs attracted many applicants for
both Clinical and Research Associate positions.   The NINDB/
NINDS Laboratory of Neurochemistry could point to a distinguished group of such "graduates."

For example, my own group included Guy McKhann, now professor and chairman of neurology at The Johns Hopkins Medical
School; John Wherrett, professor and chairman of neurology
at the University of Toronto Medical School; and Robert S.
Bourke, professor and chairman of neurosurgery at the Albany
Medical College. Similarly, Ross Brady's section had, among
others, BERNARD W. AGRANOFF, now professor of biochemistry
and head of the neuroscience laboratory at the University

of Michigan Medical School; JOSEPH D. ROBINSON, professor and chairman of pharmacology at the State University of New York at Syracuse; JULIAN N. KANFER, professor and chairman of biochemistry at the University of Manitoba in Winnipeg; and EDWIN H. KOLODNY, director of clinical research at the Eunice Kennedy Shriver Center for Mental Retardation at Waltham, Massachusetts. Wayne Albers had, among others, STANLEY FAHN, now professor of neurology at Columbia College of Physicians and Surgeons; GEORGE J. SIEGEL, professor of neurology at the University of Michigan Medical School; and FREDERICK J. SAMAHA, professor of neurology and pediatrics at the University of Pittsburgh Medical School. Many more could be named, all actively engaged in neurochemical-type research.

The intramural Clinical and Research Associate programs at NIH provide research training experiences for our country's future academic teachers and investigators. In neurochemistry most are M.D.'s, and thus are oriented to clinical neurological problems and their elucidation and management by neurochemical means. But such impressive records will remain in jeopardy as long as available positions and funds for such young people at NIH (and elsewhere) are curtailed. The infusion of new ideas and new leaders will rapidly dwindle, and experience has taught that any appreciable hiatus in the process will take decades to repair (1).

Besides responsibilities in research and research training, NIH intramural scientists are frequently asked to take on additional tasks. Many have served on editorial boards of scientific journals, some as chief editors. A number of us have had honorary academic appointments at local universities and have taught there or in the extension courses offered by the Department of Agriculture and, at NIH, by the Foundation for Advanced Education· in the Sciences. Many are active in the NIH Assembly of Scientists. And there are a variety of other special assignments and opportunities. Such activities are part of every scientist's responsibilities and reflect one's standing in the scientific community.

History in the Making

This account has necessarily been fragmentary. It has passed over many good and valuable people, especially the loyal support personnel: technical, nursing, secretarial, administrative. I have said little about the last decade, when HENRY G. WAGNER and Thomas Chase served as Scientific Directors for the periods 1968-1974 and 1975-1983, respectively, under Ted MacNichol (5), Tower (from 1973), and

MURRAY GOLDSTEIN (from 1981) as Institute Directors. Those years are still history in the making, too recent to assess properly.

But what has been recorded here by way of illustration surely attests to a vigorous and productive program of clinical and basic research in the neurosciences. In many cases the opportunities and the work have been unique. They have underscored the extraordinary worth of the research hospital and surrounding laboratories of NIH as a special place for discovery, for training, and for healing. Few of us would forgo a chance to repeat the experience.

"The larger the island of knowledge, the greater the shoreline with the unknown." John Donne could well have been referring to the neurosciences, for our knowledge of the nervous system seems to be increasing in quantum leaps while our realization of its greater complexity and newly raised questions heightens the challenge of future research. The NINCDS intramural research program is poised to meet that challenge.

References

1. Bailey, P. National Institute of Neurological Diseases and Blindness: Origins, founding, and early years (1950 to 1959). In The Nervous System. Vol. I: The Basic Neurosciences, pp. xxi-xxxii, D. B. Tower and R. O. Brady (eds.). New York: Raven Press, 1975.
2. Masland, R. L. National Institute of Neurological Diseases and Blindness: Development and growth (1960 to 1968). In The Nervous System. Vol. I: The Basic Neurosciences, pp. xxxiii-xlvi, D. B. Tower and R. O. Brady (eds.). New York: Raven Press, 1975.
3. Tower, D. B. D. Carleton Gajdusek, M.D.—Nobel laureate in medicine for 1976. Arch Neurol 34:205-208, 1977.
4. Tower, D. B. The Laboratory of Neurochemistry, IR, NINDS: History and Development of Its Program—A 20-Year Perspective, 1953-1973. (Unpublished report to the NINCDS, 1973.)
5. MacNichol, E. F., Jr. National Institute of Neurological Diseases and Stroke (1968-1973). In The Nervous System. Vol. I: The Basic Neurosciences, pp. xlvii-lii, D. B. Tower and R. O. Brady (eds.). New York: Raven Press, 1975.

Introduction

NUTRITION RESEARCH

Interest in nutrition at the National Institutes of Health had an almost accidental beginning. The main concern of the antecedent Hygienic Laboratory had been infectious diseases, and one of the serious maladies then generally regarded as infectious was pellagra. JOSEPH GOLDBERGER was assigned to investigate pellagra after solid grounding in the study of typhus and yellow fever.

NIH is the proud custodian of Goldberger's diary covering the crucial years 1914-1915, when his epidemiologic studies demonstrated that pellagra was in all probability the result of a nutritional deficiency. He later developed a treatment using yeast in the diet and showed that the amino acid tryptophan was critically related to the cure of the disease. Soon the B vitamin nicotinic acid, now called niacin, was identified as a specific pellagra preventive. From these beginnings an interest in other aspects of nutrition evolved, particularly in the Institute concerned with arthritis and metabolic diseases. Other nutrients and facts about nutrition were discovered, both in experimental animals and man.

Interest in the field waned somewhat as more promising research areas developed. Molecular biology, immunology, virology, and cell biology proved more attractive to many younger investigators. In recent years, however, there has been a resurgence of certain aspects of nutrition research, particularly those relating to specific diseases. Thus, nutritional aspects of atherosclerosis, certain cancers, diabetes and other endocrine disorders, osteoporosis, and obesity have all been subjected to important inquiries in the laboratories and clinics of NIH. Many of these investigations are narrated in Dr. Bieri's and other chapters.

D. S.

6

NUTRITION RESEARCH

John G. Bieri

Nutrition research began in the predecessor organizations of NIH, mainly the Hygienic Laboratory of the U.S. Public Health Service, during the period 1910-1930. The name principally associated with the origin of nutrition research in PHS is that of JOSEPH GOLDBERGER.

Goldberger and Pellagra Prevention

In 1914 pellagra was occurring sporadically and with increasing frequency in various southern states. Goldberger, assigned to find the cause of the disease, came early to the conclusion that pellagra was not infectious—as leading medical authorities believed—but was related instead to diet. Working with Goldberger in Georgia were a number of associates including WILLIAM F. TANNER, D. G. WILLETS, EDGAR SYDENSTRICKER, and GEORGE A. WHEELER. Epidemiological and controlled clinical studies established in 1920 that pellagra was primarily the result of a dietary deficiency.

Goldberger and his associates showed that the poor, monotonous diets common to many low-income people—diets high in carbohydrate and low in good-quality protein—induced pellagra when fed to volunteer convicts in a Mississippi penitentiary. In other public institutions where the disease occurred, these investigators demonstrated that generous amounts of milk, eggs, meat, beans, and peas prevented it. Still, many physicians who were treating pellagra at the time strongly believed that it was due to an infectious organism and would not accept Goldberger's evidence.

As a final proof that no infectious mechanism was involved, Goldberger and Wheeler injected each other with

JOHN G. BIERI, Ph.D., Guest Worker and Scientist Emeritus. Formerly Chief, Nutritional Biochemistry Section, Laboratory of Nutrition and Endocrinology, National Institute of Arthritis, Diabetes, and Digestive and Kidney Diseases.

blood from a pellagra patient. Later Goldberger and four associates swallowed capsules containing patients' wastes and skin
scrapings, and Goldberger injected blood from a pellagrous
woman into his wife, Mary. None contracted the disease, though
it is not recorded what adverse symptoms may have resulted
from these heroic experiments.

Ariboflavinosis

In 1928 the death rate from pellagra in the United States
was 6 per 100,000 population, or a total of about 7000 deaths.
Of course, the number of serious cases far exceeded the fatalities. It was in 1928 that a young medical scientist, W. HENRY
SEBRELL, Jr., was assigned to the Hygienic Laboratory in Washington as an assistant to Goldberger, with the task of conducting animal experiments that might provide clues to the
nutritional factors involved in pellagra. Within a year of
Sebrell's arrival, Goldberger died and Wheeler was assigned
to supervise the pellagra investigation. Shortly thereafter,
Wheeler retired because of disability and the nutrition work
fell on Sebrell's shoulders.

In their laboratories Sebrell and Goldberger had produced
experimental pellagra in dogs, a condition known as black
tongue, and had shown that various foodstuffs, including
yeast, would readily cure it. At that time, a vitamin B complex was known to reverse several deficiency symptoms in experimental rats. Other investigators in the Hygienic Laboratory, under the supervision of MAURICE I. SMITH, were looking
into the chemical composition of the vitamin B complex. They
established that it contained at least two components, one
heat stable, the other heat labile. A few years later (1937)
Conrad A. Elvehjem and associates at the University of Wisconsin discovered that the pellagra-preventive factor was nicotinic acid, later called niacin. It is interesting that
niacin's biochemical role as a coenzyme had been known for
several years before its pellagra-preventive property was
established.

In the earlier studies of pellagra, Goldberger and other
clinicians had noted abnormalities of the lips and angles of
the nose, as well as the predominant scaling of the skin.
This suggested that two dietary factors were operative.
Sebrell's studies with dogs over a period of years showed
that the second factor was riboflavin (vitamin B_2).

Later Sebrell and R. E. BUTLER performed a classic experiment to ascertain whether the two factors were also active in humans. Several inmates of a mental institution were
given diets very low in both niacin and riboflavin. After

the signs of pellagra appeared, treatment with niacin cleared the skin lesions in about a month, but did not correct the dry, red lips with cracked fissures or the seborrhea around the nose. Supplements of riboflavin eliminated the lip and nose lesions in one week. This was the first unequivocal demonstration of human riboflavin deficiency—ariboflavinosis. Subsequently verified by other investigators, it proved the essentiality of this B vitamin in the human diet.

PHS Nutrition Research, 1930–1947

When the Hygienic Laboratory became the National Institute of Health* in 1930, a number of divisions were formed including Pathology, Chemistry, and Pharmacology. Several of these were incorporated into the Experimental Biology and Medicine Institute (EBMI) in 1947, with Sebrell as director. During the period 1940–1947 these laboratories had carried out investigations of a multidisciplinary nature dealing with a variety of nutrients in both animals and man.

A series of studies clarified the nutritional factors involved in liver cirrhosis seen in rats fed low-protein diets. Choline and the sulfur amino acids cystine and methionine were studied by Sebrell, J. V. LOWRY, FLOYD S. DAFT,** and RALPH D. LILLIE. Lillie characterized a previously undescribed pigment, which he termed ceroid, in the livers of protein-deficient animals.

This group also worked on the effects of the B vitamin pantothenic acid in preventing the hemorrhages and atrophy that developed in the adrenal glands of rats on diets lacking the vitamin B complex but containing pyridoxine (vitamin B_6). The pathology of the adrenals in pantothenic acid deficiency was thoroughly described by L. L. ASHBURN, chief of the Division of Pathology, and A. A. NELSON.

JERALD G. WOOLEY and Sebrell conducted a series of studies to clarify the nutritional requirements of rabbits and developed one of the first satisfactory purified diets for this species. OLAF MICKELSEN was later involved, especially in working out the sodium and potassium requirements. This group also did some of the first experiments on the relation between nutrition and infection, studying the course of experimental pneumococcus infections in mice deficient in thiamine (vitamin B_1) and riboflavin. SAMUEL S. SPICER col-

---

*Renamed National Institutes of Health in 1947.

**Changed name to Doft after leaving NIH in 1962. He returned to NIH as a guest worker in 1965.

laborated with Wooley in studying dietary factors affecting
the reaction of rabbit blood cells to nitrite.

Lowry, Sebrell, and Ashburn studied experimental thiamine
deficiency in rats. They described cardiac arrhythmia, an
associated lesion, and neurological lesions related to the
deficiency—pathology analogous to that of human beriberi.
CARL VOEGTLIN, who was to become the first director of the
National Cancer Institute, investigated the effect of various
nutrients—protein, riboflavin, and biotin—on the progress
of liver tumors in rats. These studies were among the earliest on the relation between nutritional factors and cancer,
currently a very active field of investigation. In a different
area, HARRY EAGLE, a microbiologist, quantified the nutritional requirements of trypanosomes, facilitating the laboratory study of these infectious organisms. They are the causative agents of several major diseases, including Chagas' disease in South America and African sleeping sickness. Later
Eagle studied the nutritional requirements of mammalian cells
in culture.*

Studies on selenium illustrate the unpredictable directions of research. An endemic disease of cattle and horses
in specific areas of South Dakota had been known since the
late 1800s and was eventually attributed to selenium toxicity. Some plants grown on these high-selenium soils accumulate abnormal concentrations of the element, which in turn
poison grazing animals. The question whether humans in these
areas might develop selenium toxicity led to a series of
papers during 1936-1940 by Maurice Smith, Lillie, E. F. STAHL-
MAN, and B. B. WESTFALL of the Divisions of Pharmacology and
Pathology. These classic studies explored the toxicology,
pathology, and metabolism of selenium in a variety of experimental animals. Twenty-five years later, selenium was again
to be a focal point of interest at NIH, not as a toxic agent
but rather as an essential nutrient (discussed below).

Nutrition Research at NIAMD, 1950-1953

In 1950 EBMI became the National Institute of Arthritis
and Metabolic Diseases (NIAMD). JAMES M. HUNDLEY headed the
Laboratory of Nutrition. His interests centered on protein,
vitamin, and mineral requirements. In a series of studies
with rats, he showed how various amino acid supplements could
improve the protein quality of wheat and bread. With R. B.
ING and R. W. KRAUSS, Hundley demonstrated that certain dried
algae were good sources of the amino acids lysine and threo-

---

*See Eagle in chapter entitled "Tissue Culture."

nine. With G. DONALD WHEDON he studied the effects of supplements of lysine, threonine, and other amino acids in human diets based on rice. He also studied copper and niacin deficiencies in rats.

An early addition to the Laboratory of Nutrition was JOHN C. KERESZTESY, who had already achieved distinction with the Merck Pharmaceutical Company by his contributions to the isolation of pyridoxine. Keresztesy and MILTON SILVERMAN studied the chemical nature of various naturally occurring forms of the B vitamin folic acid. Associated with them were SIDNEY FUTTERMAN and ROY L. KISLIUK, who investigated the enzymatic relationships of folic acid in tissues. For a number of years BERNARD T. KAUFMAN studied a specific enzyme in folic acid metabolism, folate reductase.

The discovery of sulfonamide drugs and their rapid medical application shortly before World War II led to many studies of their side effects. Sulfonamides added to the diet of rats induced typical anemia and leukopenia. Spicer, Daft, Sebrell, and Ashburn showed that liver extracts would prevent these blood dyscrasias. At that time folic acid, a growth factor for bacteria, was being studied widely as a new member of the B complex. Since folic acid seemed to parallel the liver extracts in its properties, ARTHUR KORNBERG, Daft, and Sebrell tested folic acid in the diets of sulfonamide-treated rats. Crystalline folic acid completely prevented the blood changes. The work demonstrated a key role for folic acid in hematopoiesis—and marked Kornberg's introduction into nutritional biochemistry and later enzymology.

As a young physician at the start of World War II, Kornberg joined the Public Health Service and was detailed to NIH. A dozen years later he moved to Washington University (St. Louis) and then to Stanford University. In 1959 he was awarded the Nobel Prize for physiology and medicine. Kornberg, with HERBERT TABOR and Sebrell, showed that folic acid could accelerate blood regeneration following hemorrhage in rats. With Daft and Sebrell, he studied the vitamin K deficiency induced in rats by dietary sulfonamides. Controversy centered on whether the sulfa drugs exerted the effect solely through the intestinal flora, inhibiting vitamin K biosynthesis, or acted systemically on the clotting mechanism. The group showed that the decrease in clotting time following oral or intravenous administration of the agent closely correlated with a marked reduction of vitamin K activity in the intestinal and fecal contents, indicating that the action of the drug on the intestinal flora was the predominant factor.

Folic Acid, Methotrexate, and Choriocarcinoma

Here we digress from the work of NIAMD to mention studies on folic acid in the National Cancer Institute. ROY HERTZ and WILLIAM TULLNER had shown in the late 1940s that this B vitamin is needed in the diet for normal growth response to estrogen. Deletion of the vitamin from the diet of chicks produced a 40-fold differential in the growth of estrogen-stimulated tissues (oviduct), and like effects were obtained with antifolic acid compounds. In 1956 MIN CHIU LI, Hertz, and D. B. Spencer, pursuing analogous studies in women, reported that choriocarcinoma, a virulent cancer of the uterus, responded to the folic acid antagonist methotrexate. Complete and sustained remissions are obtained in most patients, even when the disease is widely disseminated.

Selenium Studies

With the opening of the Clinical Center in 1953, the Laboratory of Nutrition and Endocrinology of NIAMD expanded, with Hundley as Chief, shortly to be followed upon his retirement by Mickelsen. Daft, Director of NIAMD, had brought to his laboratory in 1949 a young German physician, KLAUS SCHWARZ, to study the liver necrosis of rats maintained on a low-protein diet. In addition to amino acids (cystine and methionine), vitamin E was known to prevent the necrosis, and Schwarz had shown that a third, water-soluble factor was also effective. After seven years of intensive research on the water-soluble "factor 3," Schwarz and his associate CALVIN FOLTZ isolated a substance of which the active ingredient proved to be a trace element, selenium. It was shown subsequently to be an essential component of the enzyme glutathione peroxidase.

The discovery of this nutritional role of selenium led quickly to the finding that the element would prevent three endemic diseases of livestock—exudative diathesis in chickens, white muscle disease in lambs and calves, and yellow fat disease in pigs. These nutritional deficiency diseases occurred sporadically in certain areas of the world and cost millions of dollars annually in losses to farmers. The affected areas were found to have soils with low or unavailable selenium. Fortification of soils or direct supplements to animals virtually eliminated the diseases overnight. This is a classic example of how basic research can lead to unexpected practical results.

Selenium nutrition and biochemistry again came into prominence at NIH almost 20 years later with a discovery by THRESSA

C. STADTMAN and her associates in 1972. They showed that a component of the clostridial glycine reductase complex is a selenoprotein. This heat-stable protein of low molecular weight was shown to contain one gram atom of selenium as a selenocysteine residue within the polypeptide chain. This was the first identification of a macromolecule dependent on selenium for its biological activity. Later at NIH a selenium-dependent formate dehydrogenase of *Methanococcus vannielii* was shown by J. B. JONES, GREGORY L. DILWORTH, and Stadtman to contain the same selenoamino acid. Investigators in California and Germany identified selenocysteine residues in mammalian glutathione peroxidase.

Two other selenium-dependent bacterial enzymes were identified in 1979-1980 by Dilworth and MARIS G. N. HARTMANIS in Stadtman's laboratory. These are nicotinic acid hydroxylase of *Clostridium barkeri* and thiolase of *Clostridium kluyveri*. The chemical form of selenium in these enzymes is not yet known.

The biological occurrence of selenium as a component of proteins is not limited to enzymes. As an outgrowth of studies on the mechanism of synthesis of selenoproteins, it was discovered that selenium is present in certain transfer nucleic acids (tRNAs), which serve to convey amino acids to the ribosomes in protein synthesis. Here selenium is specifically incorporated and not merely replacing sulfur (C.-S. CHEN, WEI-MEI CHING, ARTHUR J. WITTWER, and Stadtman). In one case it has been shown that the ability of tRNA to accept its cognate amino acid depends on the presence of selenium in the tRNA molecule. Thus a regulatory role of selenium in protein synthesis (or some other process controlled by an aminoacylated tRNA) is indicated.

At the present writing, the full story of selenium in human health is still unknown. Long considered to be a carcinogen, the element actually appeared in recent studies to prevent certain tumors in animals. We thus have the interesting anomaly of an essential nutrient, perhaps an anticarcinogen, that must not be introduced into human food according to the Delaney Amendment because it may be carcinogenic.

In addition to their work on factor 3 and selenium, Schwarz's group also studied the role of vitamin E in cellular metabolism. They showed that liver homogenates from rats deficient in vitamin E and factor 3 did not maintain a normal rate of respiration, whereas vitamin E and other antioxidants would prevent the respiratory decline. Active in this work were SIDNEY S. CHERNICK, G. P. RODMAN, LAURENCE M. CORWIN, and MARIE N. LIPSETT.

In association with Schwarz, WALTER MERTZ characterized a factor in yeast that enhanced glucose tolerance in rats.

This effect of the "glucose tolerance factor" was shown by
Mertz (after leaving NIH) to be due to chromium, now viewed as
an essential trace element. (Mertz is currently Director of
the Nutrition Institute, U.S. Department of Agriculture.)

An interesting anecdote about the isolation of factor 3
relates that Schwarz, who thought he had a new B vitamin, took
his most potent preparation to DeWITT STETTEN, Jr., then the
scientific director of NIAMD. Stetten sniffed the solution
and recognized a garlic odor characteristic of selenium compounds. Had Dr. Schwarz tested it for selenium? Schwarz
confirmed that the material did contain selenium and, within
a few weeks, had shown that various inorganic selenium compounds would prevent liver necrosis in rats.

Germfree Animals in Nutrition Research

In 1955 interest in the nutritional status of animals under germfree conditions led several laboratories at NIH to
begin studies with this relatively new technique. In the National Institute of Dental Research, WALTER L. NEWTON and ROB-
ERT J. FITZGERALD, with ERNEST G. McDANIEL of NIAMD, showed
that germfree animals, though immune from caries (tooth decay)
when fed high-sucrose diets, did develop calculus deposits on
the enamel surfaces.

In NIAMD Daft and McDaniel studied a number of nutritional
factors in the germfree rat. It was known that in conventional
rats penicillin or ascorbic acid (vitamin C) would prevent the
symptoms of pantothenic acid deficiency. In the germfree rat,
however, these substances were ineffective in preventing the
symptoms. This was an example of how dietary additives, in
the one case an antibiotic, in the other a water-soluble vitamin, can enhance the synthesis of a B vitamin by intestinal
flora.

Also in this laboratory B. E. GUSTAFSSON, a Visiting Scientist from Sweden, studied factors affecting the vitamin K
requirement of the germfree rat. With Daft, McDaniel, JAMES
C. SMITH, Jr., and Fitzgerald, he showed that vitamin K_1 was
much more active than simpler, synthetic forms of the vitamin,
and that the type of dietary fat could affect the rate of onset of vitamin K deficiency.

D. L. BEAVER showed for the first time that vitamin A-
deficient rats kept under germfree conditions may survive
for long periods, in contrast to deficient conventional rats,
which die rapidly when exposed to the usual microorganisms
found in animal rooms. Several years later WILLIAM E. ROGERS,
Jr., and JOHN G. BIERI expanded this observation, demonstrating that vitamin A-deprived germfree rats could indeed be

maintained without the usual signs of deficiency many months longer than littermates kept under conventional conditions, but that the germfree rats eventually developed nervous tremors. This work showed that vitamin A was essential to bone and nerve tissues during the rapid growth period, but was not critical for survival of mature rats, though complicating factors did eventually lead to death.

Subsequent studies compared the requirements for zinc in conventional and germfree rats (J. C. Smith, McDaniel, L. D. McBEAN, Daft, and J. A. HALSTED). It was found that the germfree animal has a lower requirement—that the intestinal flora sequesters zinc. This same group also explored the relationship between zinc and vitamin A, and showed that the zinc-deficient rat did not mobilize vitamin A from the liver as efficiently as the normal animal (J. C. Smith, E. D. BROWN, McDaniel, and W. CHAN). These studies were a collaborative effort between NIAMD and the Veterans Administration.

The germfree rat was used by Bieri and McDaniel to demonstrate that ubiquinone (coenzyme Q-10) was of endogenous origin in rats—that it did not have to be supplied by either the diet or the intestinal flora. A chemically defined diet free of the coenzyme was used. It was shown in other germfree studies that the fatty liver developing when rats are fed orotic acid is not dependent on the intestinal flora (HERBERT G. WINDMUELLER, McDaniel, and ALBERT E. SPAETH).

Nutrition of Experimental Animals

During the period 1951-1965, the Section on Nutrition, Laboratory of Nutrition and Endocrinology, in NIAMD, accumulated a wide body of basic nutrition information on experimental animals. GEORGE M. BRIGGS, in collaboration with MATTIE RAE SPIVEY FOX and Bieri, elucidated the requirements of chicks for several B vitamins, choline, fat-soluble vitamins, and essential fatty acids. A major effort was undertaken to improve purified diets for chicks and rats. This was important because satisfactory experiments could not be performed on new growth factors or on interrelations among known nutrients unless the basal diets were optimal for growth and performance.

Development of satisfactory mineral mixtures was primary. The existing mixtures had numerous defects, either lacking newer trace elements or having some elements in forms that interacted with one another or with other dietary components. In the latter category, destruction of vitamins and rancidity of the dietary fat were most serious. In a series of detailed studies, Briggs, Fox, and Mickelsen developed new mineral mixtures for both chicks and rats. These were nutritionally adequate and produced no adverse effects on other dietary components. The results have much enhanced the reliability of nutrition experiments.

The requirements of the guinea pig for a number of nutrients were carefully determined over a period of 20 years by MARY E. REID, long a member of the Nutrition Section. Together with Briggs, she developed a purified diet that successfully maintained infant guinea pigs. Reid retired at age 70 but continued as a guest worker, still producing publications until her death at age 83. Part of her success as a nutrition scientist was due to the meticulous attention she gave her animals. She personally fed and weighed them several times weekly, and even bathed the guinea pigs when excreta soiled their fur.

The chief of the laboratory, Mickelsen, produced a model for human obesity by feeding a diet very high in fat to laboratory rats. With RICHARD S. YAMAMOTO, he characterized changes in body composition in these obese animals and showed that only certain strains of rats would spontaneously become obese. Furthermore, obesity would only result if the high-fat diet was also relatively high in protein.

E. HAWK, Windmueller, and Mickelsen, in attempting to sterilize diets for germfree work, studied the reaction between ethylene oxide, a gas used as a fungicide for certain foods, and various components of purified diets. They showed that the gas reacted with amino acids and destroyed niacin, thus proving unsatisfactory for sterilization.

Another achievement of the Nutrition Section during the years 1954-1960 was the clarification of new growth factors. Among the compounds studied were thioctic acid and ubiquinone. These were found not to be required nutrients for rats or chicks.

The nutritional studies of the Institute were always characterized by a wide involvement in collaborative work with investigators throughout NIH. The group had the expertise to devise highly refined diets for a variety of experimental animals so that toxic agents, carcinogens, and drugs could be readily studied in a number of species.

The Cycad as Carcinogen

The Laboratory of Nutrition and Endocrinology and the Laboratory of Pathology, both of the Arthritis Institute, collaborated in a revealing study on the toxicity of cycads. The cycad nut was an occasional food item in the Pacific islands, Africa, and Japan. A neurological condition, amyo-

trophic lateral sclerosis, was suspected to be associated
with the consumption of cycads. Mickelsen obtained a supply
of the nuts through Marjorie Whiting, a PHS nutritionist who
had attempted to determine the cause of the disease on Guam.
Mickelsen and Yamamoto fed the nuts to rats. They were sur-
prised to find, instead of nerve lesions, tumors in the liver
and other organs. Together with GERT L. LAQUEUR and MARIA
SPATZ of the Laboratory of Pathology, they injected into rats
the active component of the cycad, a glycoside called cycasin.
But no tumors occurred, nor were tumors seen when the cycad
nuts were fed to germfree animals. It was determined that a
bacterial glucosidase from the intestinal flora was necessary
to convert cycasin to an active carcinogen.

Vitamin B_{12}, Protein, Calcium, Etc.

In collaborative work by HERBERT WEISSBACH of the National Heart Institute and Bieri, cobalamin (vitamin B_{12})
deficiency in chicks was found to reduce the activity of enzymes involved in forming the coenzymes of both B_{12} and folic
acid. Silverman and Fox showed in rats and chicks that vitamin B_{12} deficiency increased the metabolism of histidine associated with folic acid, but addition of methionine to the
diet reversed this effect.

Another member of the nutrition group, JESSE N. WILLIAMS,
Jr., described changes in cytochromes, intracellular catalysts, as influenced by a variety of nutritional variables,
primarily the protein level of the diet.

Windmueller showed for the first time that the primary
source of energy for the small intestine was the amino acid
glutamine. Later he quantified the amounts of lipoproteins
synthesized by the small intestine in comparison with their
synthesis by the liver.

In the area of clinical nutrition, Whedon's group in the
Metabolism Branch of NIAMD, during the late 1950s, investigated bone metabolism and osteoporosis as affected by dietary
calcium. PAUL A. di SANT'AGNESE studied nutritional requirements peculiar to children with cystic fibrosis.

Fluoridation of Water Supplies

One of the outstanding success stories of how basic nutrition research eventually led to improved human health and a
dramatic economic saving to the country is that of the relationship between the amount of fluoride in water and the incidence of dental caries. In the early 1930s H. TRENDLEY DEAN

of the Public Health Service* was assigned to determine the
factors that caused an unattractive staining of the teeth
called "mottled enamel." This condition was endemic in isolated areas of the United States, notably in Texas and Colorado. Dean and others suspected some substance in the water
supplies, and indeed it was found that the fluoride content
was abnormally high. It was also observed that the mottled
enamel was more resistant to decay (caries). Cooperative
studies by the Dental Hygiene Unit and the nutrition group of
Sebrell, Dean, ELIAS ELVOVE, and RICHARD D. BREAUX showed that
water concentrated from sources known to be high in fluoride
produced chemical changes in the teeth of rats similar to
those produced by added sodium fluoride. This led to the even-
tual elimination of mottled enamel by the removal of excess
fluoride from water supplies.

Of more importance, however, were the large-scale trials
to determine whether an adjusted fluoride content in drinking
water, insufficient to produce mottling, would reduce caries.
After many epidemiologic studies in naturally fluoridated
areas to determine the optimum concentration, the Public
Health Service in the 1940s cooperated with the local offi-
cials of Grand Rapids, Michigan, to introduce controlled fluoridation (1 ppm) in the public water supply. The nearby community of Muskegon, with nonfluoridated water, served as the
control. After 15 years FRANCIS A. ARNOLD, Jr., ROBERT L.
LIKINS, ALBERT L. RUSSELL, and DAVID B. SCOTT of the National
Institute of Dental Research issued a final report on the
striking and persistent inhibition of caries in deciduous and
permanent teeth of children born since the introduction of
fluoridation. From 1945 to 1947 FRANK J. McCLURE conducted
a series of studies on the role of fluoride and other dietary factors in the composition of teeth and bone. This work
greatly increased knowledge of the factors contributing to the
carious process. Studies on fluoride metabolism were also
conducted by ISADORE ZIPKIN and NICHOLAS C. LEONE.

The widespread adoption of water fluoridation can be
classed with pasteurization of milk, purification of water,
and immunization against diseases as among the most important
public health measures of all time. Today some 110 million
people in the United States and countless others throughout the world drink fluoridated water. Thus the benefits of

---

*Dean was Director of the National Institute of Dental
Research from 1948 to 1953.

fluoride are brought, at low cost, to all segments of the
population—rich, poor, young, and old—and extend throughout
life.*

Chemically Defined Human Diets

A significant series of experiments in basic nutrition
was conducted in the National Cancer Institute during 1957-
1959. JESSE P. GREENSTEIN, Chief of the Laboratory of Biochemistry, became interested in the effects of malignancy on
nutritional status in rats. Knowing that tumor-bearing animals
often reduce food intake, Greenstein undertook to administer
total nutrition by feeding through a tube into the stomach. A
liquid diet was necessary, and Greenstein decided to use pure
chemicals for all components in order to have better control.
Such a chemically defined diet would contain amino acids in
place of protein, fatty acids in place of natural fat, simple
sugars in place of complex carbohydrate, and all the vitamins
and mineral elements known to be required. For a dry diet,
this would not have been difficult, but considerable chemical
skill was required to keep these 50-odd compounds from interacting in a water solution. Greenstein, with the assistance
of SANFORD M. BIRNBAUM, MILTON WINITZ, and TAKASHI SUGIMURA,
formulated a chemically defined liquid diet that would sustain normal growth in rats.

This was a notable contribution to experimental animal
studies, not only in the area of cancer but in a number of
fields where accurate control of nutrient intake is essential
for meaningful results. Regrettably, Greenstein died before
he could see the wide application of his technique. Some of
his colleagues entered industry and helped pioneer the application of controlled nutrient solutions in human nutrition
studies. Known as hyperalimentation, or parenteral nutrition, the diets in liquid form are delivered directly into
the bloodstream. This technique is now used extensively in
patients with impaired ingestion or digestion, notably premature infants, children with congenital defects, and persons
who have undergone gastrointestinal surgery for cancer.*

International Nutrition Studies

During the period 1955-1960, NIAMD initiated a new effort
in applied nutrition through the Interdepartmental Commit-

---

*See also Meister section of chapter entitled "Development
of Enzymology."

tee for Nutrition in National Defense. ("Defense" was later changed to "Development.") This committee was a dual effort of NIAMD and the Department of Defense. Under the able administration of H. R. SANDSTEAD and, after his accidental death, ARNOLD E. SCHAEFER, over 30 nutritional surveys were conducted in developing countries throughout the world.

Associated with Schaefer in the administration of this program were ERNEST M. PARROTTE, ARTHUR G. PETERSON, and GERALD F. COMBS. The surveys were multidisciplinary and included physical examination, blood and urine analyses for vitamins, and measurement of dietary intake. They have had long-term effects in the developing countries through improved nutritional planning and augmented local awareness of nutritional problems. These surveys were important to the proper planning and conduct of the Ten-State Nutrition Survey by the Department of Health, Education, and Welfare in 1968-1970.

Acknowledgment

The author is grateful to W. H. SEBRELL, Jr., and OLAF MICKELSEN for reviewing this manuscript and clarifying much of the early history of NIH. Discussions with E. G. McDANIEL were helpful in identifying many of the former nutrition investigators.

Introduction

TISSUE CULTURE

In the early years of the twentieth century, Ross Harrison, followed by a number of other investigators, opened the field of mammalian cell culture. This technique has become extraordinarily important in the armamentarium of the biologist and has found many and diverse applications. Practically all types of experiments that were formerly limited to bacterial or protozoan cells can now be performed on mammalian cells.

Early on, it became necessary to define the detailed conditions for mammalian cell growth. This included not only the choice of appropriate temperature and vessel, but also the exact composition of the nutrient medium and the elimination from it, as far as possible, of all ill-defined chemical substances. In the laboratories of WILTON EARLE and HARRY EAGLE among others, these goals were achieved, and wide varieties of mammalian cells were cultivated, much as bacteria had been cultivated by earlier workers.

Such cells in culture proved to be useful for assessing carcinogenic agents and anticancer drugs. Scientists sought a definition of "malignant transformation," the change that a normal cell undergoes when it becomes cancerous. In contrast to most normal cells, transformed cells were found in many cases to be virtually immortal and to be freed from "contact inhibition." When reinjected into the host animal, they were found to produce solid tumors.

The study of cancer was but one of many areas in which cell culture proved to be valuable. The science of human genetics received a tremendous forward thrust when ROBERT KROOTH showed that cells derived from individuals afflicted with genetic diseases such as galactosemia and acatalasia still exhibited after many generations the enzyme defects characteristic of these diseases. This observation transformed human genetics from an observational science into an experimental one. It also permitted the collection and maintenance of a library of human genetic disorders in the form of frozen cells from patients, greatly advancing the mapping of the human karyotype.

An extension of this line of investigation has led to prenatal diagnosis of genetic diseases from examination of cells
present in amniotic fluid. Such fluid is readily procured by
amniocentesis—withdrawal through a needle inserted into the
pregnant uterus. The cells are cultivated and then studied
for abnormalities in their chromosomes or for the characteristic absence of certain enzymes.

In an entirely different area, the science of virology has
become highly dependent upon the technique of cell culture.
Bacteriophages, which are viruses that parasitize bacteria,
are grown in living microbes, and mammalian viruses are similarly grown in mammalian cells. Indeed, without cell culture
(also called tissue culture), it is improbable that vaccines
against such virus diseases as poliomyelitis could have been
produced.

One other development that might be mentioned in introducing the subject of tissue culture is cell hybridization,
the fusion of two cells of different types, sometimes derived
from different animal species. Such cells give rise to colonies combining the properties of two distinct lines in each
constituent cell. Grown in small clusters, such cells can be
the source of pure monoclonal antibodies, which are now dramatically transforming biological and medical research.

D. S.

7

TISSUE CULTURE

I. The Tissue Culture Section, NCI

Virginia J. Evans

Katherine K. Sanford

The opening of the National Cancer Institute in October 1939 brought together at Bethesda two groups of Public Health Service investigators engaged in cancer research. One group had been housed at Harvard University under the direction of JOSEPH W. SCHERESCHEWSKY, the other employed at the Hygienic Laboratory under CARL VOEGTLIN. Voegtlin, who became the new Institute's first director, had early recognized the potential of tissue culture for cancer research.

The Tissue Culture Section expanded under WILTON R. EARLE's leadership. Through the years, doctoral co-workers included J. C. BRYANT, V. J. EVANS, C. H. FOX, R. R. GANTT, J. T. MITCHELL, K. K. SANFORD, W. G. TAYLOR, R. W. TUCKER, and B. B. WESTFALL, and there was also an ever-changing group of research fellows and assistants, including Earle's senior technologist E. L. SCHILLING. The section collaborated with both NIH and outside investigators, including the cytogeneticist Ram Parshad of Howard University College of Medicine. Evans became head of the section at Earle's death in 1964, and Sanford became head on Evans' retirement in 1973.

Background

Earle developed tissue culture into a precise tool for cancer research. Among his first findings was a degeneration

VIRGINIA J. EVANS, Sc.D., retired. Formerly Head, Tissue Culture Section, Laboratory of Biology, National Cancer Institute. KATHERINE K. SANFORD, Ph.D., Chief, In Vitro Carcinogenesis Section, Laboratory of Cellular and Molecular Biology, NCI.

of cells resulting from short exposure to visible light in the presence of photosensitizing substances from red blood cells. At the Hygienic Laboratory, he improved both the hanging-drop and the Carrel flask techniques of cell culture through adjustment of pH (alkalinity/acidity), oxygen, and carbon dioxide. There was an approximately direct relationship between explant size and area of outgrowth, though explants below a certain size did not survive for reasons unknown. Another of his early contributions was "Earle's saline," an isotonic, balanced solution widely used in culture media. Later he showed that horse serum with chick embryo extract and chicken plasma clot would support the continued proliferation of epithelial cells from rat mammary carcinoma.

Earle's primary goals were to convert normal to malignant cells in vitro by means of a chemical carcinogen and to study the sequential changes occurring during the transformation. He carried out several exploratory studies with rodent cells to select a suitable tissue type and carcinogen dose and to develop procedures for solubilizing the carcinogen and preventing its photodecomposition. In addition, he designed photographic apparatus and staining procedures that enabled him to observe a gradual but radical morphologic alteration in plasma clot cultures of carcinogen-treated C3H mouse cells.

Spontaneous Malignant Transformation

At NCI, in 1940, Earle cultured a line of cells from normal subcutaneous connective tissue of a C3H mouse. The carcinogen methylcholanthrene was applied to the cultures. Using microphotographic instrumentation, motion and still, Earle recorded morphologic changes associated with carcinogen dosage. When carcinogen-treated and untreated cells were implanted in mice, both resulted in malignant tumors. One of the carcinogen-treated cell lines, designated strain L, was cultured continuously for many years.

The results of these experiments and those on rat fibroblasts by George O. Gey, at Johns Hopkins Medical School, showed clearly that malignant transformation could take place in vitro. The question still remained whether the transformation was induced or spontaneous. Did it result from the carcinogen, from some undefined environmental factor(s), or from intrinsic instability of cells during culture? Further studies on C3H mouse fibroblasts led to the conclusion that the transformation does not require a carcinogen but is a reproducible response to the culture conditions. Rodent cell lines derived from a wide variety of normal tissues were found to undergo malignant transformation during long-term culture.

Advances in Cell Culture Technology

The transformation could have been induced by some environmental factor—such as unidentified chemical carcinogens, hormones, or viruses—introduced through the complex biologic culture medium. To eliminate these potential causes, efforts were directed toward developing a medium that could be chemically characterized. The first step was to replace the undefined plasma clot with a sheet of perforated cellophane, permitting the ready dispersal of cells for culturing single-cell clones and cell suspensions.

To culture a homogeneous cell population required that a clone, or pure culture, be grown from a single tissue cell. Single cells were isolated in glass capillary tubes, which restricted the rapid diffusion of metabolites and thus conditioned the surrounding medium. In 1948 the first pure clone, NCTC 929L, was developed. This "monoclone," derived from strain L, is widely used in research today. The capillary cloning procedure was successfully applied to many other cell types.

With the cellophane substrate, cultures of increasingly larger surface area were grown. The development of three-dimensional substrate cultures incorporating a matrix of either multifolded perforated cellophane sheets or Pyrex helices yielded even greater numbers of living cells. These three-dimensional cultures were forerunners of today's substrate-dependent cultures produced commercially in bulk.

Our numerous studies to induce malignant transformation by tumor viruses or chemical carcinogens were invariably complicated by the spontaneous transformation of control (untreated reference) cultures. Therefore, we directed our attention toward controlling environmental factors. Numerous technologic advances were required. Methods and instrumentation were developed for preparing replicate cultures, for renewing medium without cell loss, and for quantifying proliferation rates by enumeration of isolated cell nuclei. To prevent loss of cells during renewal of nutrient fluid, a new culture vessel with a conical tip for centrifugation—the T flask—was designed.

These advances in technology permitted quantitative growth assays for evaluation of factors influencing cell proliferation. In one such study we found that malignant cells of fixed-tissue origin can proliferate in suspension. With suspension culture, large quantities of cells could be obtained for production of viruses and other biologics.

The figure portrays Wilton Earle surrounded by cell culture vessels designed and used in the Tissue Culture Section.

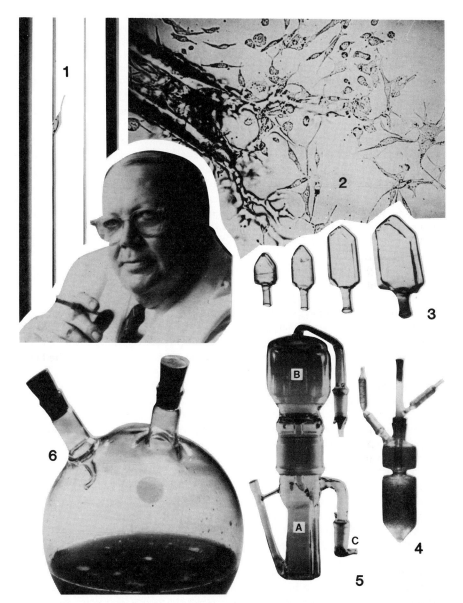

WILTON EARLE and cell culture vessels. 1. Tissue cell iso-
lated in glass capillary tube. 2. Proliferating cells emerging
from tube. 3. Pyrex flasks for quantitative growth studies.
4. Three-dimensional substrate culture on glass helices in
aerated medium. 5. Substrate culture on multifolded perfo-
rated cellophane sheet in medium intermittently forced from
A to B by CO_2 in air through C. 6. Shaker flask for propa-
gating multimillion-cell culture in agitated fluid suspension.

Maintenance of Differentiation in Culture

From suspension cultures and large surface-substrate cultures, adequate numbers of cells were obtained for analyses of biochemical properties, including enzyme patterns. The objectives were to identify the type of cell and tissue of origin, to determine whether the cells would maintain differentiated function and structure, and to establish any effects of environment on biochemical behavior. With some cell lines, structural or functional differentiation was maintained for long periods. In contrast, other lines lost certain differentiated properties of the tissue of origin. This loss may be associated with random mutation, induced changes in DNA, or quantitative changes in enzyme activities. It has not yet been rigidly correlated with malignant transformation.

Development of Chemically Defined Media

Further studies were directed toward control of the physicochemical microenvironment of the cells by development of a chemically defined culture medium. Both analytic and synthetic approaches were used, together with deletion techniques. Clone 929L provided assay cells. The serum and embryo extract components of the medium were fractionated and analyzed chemically. When tested on the cells, two fractions together—the ultrafiltrate of embryo extract and the large molecular protein fraction of horse serum—yielded cell numbers approaching those obtained with complete medium. The serum proteins were further fractionated, but all protein fractions stimulated growth.

Our synthetic approach was to add defined components to the protein fraction of horse serum and/or the ultrafiltrate of chick embryo extract. These supplements included an amino acid mixture based on chromatographic analyses of the free and conjugated amino acids in the complex biologic medium. Earle's saline formed the diluent, and vitamins with certain other components (from Morgan, Morton, and Parker's mixture 199) were tested in groups. By 1954, fractionations, analyses of the fractions, and exploratory nutritional experiments made possible the formulation of a chemically defined medium, later designated NCTC 109. In 1955 a line of clone 929L was initiated in this serum-, protein-, and antibiotic-free medium and cultured continuously for 24 years. NCTC 109 and Healy, Fisher, and Parker's synthetic medium 858 were the first chemically defined media to support continuous proliferation of an established mammalian cell line.

Subsequently some 30 additional cell lines from diverse tissues of five species were adapted by gradual serum depletion to serum-free chemically characterized medium NCTC 135 (differing from 109 in lacking cysteine). Few if any failures occurred. Cells could be successfully grown in chemically defined medium following adaptation or selective multiplication of variants of the original cells. We further demonstrated that normal cells could be explanted directly from mouse and rat embryos to chemically defined medium and grown continuously without exogenous serum or protein.

In short-term studies Fischer and Eagle identified the amino acids, and Eagle the vitamins, essential for cell survival and proliferation in a medium containing dialyzed serum. We found, however, that small amounts of dialyzed serum can prevent certain nutritional deficiencies. In defining the nutritional requirements for long-term proliferation in serum- and protein-free chemically defined medium, some additional requirements for survival and/or maximal growth became apparent, such as the nonessential amino acids and biotin. Simpler media were formulated, all components of which were shown to serve some function or to be necessary for cell survival, maximal proliferation, or prevention of cell fragility.

Recently a new formulation has been developed for human skin epithelial cells. This is an important type for in vitro studies on carcinogenesis because skin is a primary target for ubiquitous carcinogens such as benzo(α)pyrene.

The successful growth of cells in serum-free chemically defined medium by the mid 1950s can be attributed to several factors, including the commercial availability of high-quality chemicals, instrumentation for obtaining pure water, and equipment and procedures to ensure chemically clean glassware. Such defined media have been useful for growing cells in agitated fluid suspension as well as stationary culture. Mechanical stresses imposed by fluid agitation, however, sometimes caused cell deterioration unless Methocel, a chemically characterized, nutritionally inert polymer (first used by Kuchler and Merchant), was added to the medium. The observation that Methocel substitutes for serum in agitated suspension culture suggests that one role of the large serum protein molecules is to protect cells from mechanical stress. Methocel also enhances growth of cells in serum-free stationary culture.

Our primary objective in developing a chemically characterized culture medium was to determine whether cells initiated and grown in this better-defined environment would still undergo malignant transformation. All mouse lines in serum-free medium did transform after a prolonged interval. The experiments ruled out exogenous viruses, known chemical carcinogens, and hormones as causative agents. It has been suggested that so-called spontaneous malignant transformation is due to intermittent anaerobiosis, activation of endogenous viruses, or high population density with 'extensive cell-to-cell contact. Our experiments did not support any of these hypotheses.

Influence of Serum Type on Transformation and Chromosomal Stability

The discovery that the type of serum in the culture medium can influence the frequency of malignant transformation provided the first evidence that these transformations are not strictly spontaneous. Mouse cells cultured in chemically defined medium supplemented with horse serum (HS) transformed after relatively short periods, whereas cells cultured with fetal bovine serum (FBS) transformed after variable and considerably longer periods, sometimes extending to more than two years. It appeared that some influence in HS initiates malignant conversion and/or that some influence in FBS protects against it. We were unable, however, to control the transformation reproducibly in our assays of various serum fractions.

The type of serum also influenced karyotypic (chromosomal) stability. The chromosomes of mouse cells grown in HS- as compared with FBS-supplemented medium were less stable, shifting rapidly from the diploid number (full complement) and altering in morphology as a result of breaks and rearrangements. A large molecule fraction of HS was found to produce breaks and exchanges of chromatids (strands of the dividing chromosome). Chromosomal alterations occurred early in culture, and the incidence of abnormal chromosomes tended to increase at about the time of overt demonstration of malignant transformation; but no specific chromosomal aberration could be correlated with the onset of transformation in mouse or rat cells in vitro. Nonetheless, the apparent association between serum-induced accelerated malignant transformation and karyotypic instability suggests that agents in culture that damage chromosomal DNA may also initiate carcinogenesis. Furthermore, in comparisons of mouse, hamster, rat, and human cells in culture, the more stable the karyotype, the less frequent was the occurrence of spontaneous malignant change.

Influence of Oxygen Concentration and Visible Light

In addition to the type of serum, oxygen concentration and visible light were found to influence karyotypic stability. Reducing the oxygen in the gas phase of the culture from atmospheric concentration (18 percent) to 0-1 percent decreases the number of chromosomal aberrations and the rate of shift from diploidy. The lowered oxygen concentration also enhances survival and growth of single cells. It is noteworthy that cultures with 0-1 percent O_2 in the gas phase have a concentration of oxygen dissolved in the medium comparable to that of intercellular fluids in vivo.

A single 3- to 20-h exposure of cultures to low-intensity, cool-white fluorescent light (4.6 W/m^2, effective wavelength in the visible range 405 nm) at 37°C produces chromatid breaks and exchanges in both mouse and human cells. Experimental results indicate that the chromatid damage is caused by hydrogen peroxide (H_2O_2) or free hydroxyl radicals (OH) generated within the cell during light exposure.

In addition to chromatid damage, three other cellular responses to light were observed. Fluorescent light was found to produce DNA-protein cross-links in mouse or human cells. A single exposure (20 h at 37°C) to low-intensity light (4.6 W/m^2, effective wavelength 450-490 nm) suffices, and the effect is proportional to the intensity of illumination. Further, it is medium-mediated, enhanced by oxygen, decreased at high-cell density, and catalase-insensitive. Such damage at the molecular level could lead to important biologic aberrations, such as mutations, chromosome damage, and malignant transformation.

A second effect of light exposure is a proliferative response. Whereas long exposure (>8 h) of medium and cells to low-intensity light produces toxic and/or growth-inhibitory photoproducts, especially for low-density cell populations, short exposures (3 to 4 h) reproducibly enhance the proliferation rate and significantly extend the life span of human fibroblasts in culture. This effect is reversible and mediated through the chemically defined portion of the culture medium.

Finally, light affects the malignant transformation. Repeated exposure of mouse cells to low-intensity fluorescent light (4.6 W/m^2) and continuous exposure to oxygen at atmospheric concentration causes or enhances transformation of mouse cells in culture.

The Aberrant Methylation Hypothesis

Among the biochemical theories advanced to explain the transformation of normal to cancer cells is the aberrant methylation hypothesis of Srinivasan and Borek. The observation that extracts of certain tumor tissues have a greater capacity for methylating (introducing CH_3 groups into compounds) than those of normal tissues led to the concept that altered nucleic acid methylation may be the initiating or necessary chemical event in at least certain types of malignant change. Some support for this hypothesis was obtained from experiments with mouse cells transformed spontaneously in culture. The malignant cell extracts had a greater methylating capacity than extracts of their normal counterparts.

The discovery of methyltransferases (enzymes that transfer methyl groups between compounds) in all RNA tumor viruses examined lent further support to the methylation hypothesis. Although these viruses alter methylation of nucleic acids, it is still uncertain whether the alterations are primary, secondary, or concomitant to malignant transformation.

Markers of Malignant Transformation in Culture

Cytology and Colony Morphology. The distinguishing feature of malignant neoplastic cells in vivo is their capacity for uncontrolled invasive growth leading to destruction of normal tissues, sometimes to metastasis, and ultimately to death of the host. Thus the test for malignant transformation in cultured cells was their capacity to grow continuously as invasive neoplasms when implanted into compatible animals. The many disadvantages of this time-consuming approach led us to seek reliable criteria of malignancy that could be applied directly to cells in culture.

Using paired lines of malignant cells and their normal counterparts, we found that certain cytologic changes detectable with the light microscope correlate with the onset of tumorigenicity. Thus they can serve as in vitro criteria for neoplastic transformation of fibroblasts or epithelial cells. These criteria include increased staining capacity (cytoplasmic basophilia), reduced spreading of cytoplasm on solid-surface substrate, increased separation of cells, cell underlap or crisscross growth, random orientation, heterogeneity in the size and shape of nuclei, increased nuclear-to-cytoplasmic ratio, increased size and number of nucleoli, and tendency of cells to form cords or clumps.

A measure of reduced cytoplasmic spreading was used successfully to assay the transition of rodent cells from the normal to the oncogenic state. The distribution of cells in clumps and cords and their loss of parallel orientation were also diagnostic. Experiments directed to an understanding of these phenomena have been reported.

Cytologic diagnoses were consistent with results of in vivo assay in 92 percent of the numerous cultures examined. The cytologic and morphologic changes, even in populations derived from a single cell, appear to be direct manifestations of malignant change, as indicated by their reproducibility and regular association with tumorigenicity when the cells are returned to the host.

Loss of Anchorage Dependence. Normal tissue cells require a solid surface for attachment and growth, whereas malignant cells can grow suspended in a semisolid medium. This loss of anchorage dependence has been considered a criterion of the malignant state. In our studies with rodent cells, capacity to grow in a semisolid agarose medium consistently discriminated between malignant and normal cells.

Susceptibility to Killing by Activated Macrophages. Still another property characterizing malignant cells is an enhanced susceptibility to killing by activated macrophages (a type of cell-destroying cell of the reticuloendothelial system). The macrophage reaction discriminated between our paired normal and malignant cell lines derived in vitro from the same cell or cell pool.

Deficiency in DNA Repair. Mouse cell lines that underwent malignant transformation during long-term culture also developed a concomitant increase in susceptibility to chromatid damage by light. Cell lines were monitored for light susceptibility by enumerating chromatid breaks and exchanges after a 20-h exposure to low-intensity (4.6 W/m^2) fluorescent light. Transformation was associated with a significant increase in these light-induced changes.

In contrast to mouse cells, normal human cells are difficult to transform by carcinogenic agents, maintain a stable karyotype, do not develop an increased susceptibility to light-induced chromatid damage during culture, and have not been reported (with one possible exception) to undergo spontaneous transformation in vitro. However, human skin fibroblasts transformed by chemical carcinogens (and cells derived from a human adenocarcinoma) showed a significant increase in light-induced chromatid damage as compared with normal controls. Moreover, cultured skin fibroblasts from patients with xeroderma pigmentosum and ataxia telangiectasia, inherited conditions predisposing to cancer, developed a greater susceptibility to such light damage than numerous lines of skin fibroblasts from normal donors.

Experiments were performed to determine the mechanism(s) of action in the light-induced chromatid damage associated with malignant transformation. The results suggest that the susceptible cells have decreased DNA repair capacity during a phase (G_2) of the cell cycle. Similar results were obtained with X-irradiated cells: malignant cells, but not normal ones, showed a defect in repair of DNA damage during the G_2 phase, or within 1.5 h of metaphase.

Summary and Conclusions

The Section's early work was focused on tissue culture technology with a view to investigating malignant transformation. Our advances fashioned cell culture into a precise quantitative tool for many problems in biomedical research. Postulated criteria to identify malignant cells in culture were examined, and additional criteria were developed and evaluated. From our experimental findings through the years, "spontaneous" transformation in culture appears to be induced by specific environmental factors. These include a chemical component(s) of serum, visible light, and a high concentration of oxygen. The progression of mouse and human cells to malignancy in culture appears to be associated with an impaired capacity to repair chromosomal DNA damage produced by these agents.

TISSUE CULTURE

II. Studies in Cell Biology, NIAID

Harry Eagle

Growing out of previous studies on the nutritional requirements of cultured treponemata, studies on the growth and metabolism of animal cells in vitro were conducted from 1949 to 1961 under the direction of HARRY EAGLE in the Laboratory of Cell Biology, National Institute of Allergy and Infectious Diseases (and predecessor organizations). The initial objective was to define the nutritional requirements of mammalian cells in the hope that simplified media would permit more penetrating research on metabolism. Secondarily, it was hoped that differences would emerge between normal and cancer cells that would provide insight into the nature of the malignant transformation.

In defining the nutritional requirements, a minimal essential medium was developed, every component of which was demonstrably requisite to survival and growth. After 25 years, that medium and its modifications continue to serve as a basic tool in a broad spectrum of investigations of cell structure, metabolism, and function. The growth factor studies permitted Eagle and his colleagues to investigate requirements for viral propagation and facilitated an analysis of the time course of viral synthesis.

It was established that blood serum contained, over and above the defined growth requirements, nondialyzable factors essential for the sustained propagation of most animal cells, and that these factors, liberated from serum protein by tryptic digestion, permitted growth of cells in a protein-free environment. These findings led 20 years later to Gordon H. Sato's classic demonstration of a major role for serum

HARRY EAGLE, M.D., Director, Cancer Research Center, and Associate Dean for Scientific Affairs, Albert Einstein College of Medicine. Formerly Chief, Laboratory of Cell Biology, National Institute of Allergy and Infectious Diseases.

ISBN 0-12-667980-0
121

protein as a carrier of essential hormones and polypeptides and to the development of serum-free media for the propagation of certain hormone-dependent cell lines. The extensive cellular studies of the past two decades on "inborn errors of metabolism" began in Eagle's laboratory with ROBERT S. KROOTH's cultivation of cells from humans with genetic defects and his elucidation of the biochemical deficiency in those cultures.

These and other studies involving the use of cultured animal cells in a wide variety of metabolic and medical problems are detailed below.

Nutritional Requirements

Amino Acids

Initially, 13 amino acids were shown to be required for the sustained propagation of animal cells: *lysine,* arginine, cystine, glutamine, *histidine, isoleucine, leucine, methionine, phenylalanine,* tyrosine, *valine, threonine,* and *tryptophan.* The nine indicated by italics were known to be nutritionally required for nitrogen balance in man or rat and for the survival of the whole animal. The additional in vitro requirement for cystine, arginine, and tyrosine reflected their active biosynthesis in vivo by the liver. The limited synthesis of glutamic acid and glutamine in some primary cultures probably explains why neither is required in short-term studies on nitrogen balance in man. The glutamine requirement in culture could be met by high concentrations of glutamic acid; and it was shown by ROBERT I. DeMARS, then a postdoctoral fellow in Eagle's laboratory, that glutamic acid at those high concentrations induced the synthesis of glutamine synthetase. Once the enzyme had been induced, cells could grow at relatively low concentrations of glutamic acid in lieu of glutamine.

Particular interest attaches to the in vitro requirement for cystine (or cysteine, its reduction product). Although cyst(e)ine was generally required for cell survival in culture, definite if limited initial growth sometimes occurred in a cyst(e)ine-free medium, indicating the presence of a mechanism to provide it. Tracer studies revealed that cells could mobilize cystine residues bound to serum protein in disulfide linkage. Upon removal of those residues—e.g., by treatment with thioglycolate—cyst(e)ine became essential for growth.

Of the six amino acids synthesized by the cells and thus not required in the culture medium, the carbon skeletons of glycine, serine, and alanine were shown to derive from glucose, while those of proline, aspartic acid, and asparagine came largely from glutamine. The amino groups derived primarily from glutamine via glutamic acid. Interestingly, when cells were grown in a medium containing ribose and pyruvate instead of glucose, alanine derived almost wholly from pyruvate, while serine and glycine came from ribose.

At physiological concentrations, the amino acids provided in the medium were shown to be concentrated 3- to 30-fold in the cellular pool. The minimum pool concentrations necessary for protein synthesis were also determined.

Vitamins

Seven vitamins proved to be essential for the growth of animal cells: choline, folic acid, nicotinamide, pantothenate, pyridoxal, riboflavin, and thiamine. Five to fifteen days after any of these was omitted from the medium, degenerative changes developed that led eventually to death of the culture. Most conjugates and precursors were almost as effective as the vitamins per se. Subsequently, myoinositol also proved to be an essential vitamin for 16 of 19 cell lines. One line was shown to synthesize inositol from glucose and to release small amounts into the medium, which could then serve as a feeder for inositol-dependent strains.

Salts

Ions of six types were shown to be essential for the survival and growth of animal cells: Na^+, K^+, Ca^+, Mg^{++}, Cl^-, and $HPO_4^=$. A rigorous requirement for HCO_3^- is normally met by the metabolism of glucose and is evinced only at low population densities. (See below.) The minimal and optimally effective concentrations for each ion were determined.

Carbohydrates

Glucose was shown to be required for the survival and growth of cells. In a medium containing only the minimal essential components, glucose is needed for energy and for the carbon entering the biosynthesis of all the nutritionally nonessential amino acids, purines, pyrimidines, lipids, and other compounds requisite for cell growth and function.

MINIMUM ESSENTIAL MEDIUM FOR CULTIVATION OF MAMMALIAN CELLS IN MONOLAYER OR SUSPENSION*

Compound	Concentration (mM)	Concentration (mg/l)	Compound	Concentration (mg/l)
L-Amino acids			Vitamins	
Arginine	0.6	105	Choline	1
Cystine	0.1	24	Folic acid	1
Glutamine	2.0	292	Inositol	2
Histidine	0.2	31	Nicotinamide	1
Isoleucine	0.4	52	Pantothenate	1
Leucine	0.4	52	Pyridoxal	1
Lysine	0.4	58	Riboflavin	0.1
Methionine	0.1	15	Thiamine	1
Phenylaline	0.2	32	Serum protein	
Threonine	0.4	48	(whole or dia-	
Tryptophan	0.05	10	lyzed serum,	
Tyrosine	0.2	36	5-10%)****	
Valine	0.4	46		
Carbohydrate				
Glucose	5.5	1000		
Salts				
NaCl	116	6800		
KCl	5.4	400		
$CaCl_2$	1.8(0)**	200(0)**		
$MgCl_2$ $6H_2O$	1.0	200		
NaH_2PO_4 $2H_2O$	1.1(11)**	150(1500)**		
$NaHCO_3$***		2000		

   *The concentrations of most of the amino acids are greater than those originally recommended, and the relative amounts conform more closely to the protein composition of cultured human cells. This permits the cultures to be kept for some-what longer periods without refeeding. The concentration of some of the salts has been rounded off. In using this medium for the growth of cells in suspension, Ca^{++} should be omitted or greatly reduced in order to minimize clumping, and the concentration of NaH_2PO_4 may be increased 10-fold for more effective buffering.

   The fact that some of the amino acids can be replaced by such immediate precursors as the corresponding keto acids, the vitamins by the corresponding cofactors, or the glucose by a number of carbohydrates does not change the minimum number of essential growth factors but relates only to the

For a number of cell lines, several carbohydrates, including D-fructose, D-galactose, D-mannose, D-ribose, trehalose,
and turanose, could substitute for glucose to varying degrees.

A Minimum Essential Medium

The demonstrably essential components described above
were combined at their most effective concentrations into a
minimum essential medium (MEM) for the propagation of animal
cells in vitro (see table). MEM was first described in 1955,
and various modifications continue to be used worldwide for
cell culture.

Population-Dependent Requirements for Growth

Many metabolites that cells can synthesize to a limited
degree were shown at low population densities to be lost to
the medium in amounts that precluded the cells' survival.
For such metabolites, there are population-dependent nutritional requirements. Thus, serine becomes an essential amino
acid for some cell lines at low densities (e.g., 10^2–10^3
cells/ml), varying with the cell strain. Similarly, asparagine and pyruvate, which do not ordinarily have to be supplied
to the medium, become essential for certain cells at low-
density cell populations. At the other extreme, compounds
normally added for growth but synthesized by the cells in
small amounts, such as glutamine and inositol, may become nutritionally nonessential at higher population densities.

---

*form in which they may be supplied. Conversely, the fact
that $NaHCO_3$ is not assigned a mimimum concentration means
that CO_2 is formed in adequate amounts from other components,
such as glucose.*
   ***In suspension cultures.*
   ****With small cell populations, $NaHCO_3$ may be reduced
from 0.2 percent to as little as 0.04 percent in order to
minimize alkalinization of the medium in the early stages
of growth.*
   *****Optional supplementation is as follows: (a) "non-
essential" amino acids (alanine, asparagine, aspartic acid,
glycine, glutamic acid, proline, serine), each at 0.1 mM;
(b) sodium pyruvate (1 mM). Of these, asparagine, serine,
glycine, and pyruvate have proved necessary for the growth
of certain cell lines in a dialyzed serum medium, and serine
is similarly required for the growth of single cells.*

These findings point up a major difference between the conditions of cell growth in vitro and in vivo. In the former, the volume of medium may be thousands or millions of times greater than that of the cells; in the latter, cells may constitute more than half the volume of a compact organ. The critical population density in vitro is that at which the cells are able to "condition" the medium—i.e., to build up a concentration of the specific factor in equilibrium with the minimum effective intracellular concentration—before the cells die of the specific deficiency.

Some Research Applications of Cultured Animal Cells

Use of Cell Cultures for Screening Possible Tumor Agents

The ready induction of specific amino acid and vitamin deficiencies in cell cultures, and their reversal by restoration of the missing metabolite, suggested that the cell culture system might facilitate the study of carcinolytic, or cancer-destroying, agents. Favoring this approach was the availability of a test system in which cells could be grown as a monocellular layer adherent to a glass surface, in immediate contact with a relatively defined growth medium, and in which the effect of the agent on growth could be determined quantitatively by simple chemical methods.

Initially, studies were carried out in collaboration with George E. Foley of the Sidney Farber Children's Cancer Research Foundation in Boston. Thirteen compounds known to have antitumor activity in experimental animals proved to be highly cytotoxic in vitro, while two inactive compounds were relatively nontoxic. In a larger group of 180 compounds, the tumor-active ones were significantly the most cytotoxic; and all 11 that were cytotoxic at 10^{-7} gm/ml or less had an antitumor effect in vivo. In general, compounds were equally cytotoxic against both normal and malignant cells. However, in a series of antifolic agents, there was a high degree of correlation between cytotoxicity in vitro, acute toxicity in mice, and carcinolytic activity in vivo.

Can determination of cytotoxicity in cell cultures serve as a primary screen for detecting new carcinolytic agents? In the intervening 25 years, several laboratories have conducted a number of studies, with a variety of cell lines, in which cytotoxicity in cell cultures has indeed been shown effective for this purpose. The approach is currently being pursued

in the National Cancer Institute. Among other advantages, it
can reduce the number of experimental animals used in screening.

Protein Turnover

The proteins of animal cells in culture were shown to
turn over at an average rate of more than 1 percent per hour,
in agreement with the half-life of cellular proteins in vivo.
That finding served as the takeoff point for studies by ROBERT
T. SCHIMKE and others on the turnover of specific cellular
proteins.

Viral Biosynthesis

Extensive investigations by JAMES E. DARNELL, Jr., NORMAN
P. SALZMAN, LEON LEVINTOW, and WOLFGANG K. JOKLIK contributed
importantly to an understanding of the time course and metabolic pathways involved in the synthesis of poliovirus and
vaccinia virus in cultured cells. These four investigators
began their distinguished careers as Research Associates at
NIH, working with Eagle in the Laboratory of Cell Biology.
Some of their major findings at NIH are mentioned below in
roughly chronologic sequence.

- When poliovirus is adsorbed onto cells preliminary to
  its migration through the membrane, it is largely inactivated. Conversely, at the end of the biosynthetic
  process, after an eclipse phase, the infectious virus
  accumulates in the cells before entering the medium.

- Essentially maximum yields of poliovirus could be obtained when the cells were in a medium containing only
  salts, glucose, and glutamine during the period of virus
  replication. Protein synthesis and turnover are inhibited within two hours after infection, and poliovirus
  proteins are synthesized from the free amino acid pool.
  The critical role of glutamine, the only amino acid that
  must be supplied to allow virus production, probably relates to its rapid disappearance from the cellular pool
  in a glutamine-free medium, presumably because of the
  high glutaminase activity of the cell.

- Poliovirus produced in suspension cell culture was
  easily concentrated by removal of the cellular debris
  by low-speed centrifugation, then centrifugation at

high speed in a cesium chloride gradient, and finally anion-exchange chromatography of the band containing the virus.

● Studies with ^{32}P-labeled poliovirus permitted a detailed analysis of the cellular adsorption and early fate of purified poliovirus.

● The early inhibition of net synthesis of RNA, DNA, and protein in poliovirus-infected cells is followed six hours later by a sharp loss of cellular material into the medium and, over three to nine hours, by a progressive increase in the acid-soluble nucleotide pool. Viral RNA is derived from this pool and not from the breakdown products of cellular RNA. Synthesis of poliovirus RNA precedes the first appearance of mature virus by only a half hour, and at no time is there a large amount of free viral RNA. Clearly, the viral macromolecules, once formed, are promptly assembled into virus particles. In the case of vaccinia, viral DNA synthesis precedes by two to four hours the formation of infectious virus.

● In strains of cultured cells varying in susceptibility to poliovirus, the basis for resistance appears to be cellular inefficiency in effecting the release of the infecting poliovirus RNA from its protein coat.

Biosynthetic Processes

The fact that animal cells could be propagated in a culture medium containing a limited number of nutrients—amino acids, vitamins, glucose, and salts—supplemented by dialyzed serum, meant that intermediates necessary for the biosynthesis of proteins, nucleic acids, carbohydrates, and lipids were being synthesized from the medium. Thus the carbon chain of glutamine was shown to serve as a precursor for aspartic acid, asparagine, and proline, probably via glutamic acid. Similarly, the carbon skeleton of alanine, serine, and glycine derived largely from glucose. For all these nutritionally nonessential amino acids, the α-amino group was shown to derive primarily from glutamic acid rather than free ammonia, perhaps by way of aspartic acid. Glutamic acid was subsequently found to be 9 to 16 times more effective than glutamine as an amino donor in a variety of transamination reactions. Leucine and isoleucine also had moderate activity, but the other amino acids tested showed none.

In a minimal medium containing neither purines nor pyrimidines, the carbon skeletons of the pyrimidines (but not the purines) derive in large part from those of glutamine and glutamic acid. The amide nitrogen of glutamine enters biosynthesized purine, pyrimidine, guanine, and cytosine. To varying degrees, different cell lines could use the preformed bases when these were added to the medium, as well as a variety of purine and pyrimidine precursors.

Genetically Determined Biochemical Diseases

Over the past two decades, cells derived from patients with a wide variety of genetically determined biochemical diseases have been used in hundreds of studies to provide major and often dramatic new insights into the specific genetic aberration and the biochemical basis for the deficiency. Robert S. Krooth's studies in the Laboratory of Cell Biology constituted a seminal approach. He was the first to culture cells from patients with galactosemia and acatalasia and to show that the biochemical defect characteristic of those diseases was expressed in cell culture. This has since been accomplished for dozens of similar biochemical deficiencies of genetic origin.

TISSUE CULTURE

III. The Nervous System in Vitro

Phillip G. Nelson

Tissue culture techniques lend themselves well to studies of biologic properties of cells in general, and much attention has been paid to control of cell division, nutritional requirements of cells, secretion of synthesized proteins, and other processes. In the past decade or so, more work has been done on highly differentiated properties of specialized cell types. Many important biological relationships are difficult or impossible to analyze unless the significant elements can be isolated from the multiple extraneous phenomena that characterize the intact functioning organism. Hence, it is important to be able to isolate components of the organism into more or less simplified systems in which matters of interest can be analyzed in detail. The large recent literature on the nervous system in culture is representative.

The first culture experiment, by Ross G. Harrison in 1904, was done to explicate the nature of the neuron (nerve cell) extensions that were so characteristic of the nervous system. The complexity of the system, however, lent uncertainty to the results. It was even unclear whether the fibrous component was connected to the nerve cell bodies. Tissue culture methods played a decisive role in resolving this basic question.

While today's methods are far more sophisticated, the general strategy and many of the major problems remain. Culture media must support cellular growth and differentiation. Culture substrates must promote cell adhesion. One must be constantly careful that the phenomenon studied in vitro has relevance to the in vivo phenomenon one seeks to model.

Studies on the nervous system in vitro can be divided

PHILLIP G. NELSON, M.D., Ph.D., Chief, Laboratory of Developmental Neurobiology, National Institute of Child Health and Human Development.

readily according to the types of neuronal tissue studied.
One area of study utilizes cells from neuronal tumors, including cloned and hybrid lines. Another major area utilizes
primary normal neuronal tissue, usually dissociated or explanted from the fetus (see figure). Interesting attempts by
HAYDEN G. COON to obtain transformed neuroblasts (embryonic
nerve cells that have undergone malignant change) from the
normal nervous system should also be mentioned.

In 1969 MARSHALL W. NIRENBERG was among several investigators who independently developed cell lines from a mouse
neuroblastoma (a cancer derived from neuroblasts). B. WINFRED
RUFFNER, JOHN H. PEACOCK, and PHILLIP G. NELSON, working with
Nirenberg, showed that these neuroblastoma cells in culture
were electrically excitable, an important neuronal property.
A number of young workers in Nirenberg's laboratory quickly
demonstrated morphologic and biochemical properties of the
cells, confirming their striking neuronal identity. TAKEHIKO
AMANO generated and maintained a large number of clonal lines
from the parent material so that a broad and fairly stable
spectrum was available. JOHN D. MINNA was successful in producing and cloning somatic cell hybrids between the neuroblastoma cells and a variety of neuronal and nonneuronal cell
types. Patterns of gene expression, such as reciprocal regulation of cholinergic and adrenergic functions, were discerned,
but with difficulty.

The neuroblastoma cells expressed a variety of receptors
—i.e., specialized structures excited by specific stimuli.
S. SHARMA, WERNER A. KLEE, and Nirenberg conducted a series of
experiments involving the opiate receptors, which could be
measured in some clones. An alteration in responsiveness to
opiates occurred with chronic exposure to these agents, which
may well bear some relationship to the striking tolerance or
habituation phenomenon seen in vivo.

The mechanism involved in the formation of synapses (nerve
junctions) constitutes one of the major areas of interest in
neurobiology, and it was clearly important to demonstrate any
synapse-forming capability of the cloned material. In 1974
CLIFFORD N. CHRISTIAN and Nelson (NICHD) joined forces with
Nirenberg (NHLBI) on this question. They were able to show
that hybrids of tumor cells—neuroblastoma and glioma cells—
liberating acetylcholine (a major transmitter of nerve impulses) would form functional synapses with primary mouse and rat
muscle cells in culture. A fully clonal system was achieved
with a muscle cell line developed by Peacock.

A critical feature of neuromuscular synapse formation is
the aggregation of acetylcholine (ACh) receptors on the muscle fiber under the neurite that innervates the muscle cell.
Christian and co-workers found that synaptically competent

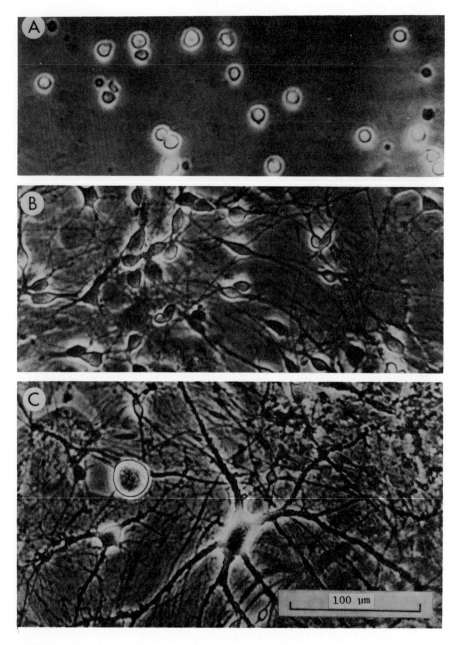

NEURONS in dissociated cell culture prepared from fetal mouse spinal cord. A. Immediately after dissociation and plating. B. One week later. C. After 4-5 weeks in vitro.

neural cell lines secrete material that, when applied to muscle cells, induces ACh receptors to aggregate. A large number of clones have been examined with regard to their capacity to form synapses. As expected, many negative clones could be shown to lack some critical component of the synaptic apparatus, such as the ability to synthesize, store, or release ACh.

One interesting clone exhibits properties that tie in with the findings on secretion of a factor for aggregation of ACh receptors. In studies by NEIL A. BUSIS and co-workers in NHLBI and NICHD, this clone revealed a capacity to make and release ACh when depolarized. It does not make synapses, however, and appears to lack the capacity to release the receptor aggregation factor. Thus, the clonal approach has provided a deficient cell line that could help to clarify a previously unknown step in the process of synapse formation.

Concurrently with studies of continuous neuronal lines, primary cultures of nervous system origin were established. GERALD D. FISCHBACH in NICHD found that electrophysiologic techniques could be used to study developing muscle cells in culture. He succeeded in co-culturing chick spinal cord neurons with muscle cells. The pioneering work of Fischman and Shimada had shown that dissociated single neurons of spinal cord exhibit impressive morphologic development in culture and establish numerous contacts with muscle cells cultured with them. Fischbach showed that many of these contacts were physiologically functional. This meant that a critical neurobiological process could be studied in the much simplified circumstances of cell culture technology. Subsequent experiments by Fischbach and others have, in fact, supplied a high-resolution description of the process. Interactions between nerve and muscle, both in terms of neural regulation of muscle properties and the retrograde effect of muscle on nerve, are made possible by this methodology.

Essentially all regions of the central nervous system have been successfully cultured, both in explants and in dissociated cell preparations. This makes available for rigorous biophysical analysis the specialized membranes of a wide variety of central neurons.

The mechanism of action of a number of anticonvulsant agents has been studied by Fischbach and by JEFFERY L. BARKER, ROBERT L. MACDONALD, and co-workers. The importance of the gamma aminobutyric acid receptor as a target for barbiturates and benzodiazepines has been demonstrated. Modulation of the mechanism for calcium action potential (whereby epinephrine is released into the synaptic space) by pharmacologic agents, including the opiates, has been shown in dorsal root ganglion neurons of the mouse and chick. The multiplicity of ionic

channels in neuronal membranes is becoming increasingly clear
through biophysical techniques of voltage clamping and single-
channel recordings by Barker, THOMAS G. SMITH, HAROLD LECAR,
MEYER B. JACKSON, and others.

Tissue culture as an approach to studying the nervous system is in its infancy. For instance, monoclonal antibodies are
beginning to be used in identifying cell surface components
essential for synapse formation; defective neuronal interactions related to a number of disease processes are starting
to be addressed successfully in vitro; and developmental effects of a number of neuroactive drugs in wide clinical use
have been evaluated. All this work is in preliminary stages.
It is clear, however, that many of the critical questions confronting neurobiology are yielding to tissue culture systems.
This powerful tool should continue to contribute to experimental efforts to understand neurodifferentiation and neuronal
function.

Introduction

BACTERIOLOGY AND MYCOLOGY

It must be more than 50 years since Paul de Kruif cate-gorized medical scientists as "Microbe Hunters." Indeed, modern medical science had its origins in the work of Robert Koch and Louis Pasteur, and the National Institutes of Health arose from laboratories largely engaged in research on bacte-rially transmitted diseases.

This chapter treats of NIH's microbe hunters, and there were many. Until the 1940s almost all of the diseases that attracted the attention of the Public Health Service were di-rect results of bacterial invasion. Isolation of the causa-tive agent, identification of the mode of transmission, in-vestigation of host immunity to each invading organism—these were the mainstream of biomedical advance.

The work was not devoid of danger or drama. It is note-worthy that the investigators frequently contracted and occa-sionally died of the disease under study. And there was drama enough in discovery, particularly in the face of prevalent misconceptions. The idea took hold that every disease resulted from invasion by a microorganism. So firm was this view that early investigators of pellagra, as the disease spread through the South in the early 1900s, assumed that it was infectious. This was confirmed by the highly respectable Thompson-McFadden Commission, and Surgeon General Rupert Blue ordered JOSEPH GOLDBERGER to identify the causative agent. It was many years before the medical profession fully accepted Goldberger's demonstrations that pellagra resulted not from a pathogenic invasion but rather from the absence of an essential nutrient.

This chapter will introduce many of our own microbe hun-ters and their quarry. Incidentally, the pursuit has been so successful that the vast majority of physicians entering prac-tice today may never encounter a single example of most of the classical infections. Bacteriologists are turning their attention to new challenges: microbial genetics, resistance to antibiotics, the frontiers of immunology and allergy, and devastating new diseases.

D. S.

8

BACTERIOLOGY AND MYCOLOGY

Roger M. Cole

Introduction

In 1887 JOSEPH J. KINYOUN established, in a room at the Staten Island Marine Hospital, what would later become known as the Hygienic Laboratory. The purpose was to control infectious disease, and the problems of the time were largely bacteriologic: cholera, typhoid, tuberculosis, plague. The need for research was clear to Kinyoun from his visits to the laboratories of Koch and Pasteur, where the young science of bacteriology was developing. His foresight initiated intramural research in the Public Health Service (then the Marine Hospital Service), gave rise eventually to the National Institutes of Health, and established the line of descent that culminated in today's National Institute of Allergy and Infectious Diseases (NIAID).

In light of these developments, a thoroughgoing history of NIH's intramural research in bacteriology and mycology would encompass nearly a century of effort—a monumental task. The period covers the youth and flowering of bacteriology and the transition from disease orientation to biochemistry and molecular biology. Major discoveries, such as the etiologies of important microbial diseases, are easily documented. More difficult is the tracing of laboratory discoveries back to basic research, which is hard to place in perspective and seldom sees the light of public exposure. In this category are all the taxonomic classifications, laboratory methods papers, unraveling of microbial metabolism, clarification of microbial antigens and immunity, and early microbial genetics underlying today's well-publicized recombinant DNA technology.

At NIH, intramural research in bacteriology and mycology has always had a disease-oriented emphasis, influenced by the

ROGER M. COLE, M.D., Medical Director, U.S. Public Health Service (retired). Formerly Chief, Laboratory of Streptococcal Diseases, National Institute of Allergy and Infectious Diseases.

NIH: AN ACCOUNT OF RESEARCH
IN ITS LABORATORIES AND CLINICS
ISBN 0-12-667980-0

need for accountability in a public organization with "Health" in its name. Basic research, of course, is done, but is not often cited as a prime justification for funding. In the beginning, most of the activities clearly involved disease recognition, epidemiologic studies, and development and testing of control measures. For example, Kinyoun made the first diagnosis of cholera in the United States in 1888.

The scope of the studies at the small original laboratory is impressive. Kinyoun developed facilities for the diagnosis of diphtheria and the production of antitoxin in horses. With M. J. ROSENAU, after the laboratory had been moved to Washington, D.C., in 1891, he experimented with pneumococcal immunization in mice. The laboratory was prepared to diagnose and vaccinate against bubonic plague prior to the San Francisco outbreak of 1900. Most of the activities were directed against the major bacterial diseases then prevalent. Personnel often engaged in field studies to clarify epidemiology, pinpoint potential trouble spots, and apply, with local and state health authorities, whatever control measures were available.

Passage of the first Biologics Control Act in 1902 gave emphasis to a major activity of the Hygienic Laboratory. The Act provided authority for the supervision of the purity and potency of serums and vaccines, for the preparation of standards for their evaluation, and for the licensing of these products for sale and transport. A good deal of intramural research in bacteriology and serology was required, much of which led to contributions extending beyond biologics control per se. In 1948, when the National Institute of Health became plural and the National Microbiological Institute (NMI) was established, the latter incorporated the Biologics Control Laboratory. In 1955 NMI became NIAID, and biologics activities were transferred to a new and expanded Division of Biologics Standards. DBS became the present Bureau of Biologics of the Food and Drug Administration in 1972, and many of its scientists continue bacteriologic and related research on the NIH grounds in Bethesda.

Similar investigations constitute a major program of the National Institute of Dental Research; and scattered enclaves of research on bacteria, or utilizing bacteria, are located in other Institutes.

The Early Years: Pre-1938

During the growth of bacteriologic research around the turn of the century, when infectious diseases were the nation's major health problem, many of the classic studies were carried out by intramural workers of the Public Health Service. Although these earlier accomplishments, constituting a large part of the foundation of bacteriology itself, precede the period covered by most of this book, I feel that they should be recognized here to supply perspective and due coverage.*

Over the long span encompassing intramural research in PHS, two broad groups of bacteriologic studies can be traced. One began at Staten Island with emphasis on cholera, plague, diphtheria, typhoid, typhus, and other outstanding problems of the period. This line of work evolved into the present program of NIAID. The other studies originated in the problem of Rocky Mountain spotted fever and led to the establishment of the Rocky Mountain Laboratory at Hamilton, Montana. RML was incorporated into the Institute in 1948. Subsequently NIAID's intramural research program was enriched by RML's expertise in rickettsial and other arthropod-borne diseases.

Rocky Mountain Spotted Fever

The diseases on which PHS and NIH bacteriologists concentrated their efforts were those constituting new or important health problems of the time. After a trip to Montana at the turn of the century, JOHN F. ANDERSON, then Assistant Director of the Hygienic Laboratory, published a pamphlet entitled "Spotted Fever (Tick Fever) of the Rocky Mountains—A New Disease."** This focused national attention on a prime example of PHS/NIH research activities and accomplishments.

Efforts over more than 45 years resulted in clinical and epidemiologic definition of the disease as well as in the determination of its distribution, vectors, and causative agent. Control of tick vectors was instituted. Vaccines were prepared and tested, and some were used in human populations for at least 15 years (1926-1941). It became abundantly clear that the disease occurred elsewhere than in the western states, that it was in fact most prominent in the east and southeast. In 1973, however, the efficacy of the commercial vac-

---

*Bacteriology, as treated in this chapter, encompasses the study of any of the microorganisms listed in *Bergey's Manual of Determinative Bacteriology* (eighth edition, The Williams and Wilkins Company, Baltimore, 1974). Mycology as considered here deals with those fungi (eukaryotic microorganisms) that cause disease in man and animals.

**Bulletin No. 14 of the Hygienic Laboratory, United States Public Health and Marine Hospital Service, Washington, D.C., 1903.

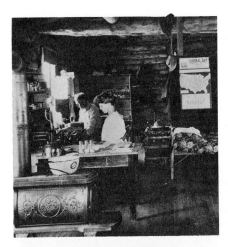
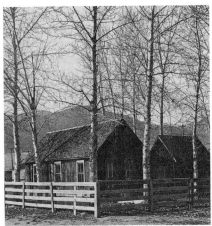

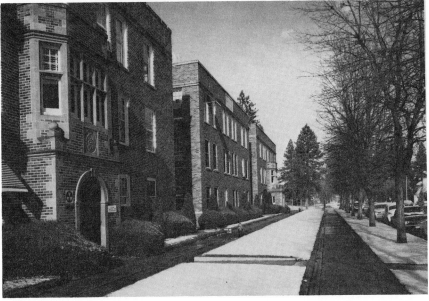

THE ROCKY MOUNTAIN LABORATORY at three stages of its history.
In June 1916 Ralph R. Parker, shown with assistant at upper
left, was investigating Rocky Mountain spotted fever in an
abandoned cabin in the Bitterroot Valley of Montana. In 1921
(the year Parker became Director of RML), the staff used
buildings (upper right) of the Montana State Board of Entomol-
ogy. The present well-equipped buildings at Hamilton, Montana,
were completed in 1945. They are located on 33 acres and con-
tain 144,000 square feet. RML is primarily concerned with
diseases transmitted to man from other animals.

cine (Lederle) was questioned, resulting in cessation of production five years later. A promising new vaccine prepared
in tissue culture (R. H. Kenyon and C. E. Pederson, 1975) is
being evaluated with an eye to future production.

The story of Rocky Mountain spotted fever is too long and
well documented to be recounted here. I will mention, however,
the principal investigators whose efforts led to our present
knowledge. Best known is H. T. Ricketts who, with W. W. KING,
found the etiologic agent, *Rickettsia rickettsii*. The work
of R. R. SPENCER and R. R. PARKER culminated in the first production and constant improvement of vaccines. IDA A. BENGTSON
and R. E. DYER first showed the feasibility of cultivating
the rickettsia in embryonated chick eggs in 1935, and H. R.
COX perfected the method between 1936 and 1941. I omit reluc-
tantly the names of many important contributors, but include
those who made the ultimate contribution: G. H. COWAN, A. H.
McCRARY, W. E. GITTINGER, L. A. KERLEE, and T. B. McCLINTIC
died of the disease in the course of their investigations.

Tularemia

Another disease with an original western flavor is tularemia, which was not named or recognized as a human health problem when G. W. McCOY and C. W. CHAPIN, in 1912, isolated the
agent *Bacterium tularense* from plaguelike lesions of ground
squirrels in Tulare County, California. The present generic
name of the agent, *Francisella tularensis,* honors EDWARD FRAN-
CIS, who contributed greatly to the knowledge of tularemia
from 1919 through 1942. His work and that of J. F. BELL, CORA
R. OWEN, and many others resulted in naming the disease, describing the pathology, defining the virulence of the agent,
showing ticks and deer flies to be vectors, establishing rabbits and other wild animals as important disease reservoirs,
and delineating the natural history and ecology of the organism.

Tularemia is now recognized in nonwestern parts of the
United States and in at least 12 other countries. Like Rocky
Mountain spotted fever, this was a "new" disease discovered
and elucidated primarily by PHS research workers, nearly all
of whom acquired the infection. In 1919 Francis had a three-
month bout after seeing his first case. He reported much
valuable clinical information from this experience, including
his acquisition of permanent immunity.

Typhus

Typhus has been known since ancient times in most parts of the world as a widespread epidemic disease associated with lice. At the Hygienic Laboratory, Anderson and JOSEPH GOLD-BERGER confirmed in 1912 that Mexican typhus ("tabardillo") was carried by the body louse. Other workers demonstrated that convalescent serum from Brill's disease patients prevented Mexican typhus, and several investigators later showed that the mild typhuslike entity found by Nathan Brill in New York City in 1910 was, in fact, a recrudescent form of epidemic typhus seen in European immigrants. In 1926 K. F. MAXCY reported epidemiologic studies on a new form of typhus endemic in the Southeast, attributing it to a rodent reservoir.

The NIH investigator most associated with typhus research was probably Dyer. Beginning in 1929, his work with L. F. BADGER, E. T. CEDER, A. S. RUMREICH, and W. G. WORKMAN clarified the confusion between rickettsiae found in southeastern ticks (causing spotted fever) and those found in rat fleas (causing endemic typhus). Dyer later served as Director, NIH (1942-1950).

He and others had demonstrated the rickettsiae of endemic typhus in both rat fleas and rats. They provided evidence of flea-borne rat-to-rat transmission and accidental infection of man by rat flea fecal contamination of skin lesions. In 1917 M. H. NEILL discovered the scrotal reaction of guinea pigs infected with typhus rickettsiae. Later called the Neill-Mooser reaction, this became the basis of a differential test. The work of many investigators, including some at RML, revealed other differences between the agents of epidemic and endemic typhus. The latter was named *Rickettsia typhi* by C. B. PHILIP in 1943, distinguishing it from the epidemic agent, *R. prowazekii*.

Of obvious importance in typhus of whatever form, besides rodent and vector control, is prevention by immunization. Bengtson and Dyer provided the key in 1935 with their cultivation of rickettsiae in chick embryos. The method was adapted to typhus, improved, standardized, and verified serologically by Cox at RML (1938-1948) and by Bengtson and N. H. TOPPING in Bethesda. Topping and others performed many studies of typhus vaccines, including those incorporating soluble antigens. What became known as Cox-type vaccine was produced at RML for the military during World War II. The United States of America Typhus Commission, established in 1942, included A. G. GILLIAM, Dyer, Topping, and W. L. JELLISON as the original PHS representatives. Gilliam conducted a field study of vaccine efficacy in Tripoli.

Psittacosis

Another disease of early interest to the Hygienic Laboratory, brought abruptly to attention in 1929 by cases occurring
in Annapolis, Washington, Baltimore, and Philadelphia, was
psittacosis, or "parrot fever." The cause was then thought to
be Nocard's bacillus (later shown to be a salmonella), but no
such organism was isolated by C. ARMSTRONG and H. ANDERSON
from impounded case-associated parrots. Both workers contracted the disease. Anderson died, and nine others in the
building (none working with parrots) became infected. The
entire Laboratory at 25th and E Streets, N.W., was temporarily
shut down.

It became clear that the agent, already shown to be highly
virulent for man, was readily and distantly airborne. It was
filterable and was shown by R. D. LILLIE (1939) to be microscopically visible. Perceiving rickettsialike inclusions,
Lillie labeled the agent *Rickettsia psittaci*. While similar
to true rickettsiae in many respects, it was later found sufficiently different to be placed in a new genus. It is now
named *Chlamydia psittaci*.

Armstrong's studies of the disease resulted in a Presi-
dential order regulating the importation and interstate traffic of parrots (1930). His convalescent serum was credited
with saving the life of Senator William E. Borah's wife when
she contracted psittacosis. This did no harm to public recognition and governmental support of PHS biomedical research
(though the efficacy of convalescent serum has often been
questioned).

Despite the stringent regulations, outbreaks occasionally
occurred, such as the one at the National Zoo described by
T. H. TOMLINSON, Jr., in 1941. Eventually widespread work like
that of D. J. DAVIS on psittacosis in pigeons (1950) implicated *C. psittaci* in pulmonic disease of goats, pigs, horses,
and cats as well as other birds. The agent has also been
shown to cause arthritis, placentitis, enteritis, conjunctivitis, and encephalitis in many of these animals. The only
other member of the genus, also widespread, is *C. trachomatis*,
which primarily infects humans, causing inclusion conjunctivitis (trachoma), lymphogranuloma venereum, and sexually
transmitted urethritis and proctitis.

Brucellosis

The classic work of ALICE C. EVANS, beginning in 1918,
distinguished the cause of Malta fever in man *(Brucella mel-
itensis)* from that of Bang's disease in cattle *(Brucella abor-*

tus) and established the relationship of the latter bacterium to undulant fever and chronic disease in humans. Evans' studies in the classification of brucellae continued for over 20 years, and her many contributions led to worldwide recognition.

When I arrived at the Institute in 1949, B. CARLE headed the Brucella Unit, B. H. HOYER was immersed in the physiology of brucellae, C. L. LARSON was identifying the antigens of *B. abortus,* and N. B. McCULLOUGH was devising laboratory tests useful in diagnosis and classification. In 1957 H. G. STOENNER and D. B. LACKMAN at RML described a new species, *Brucella neotomae,* from the desert wood rat. Later, Hoyer and McCullough confirmed and extended taxonomic relationships through DNA relatedness studies.

Evans, while still at NIH, enhanced her reputation by continuing research on the classification of meningococci and streptococci and publishing numerous articles on the nature of these bacteria. Some of her notebooks, beginning in 1919, are still in my possession. Similarly, I inherited her collection of streptococci, which became the basis for the collection I used and augmented for 30 years.

Clostridia

A new toxin-producing type of *Clostridium botulinum* (designated Type C) was isolated from limberneck of chickens by Bengtson in 1922. Her research at that time also incriminated *Clostridium tetani* on bone points and under dressings then used in smallpox vaccination. This led to new vaccination techniques that abolished post-vaccination tetanus from the United States. Bengtson devised the first complement fixation test for serologic diagnosis of rickettsial (and some viral) diseases and for determining the immunologic efficacy of vaccines. She was also active in standardization of clostridia toxins and other biologic products, in bacteriologic investigations of conjunctivitis, and in numerous studies of typhus and Q fever.

1938 and Beyond

Between 1938 and 1949, a number of other diseases and bacteria were studied at NIH. J. WATT, T. M. DeCAPITO, D. R. LINDSAY, and others completed a series of field and laboratory studies on acute diarrheal diseases in the rural South, aided by A. ELIZABETH VERDER's laboratory work at Bethesda. The

results implicated strains of *Shigella* as etiologic agents,
demonstrated the effectiveness of sulfadiazine therapy, and
showed the importance of flies in transmission. H. EAGLE and
H. G. STEINMAN investigated the cultural requirements of trep-
onemal spirochetes. B. J. OLSON, K. HABEL, and W. R. PIGGOTT
compared the efficacy of live and killed vaccines in experimental tuberculosis.

Scrub Typhus

The war in the Pacific stimulated interest in rickettsial
diseases, resulting in new studies of another such entity,
scrub typhus (mite-borne typhus, or tsutsugamushi disease).
Antigenic differences among strains of the agent, *Rickettsia
tsutsugamushi,* were defined by Bengtson and E. J. BELL. Methods for preparing antigens and testing the efficacy of immune
sera in experimental animals were devised by Cox and Topping.
Clinical, epidemiologic, and etiologic studies of the disease
in Japan and other parts of the Orient were conducted by G. M.
KOHLS, E. J. Bell, and C. B. Philip.

Q Fever

The story of Q (for *query*) fever in the United States began in 1935 with G. E. DAVIS's discovery of a filter-passing
infectious agent in ticks from Nine Mile Creek, Montana. Most
studies, however, date from 1938, when Cox and E. J. Bell cultivated the organism in chick embryo yolk sacs and tissue culture, named it *Rickettsia diaporica,* and produced a vaccine
successful in laboratory animals.

In 1938 Dyer became ill with "nine-mile fever" as a result
of a visit to RML. He later used stored samples of his blood
to show cross-immunity to the agent of Australian Q fever. Cox
and E. H. Derrick of Australia are considered codiscoverers
of the agent (which Philip would later reclassify as *Coxiella
burnetii).* In 1941 Cox improved methods for cultivating it
for vaccine production and Bengtson developed a complement
fixation test and further confirmed the immunologic relationship of the American and Australian agents.

Meanwhile, Q fever studies had been initiated at NIH in
Bethesda. Over the next 10 years (1940-1950), 80 laboratory
workers and others in Buildings 5 and 7 came down with the
disease, and one, ASA MARCEY, died. The first outbreak was
studied intensively in 1940 by Dyer, Topping, and Bengtson,
who isolated and identified the agent, and by J. W. HORNIBROOK
and K. R. NELSON, who first pointed to an atypical pneumonia

as a major facet of the disease. Lillie, T. L. PERRIN, and
Armstrong described the pathology. The 1940 outbreak and
one in 1946 gave ample, if then circumstantial, evidence of
the airborne transmission and high infectivity of *C. burnetii;*
and later studies by R. J. HUEBNER, C. G. SPICKNALL, and SARA
E. RANSOM demonstrated that the organism was more resistant
than rickettsiae to heat, formalin, phenol, etc. It was not
destroyed by heat exposure in the method then used for pas-
teurizing milk. Moreover, outbreaks were occurring in stock
handlers and slaughterhouse workers.

An outbreak in 1947 in the Los Angeles area led to the establishment there of a field laboratory and the initiation of
a three-year study by Huebner, Jellison, J. A. BELL, L. LUOTO,
C. C. SHEPARD, and others. Their results showed the previously unrecognized prevalence of Q fever in the region
and defined its relation to infected cattle and ingestion of
raw milk. Isolates and sera were sent to Bethesda for further
testing. By this time, personnel in infectious disease study
areas were required to receive the RML vaccine, and I recall
getting my share. There were no further cases, but maintenance personnel long remained reluctant (to say the least)
to enter Building 7. In addition, studies by J. W. OLIPHANT,
E. A. BEEMAN, Parker, and others revealed a hazard of contracting Q fever from infected clothing, inanimate objects,
etc. This was later emphasized when Beeman's landlady, who
regularly did his laundry, contracted the disease.

After the mid 1950s, work on *C. burnetii* at Bethesda gradually ceased as interest in viruses grew. The agent, however,
has remained an important research subject at RML. It is of
interest that no commercially produced *C. burnetii* vaccines
are yet available in the United States.

Louisiana Pneumonitis

What turned out to be a human disease related to psittacosis, but with some distinctive differences, began in late
1942 in a coastal area of Louisiana. This was a highly fatal
pneumonitis that was spread by personal contact with fatal
cases. Its occurrence engendered some of the most stringent
control measures, quarantine requirements, and laboratory precautions ever applied by the Public Health Service. Epidemiology, clinical features, etiology, and pathology of the disease
delineated during intensive field and laboratory studies were
reported by Olson, Larson, W. L. Treuting, and G. L. FITE in a
series of papers published from 1944 to 1946.

The disease was attributed to what were then called the
"viruses" of lymphogranuloma and psittacosis. The first of

these agents, now known as *Chlamydia trachomatis,* causes trachoma and some urogenital infections. However, neither that
organism nor *Chlamydia psittaci* has ever been definitively
identified as the agent of Louisiana pneumonitis. Nor, to
the best of my knowledge, has the disease ever reappeared in
Louisiana or elsewhere. Hence, opportunities for further study
are absent, speculations regarding transmission from marsh
birds or other wildlife are unsettled, and a protective vaccine said to have been developed by Olson and Larson was never
given the acid test and no longer exists.

Rickettsialpox

One of the more exciting events of this period was the
finding of a new rickettsial illness in New York City residents, the so-called "Kew Gardens mystery disease." In 1946–
1947 Huebner, Jellison, Armstrong, C. Pomerantz, and P. Stamps
discovered and completely elucidated the infection, which had
been confused with typhus. From the human cases, marked by
fever and rash, they isolated the etiologic agent and characterized it as a new species, *Rickettsia akari.* The same organism was isolated from a rodent mite, in which it was found
to be passed transovarially (from generation to generation
through the eggs), and from the mite's host, the common house
mouse.
These findings solved the cycle of transmission from the
mouse reservoir to humans through contamination with infected
mites. The disease was named rickettsialpox. Its elucidation,
recognized as a modern classic of investigative microbiology,
was duly celebrated in the *New Yorker.* The rickettsia has
since been found in other urban areas of the United States and
Russia and in wild rodents of rural Korea.

Investigations Spanning the
Previously Described Periods

Because some intramural investigations began well before
1938 and continued well beyond, they cannot be properly placed
in either time frame. Two researchers whose work spanned the
two periods and who were active and well known when I arrived
at NIH in 1949 were SARA E. BRANHAM and MARGARET PITTMAN.
Their areas of specialization, respectively, were *Neisseria*
infections and pertussis (whooping cough).

Neisseria

For nearly three decades, Branham investigated the gram-negative cocci of the genus *Neisseria* that cause gonorrhea and meningitis. Her name is particularly associated with the agent of epidemic meningitis, *Neisseria meningitidis,* or meningococcus. She was instrumental in distinguishing the three serotypes known today (A, B, and C). She established and characterized reference strains, explored protective properties of immune sera, and described many other characteristics of the bacteria. In 1930 she identified a new species, *Neisseria flavescens,* as a rare cause of meningitis and septicemia in humans but one requiring careful differentiation from the meningococcus. Her numerous contributions to knowledge and taxonomy of the family Neisseriaceae—too many to describe here—were honored posthumously in the name of a new genus, *Branhamella* (1970).

Pertussis and Haemophilus

Pittman, though officially retired, is still active. Both she and Branham were originally in the Laboratory of Biologics Control, NMI. This group entered the Bureau of Biologics, Food and Drug Administration, as a result of the reorganization of 1972, and Pittman became Chief of the Laboratory of Biologics Products. Although involved in many control studies and oversight responsibilities for vaccines, such as those for cholera, typhoid, and tetanus, she achieved her early international reputation through investigations of haemophilus and pertussis. (Originally, the agent of whooping cough was designated as *Haemophilus pertussis,* but was removed to a new genus, *Bordetella,* in 1952.)

Haemophilus remains a valid genus in which Pittman, with D. J. Davis, described a putative new species, *H. aegyptius* (1950), and the species *H. parahaemolyticus* (1953). The former organism, commonly called the Koch-Weeks bacillus, is transmitted by gnats and causes an acute infectious conjunctivitis in humans in the Southeast and other hot regions. The latter organism, found in the human upper respiratory tract, can cause pharyngitis and endocarditis.

In the 1930s Pittman carried out important investigations of variation and type specificity in *Haemophilus influenzae,* once associated with pandemic influenza but now known to cause a variety of respiratory infections, epiglottitis, and meningitis. She distinguished six antigenic types, now identified with differences in capsular polysaccharide.

Pertussis, though controlled by immunization, remains a

potentially serious and even fatal illness. A variety of vaccines are used widely in the major countries; none is ideal.
Pittman developed a potency assay in the late 1940s, and she
and J. E. LIEBERMAN devised a new method for determining the
median effective dose of vaccines in trials. A well-controlled
field trial, showing substantial protection of children in
Norfolk, Virginia (1941), was reported by J. A. Bell. Recently, infrequent severe reactions to pertussis vaccines have
aroused public interest and renewed the clamor for an improved
vaccine. J. J. MUNOZ at RML is investigating "pertussigen,"
a histamine-sensitizing factor of *B. pertussis* discovered by
Pittman in 1951, and other protein toxic factors of the bacterium.

Mycology

The Mycology Section, of which C. W. EMMONS was a member
and later the head (1936 to 1966), was one of few groups in
the United States with wide mycological expertise. Even before 1949 Emmons was recognized as a world authority in medical mycology. His laboratory attracted many collaborators,
fellows, and Visiting Scientists. Although much of his early
work dealt with dermatophytes (fungi causing infections of
the skin, hair, or nails), his later studies were largely concerned with the systemic mycoses and their causative agents.
He made the first isolations of *Coccidioides immitis* (1942)
and *Histoplasma capsulatum* (1949) from soil and rodents, and
of *Cryptococcus neoformans* (1951) from soil and pigeon droppings. From 1947 to 1955, with J. A. Bell, Olson, H. F. HAS-
ENCLEVER, Piggott, and others, he established the importance
of rodents, birds, bats, animal droppings, and soil as natural
reservoirs that served to maintain and disseminate both *Histoplasma* and *Cryptococcus*. In 1963 he explored methods for
eradicating *Histoplasma* from soil.

Later Emmons wrote or revised several authoritative manuals on mycological identification and taxonomy. With C. H.
BINFORD and J. P. UTZ, he coauthored a widely used textbook
on medical mycology. Further research identified obscure
fungi causing rare diseases and resulted in the description
and naming of new species. With several members of NIAID's
Laboratory of Clinical Investigations (LCI) and other workers,
he described the earliest studies of efficacy, toxicity, bioassay methods, and clinical results for various antifungal
antibiotics.

Utz and J. E. BENNETT continued to investigate and treat
cases of fungal disease brought to or occurring in the Clini-

cal Center.   Bennett became head of LCI's clinical mycology
department.

On Emmons's retirement from the Mycology Section in 1967,
Hasenclever became head. In 1974 Hasenclever moved to RML and
the section became a part of my Laboratory of Microbiology,
as it was then called. Many other members, including fellows,
came and moved on. One who remained was KYUNG JOO KWON-CHUNG,
who had come as a Visiting Fellow in 1966. Her early and continuing interest in the reproduction and genetics of fungi
later resulted in revolutionary discoveries in medical mycology. These included the findings that both *Histoplasma* and
Cryptococcus, long considered to be "fungi imperfecti," did
in fact possess a previously unrecognized sexual, or perfect,
state and thus unsuspected possibilities of genetic variability. In 1972 Kwon revealed the sexual stage of *Histoplasma*
capsulatum (thereon renamed *Emmonsiella capsulata)* and in 1974
demonstrated the widespread occurrence and distribution of two
mating types. Later she discovered the perfect state of *Cryp-*
tococcus neoformans (renamed *Filobasidiella neoformans)* and
C. uniguttulatus. These and other findings, too numerous to
describe here in detail, have not only placed Kwon in the
forefront of internationally recognized authorities in her
field, but have perpetuated the tradition of excellence established by Emmons.

Mycoplasmology

One of the more significant developments in bacteriology
at NIAID began with investigations of a disease common in
young people and known clinically as primary atypical pneumonia. R. M. CHANOCK and his associates in the Respiratory
Virus Unit began studying the disease about 1959. Others
had presented evidence that the cause was a virus (called the
Eaton agent, after its discoverer) that could be propagated in
embryonated eggs or tissue culture. In 1962 Chanock, L. Hay-
flick, and M. F. BARILE grew the agent on artificial media
and identified it as a pleuropneumonialike organism. These
wall-less microbes, now recognized as bacteria called mycoplasmas, had long been known to cause serious pulmonary and
other disease in domestic animals but had not been implicated
in human disease. Chanock and 14 other national and international experts named the new microorganism *Mycoplasma pneu-*
moniae in 1963.

This discovery, which marked the beginning of mycoplasmal
research at NIH, initiated a period of vigorous activity extending over 15 years. It engaged at least 40 researchers
at one time or another and resulted in nearly 200 publications

from NIAID. *Mycoplasma pneumoniae,* first cultivated in chick entodermal and monkey kidney tissue cultures, was later shown to grow in broth as well. There, its adherence to glass surfaces, as demonstrated by N. L. SOMERSON and others, facilitated the yield for vaccines. Distinction from other mycoplasmas was shown by DNA-DNA hybridization as well as by serologic tests. Its adsorption to vertebrate cells was demonstrated by O. SOBESLAVSKY and others to be mediated by cell receptors containing neuraminic acid. This latter phenomenon, which also occurs in other mycoplasmas, has been studied by many investigators. Recent work (1981-1982) by non-NIH scientists, with whom I collaborated, has shown that cytadherence largely derives from the relation of a terminal surface layer on *M. pneumoniae* to a protein, P1.

After its sensitivity to tetracycline antibiotics had been shown, *M. pneumoniae,* artificially propagated, was used by members of the mycoplasma group to infect human volunteers. Several studies of primary atypical pneumonia were conducted in military recruit populations, where it was a common problem. A number of serologic tests of antibody response, including complement fixation, gel diffusion, and indirect hemagglutination, were developed and applied. The most successful method, now widely used, was the metabolic inhibition test (MIT), developed in 1966 by R. H. PURCELL, Chanock, and associates. A radioimmunoprecipitation test was developed some years later. The MIT, in which a pH indicator fails to turn from pink (alkaline) to yellow (acid) as a result of antibody inhibition of mycoplasmal growth, was later applied also to T strain mycoplasmas (see below). Serologic testing established the occurrence of antibodies to *M. pneumoniae* in respiratory tract secretions of infected human volunteers and led to the demonstration that such antibodies were protective.

Prevention of the disease was given early emphasis. An inactivated vaccine was prepared and tested in animals by K. E. Jensen, L. Senterfit, and associates in 1965, and in human volunteers by Chanock and others in 1967. Subsequently Sobeslavsky and others prepared and characterized various chemical fractions of *M. pneumoniae* and showed the importance of glycolipid haptens (partial antigens). Several workers (SHMUEL RAZIN, BENJAMIN PRESCOTT, and I) later showed that the haptens reconstitute membranes when reaggregated with membrane proteins from a nonpathogenic mycoplasma and are immunogenic in that form. On the other hand, immunization was not achieved with artificially prepared glycolipid-protein aggregates, nor have inactivated vaccines been found sufficiently effective or free of problems. Similarly, the potential of temperature-sensitive mutants—which can grow in the nasopharynx but not at the higher temperature of the lower respiratory tract—was not realized in human immunization, despite their discovery and extensive testing for eight years by P. STEINBERG, H. BRUNNER, H. GREENBERG, C. M. HELMS, M. B. GRIZZARD, W. D. JAMES, R. L. HORSWOOD, and Chanock.

The discovery of *M. pneumoniae* stimulated other mycoplasmal research, for it became necessary to maintain and work with a collection of known mycoplasmas and antisera for purposes of comparison. There developed a great deal of experience with cultivation and serologic identification of mycoplasmas in general. During this time, *M. hyorhinis* was identified as the long-troublesome acid-producing agent most frequently contaminating tissue cultures, and several new mycoplasmas—*M. orale,* its three serologic types, and *M. lipophilum*—were described.

Mycoplasmas recovered from patients with urethritis were characterized. Some of these, the so-called T strains, were subjected to electrophoretic analysis of their proteins. After it was found elsewhere that these strains uniquely metabolize urea, studies were instituted in 1974 that led to description of the T strains as a new mycoplasma genus and species, *Ureaplasma urealyticum.* But as the staff of LID took on newer virological problems, their mycoplasma research gradually ceased.

The gap was filled, however, by the ongoing work of the Mycoplasma Section, now a part of the Laboratory of Molecular Microbiology at Fort Detrick, Maryland, but formerly in the Laboratory of Microbiology. Headed by J. G. TULLY, the Section maintains a complete bank of strains and antisera. These, together with the Section's expertise, make it a frequent site of collaborations and reference center activities. Since 1970 Tully and colleagues have described 1 new genus and 10 new species of mycoplasma. A marked stimulus to mycoplasmal research was the finding in 1972 of an entirely unsuspected group of helical mycoplasmas, some of which had been seen before but characterized as spirochetes. Their correct identification and classification is largely attributable to Tully, together with colleagues from the Department of Agriculture and from France. In 1973 this collaboration resulted in the description and naming of a genus and species, *Spiroplasma citri,* and later of two other species.

Investigation showed the genus to be a worldwide cause of economically important diseases in plants. It also causes disease in honeybees and fruit flies and infests other plants and insects. A serologic classification, devised with the aid of new methods developed in these investigations, already consists of 8 to 10 distinct serovars (substrains distinguishable antigenically). In addition, I and members of my laboratory (T. J. POPKIN, A. LISS, W. O. MITCHELL, J. M. RAN-

HAND, and others) ultrastructurally characterized spiroplasmas and other mycoplasmas. We also found and characterized spiroplasma viruses, detected the first virus of *Mycoplasma pulmonis,* and discovered the plasmids of spiroplasmas. The Bureau of Biologics, FDA, at Bethesda, continues to conduct mycoplasma research in the Mycoplasma Branch, headed by Michael F. Barile.

Constant searching for improved techniques led to the development of new spiroplasma media. One of these, in an unexpected spinoff, was shown by Tully and colleagues to be better than conventional media for many mycoplasmas. It was used for primary isolation from human urethras of a new species of mycoplasma, *M. genitalium* (Tully, D. TAYLOR-ROBINSON, D. L. ROSE, Cole, and J. M. Bove, 1983), which may be found in field studies now under way to be a cause of so-called nonspecific (nongonorrheal) urethritis.

Streptococci

Streptococci were recognized and named 100 years ago. It became common medical knowledge that they cause puerperal fever, scarlet fever, and erysipelas. In the light of our present knowledge, however, most early case reports and other studies are flawed by lack of agreement on identification of the bacteria. It was realized only gradually that there are many different streptococci, that they cause (or may not cause) different diseases, and that they infect animals other than man.

By the early 1930s, Griffith in England and Lancefield in New York had identified serologic groups of streptococci. For example, the common human pathogen causing scarlet fever and related conditions was classified as *Streptococcus pyogenes* of Group A. In addition, serotypes within Group A were established on the basis of protein antigens. Today these types, numbering at least 60, are useful guides in following and defining disease outbreaks. They may have different epidemiologic and pathologic implications.

Alice Evans was the first to study streptococci at NIH. Her contributions nearly equaled those she made to the understanding of brucellae and meningococci. Her notebooks show that she was collecting streptococci as early as 1918 and that she continued to do so until her retirement in 1945. Her early publications include a number of papers on enterococci, now known as Group D streptococci.

At that time, streptococci-attacking bacteriophages (bacterial viruses) were known but little studied. Evans investigated them from 1933 to 1942. Finding and propagating phages that were active on different streptococci, she initiated standard methods of characterization by defining their lytic spectra, heat sensitivities, and serologic specificities. One far-reaching discovery was a phenomenon, in a Group C phage system, called "nascent phage lysis," which meant that streptococci not susceptible to the phage were nevertheless lysed when added to a lysing phage culture. She recognized, but did not define, a lytic principle other than the phage. Some 20 years later, Maxted in England showed that this was an enzyme —"phage-associated lysin." It was subsequently shown by others to attack specific linkages in the basic material (peptidoglycan) of the cell walls of many streptococci. It was once prepared commercially and has been used by investigators to disrupt streptococci in preparing cell fractions.

Evans also published numerous studies (some with E. Verder) contributing fundamentally to the recognition and differentiation of animal and human strains of hemolytic streptococci, especially those of Groups A and C. Unaccountably, streptococcal phage studies virtually ceased, worldwide, from 1942 until 1952. Then investigators in England and Denmark, aided and stimulated by Evans' original work, initiated them once again. Considerably later (see below), the early NIH interest in these phages was renewed in my own laboratory.

In 1949, streptococcal research was centered in the Rheumatic Fever Unit of NMI. MARK P. SCHULTZ was Head, and EDYTHE ROSE and RICHARD WHITT supplied technical expertise. By that time the research community at large had clarified much of the confusion originally surrounding streptococci. *Streptococcus pyogenes* was known to possess at least two type-specific proteins, a polysaccharide group antigen, and a polysaccharide capsule, and was known to produce such extracellular substances (some also antigenic) as erythrogenic (rash-producing) toxin, two hemolysins active on red blood cells, a fibrinogen-lysing factor designated as streptokinase, a capsule-destroying enzyme (hyaluronidase), and vague leukotoxic factors that inactivated white blood cells.

Studies in the armed forces during World War II had unequivocally demonstrated the suspected relationship of rheumatic fever and acute glomerulonephritis to antecedent infections with *S. pyogenes*. They had shown the occurrence and spread of sulfonamide-resistant strains, had extended epidemiologic and geographic information, and had verified in large-scale trials the efficacy of penicillin in curtailing "strep" outbreaks and preventing subsequent rheumatic fever. However, the mechanism of production of rheumatic fever and of glomerulonephritis was unknown, and interest centered on the streptococcal antigens as possible culprits.

Schultz followed many cases of rheumatic fever clinically,

especially in families and twins, and attempted unsuccessfully
to reproduce the disease in laboratory animals by the use of
ill-defined combinations of streptococcal components and proteins ("bacterioplasma conjugates"). Rheumatic fever and
acute diffuse glomerulonephritis have not yet been produced
in animals, despite some promising new immunologic approaches,
nor have the mechanisms of these two poststreptococcal se-
quelae been satisfactorily resolved.

My primary bacteriologic interest, stimulated by experiences in Boston with Louis Weinstein and Chester Keefer, was
in streptococci. When Schultz died unexpectedly in 1951, I
was appointed Head of the Rheumatic Fever Unit and left the
Epidemiology Unit of Joseph Bell. Studies relating to streptococci, encompassed in several successive Laboratories (Infectious Diseases, Microbiology, Streptococcal Diseases), continued for 30 years. Altogether, our main contribution, I
think, was to enlarge usefully the basic knowledge of streptococci.

At first we continued to identify streptococci by serologic grouping and typing tests, and titrated antistreptolysin
O-levels in human sera. These tests, as well as initial throat
cultures, were in considerable demand by local physicians,
hospitals, and (for some time after it opened in 1953) the
NIH Clinical Center. While continuing these services and engaging in some related collaborative studies, we abandoned
the Schultz approach and instead began to explore the composition and characteristics of the streptococci themselves.
This new direction led to various immunogenic preparations,
verification of a group-specific test using autoclaved streptococci as agglutinogen, and use of the supernatant fluid of
the autoclaved cultures as antigen for precipitin grouping.
The latter, found independently by Lowell Rantz in California,
became known as the Rantz-Randall method.

With EMILY EMMART and others in NIAMD, we showed the im-
munogenicity of Group C streptococcal hyaluronidase in rabbits, the antienzymatic activity of the antibody, and the
wide distribution of the enzyme in tissues of injected mice.
The latter study, employing the new "Coons technique," was
my introduction to this fluorescent antibody method, which
we later used to follow the replication of bacterial cell
walls.

Meanwhile, we did the respiratory bacteriology for a
three-year study (with Joe Bell and others) of illnesses and
microbial agents in a nursery population. Other groups were
assigned the enteric bacteria and viruses. In all, 55 virus
and 54 bacterial serotypes were identified. Although staphylo-
cocci, Type B *Haemophilus influenzae,* and pneumococci were
nearly always present in these young children, the only bac-

teria associated with defined outbreaks of acute febrile illnesses were serotypes of Group A streptococci and *Shigella
sonnei I.* Similar data were obtained for certain respiratory
viruses and poliovirus.

With the establishment in 1956 of the NIH Research Associate Program, we were able to attract a succession of young
investigators and thus expand our research activities. In 1958
FRED KANTOR discovered the fibrinogen-precipitating activity
of Group A streptococcal M protein, and later showed (at Yale)
that it complexed with fibrinogen in renal glomeruli of mice—
though the lesions were unlike those of acute glomerulonephritis in humans. We also reported a different method, lately
reintroduced, of releasing antigenic M protein from streptococcal cell walls by the use of phage-associated lysin first
noted by Evans.

Beginning in 1960, JEROME HAHN and I improved the performance and evaluation of the type-specific "long-chain reaction"
of Group A streptococci grown in appropriate anti-M antisera,
and showed that the chaining resulted from end-to-end binding
of daughter cocci by divalent antibody. These results aroused
our interest in replication and division of the streptococcal
cell. Since growth obviously continued in the presence of
antibody, we conceived the technique of microscopically observing cells made visible by prior labeling with fluorescein-
tagged antibody and then allowed to grow in long chains in the
presence of unlabeled antibody. The method was successful, and
the results, published in *Science* in 1962, aroused a great
deal of interest, since a fixed marker applicable to growing
and dividing bacteria had not been known.

Shortly thereafter, I applied the method to wall replication in *Salmonella typhi*. EDWIN BEACHEY, a Research Associate,
extended it to *Escherichia coli* after his arrival in 1963.
These studies showed that gram-positive cocci form new wall
hemispheres as they divide, but that the new outer envelope
of gram-negative daughter cells is formed in a diffuse fashion
by apparent intercalation of new segments among the old. The
findings engendered an American Association for Microbiology
Symposium in 1964 and have been reproduced in numerous textbooks and reviews. Indeed, they have engendered a new subfield
of investigation. Although the findings for gram-positive
cocci have been confirmed and extended by many more elegant
and ongoing studies, the situation in rod-shaped bacteria
is still a matter of some debate and continuing exploration.*

---

*An article, however, that appears to confirm the diffuse
intercalation hypothesis in *E. coli* by the use of radiolabel-
ing methods has recently appeared. See Burman, Raichler, and
Park, *J Bacteriol* 155:983-988, 1983.)

Intrigued by the possibilities of immunofluorescent labeling, Jerry Hahn and I used it to show that type-specific
M protein is a cell wall component external to the group-
specific polysaccharide. Once removed enzymatically, it is
not resynthesized on the same wall surface, as once believed,
but appears only at sites of new wall formation. Adjunct
studies by electron microscopy, which I was then just starting, demonstrated the external fimbriae (fringes) of M protein
and their absence after treatment with proteolytic enzymes—
thus antedating the more precise and better-known work of John
Swanson in New York.*

FRED GILL, who became a Research Associate in 1963, used
specific immunofluorescence to study the fate of M protein on
antibody-coated streptococci after their phagocytosis by mouse
macrophages. This work showed that the labeled M protein was
removed early from the streptococcal surface and pooled within
phagocytic vacuoles, thus suggesting a macrophage mechanism
for making antigens more available for induction of antibody
synthesis.

Thereafter, research on phagocytosis of Group A streptococci was nonexistent until Research Fellow Jon Ranhand
(1968), Research Associates RICHARD GETNICK (1969) and ALAN
GLICK (1970), and I attacked the problem by enzymatic and ultramicroscopic methods. The microscopy showed rupture of
phagocytosed streptococci—but no destruction of cell wall.
This confirmed the persistence of walls and their sequestra-
tion by phagocytes in certain tissues, as ISAAC GINSBURG,
Visiting Scientist from Hadassah University, had shown by immunofluorescence in 1968. A subsequent study demonstrated
that native Group A walls are insusceptible to lysozyme or
phagocyte lysozymal enzymes, thus accounting for their intraphagocytic persistence. Appropriate chemical treatments of
walls that made them sensitive to lysozyme rendered them sensitive also to rapid intraphagocytic degradation.

New approaches to the study of streptococci were initiated
when CARMEN LEONARD became a staff member of the laboratory
in 1965. Her prior experience in genetics of bacilli facilitated a rapid adaptation to the Group H streptococcus, in
which a system of DNA-mediated transformation had been described by workers in Poland. In those studies, only antibiotic resistance had been used as a genetic marker. Leonard

---

*It is now known, largely from the later work of Ed Bea-
chey in Memphis, that the surface fimbriae of Group A streptococci contain other proteins and lipoteichoic acid, which
function in adherence of the bacteria to mammalian cells.

showed that auxotrophic* mutants could be transformed to the normal (or prototrophic) state by DNA from the latter. She also demonstrated that such transformation could take place in a chemically defined medium, but that noncompetent (nontransformable) cells in the same medium still produced a soluble factor essential for competence development. She compared, purified, and characterized factor produced in defined and in complex media.

A notable achievement was the demonstration in 1968 that Group A streptococci, in which no system of genetic transfer had ever been discovered, could be genetically altered by transduction.** This discovery opened the way for genetic studies of these streptococci and stimulated the development of a field that has become more and more active.

Meanwhile, Ranhand expanded knowledge of the Group H transformation system by demonstrating differences between genetically competent and incompetent cells, including the appearance of new proteins, autolysis, and liberation of transforming DNA in the competent population. He went on to studies of binding, entry, and integration of transforming DNA, and eventually to ongoing investigations of streptococcal plasmids.***

The finding of streptococcal transduction increased our interest in streptococcal bacteriophages. Many were isolated and purified by ALBA COLON, who showed (with Leonard) that ultraviolet irradiation improved transduction frequency and that, contrary to old ideas of group specificity, phages from streptococcal groups A, C, and G could interchangeably lyse, lysogenize, and transduce among the several groups. We found, by electron microscopy and plaque formation on indicator strains, that 99 percent of Group A streptococci are lysogenic (i.e., carry largely unexpressed phage, or prophage). This discovery led indirectly to Colon and Whitt's observation that some of the rare nonlysogenized strains produce an erythrogenic toxin (Type B), amending the generally accepted concept that lysogeny was always required for toxin production.

Our curiosity was extended to the likelihood, not previously verified, that bacteriophages infest Group H streptococci. The group and LOWELL PARSONS (Research Associate, 1971) showed that many strains carry transformation-inhibiting

---

*Those lacking a normal attribute, such as ability to synthesize a nutrient.

**The transfer of genetic material from one bacterium to another by bacteriophage.

***Bacterial plasmids are extrachromosomal, self-replicating, circular DNA molecules.

phages, thereby explaining in part the known existence of non-transformable strains. KENNETH NUGENT (Research Associate, 1972) purified and characterized one of the long-tailed Group H phages, thus supplying data, not previously known for any streptococcal phage, on protein content and nature of the nucleic acid. The latter, a double-stranded linear DNA, was found capable of transfection—i.e., production of phage by addition of the DNA to competent cells.

Phage characteristics were confirmed and extended by DANIEL MOYNET (Visiting Fellow, 1977). With FRANK DeFILIPPES of the Laboratory of Biology of Viruses, he used restriction enzyme analysis to construct a physical map of a Group H phage genome—the first for a streptococcal phage. He also found a new phage virulent for Group H streptococci, and determined the sizes, structures, nucleotide ratios, and restriction enzyme patterns of the linear DNA genomes of eight different phages carried by streptococci of five different serologic groups. These findings are a prerequisite to the potential use of phages as vectors in streptococcal genetics.

Studies were made of some extracellular streptococcal products. GARY CALANDRA (Research Associate, 1973) investigated streptolysin S, the oxygen-stable, nonantigenic substance responsible for the surface hemolysis of Group A streptococcal colonies on blood agar plates (thus the term *hemolytic streptococci*). He found and isolated the intracellular precursor form, developed sensitive methods of assay, and discovered new techniques for activating the hemolysin.

In this subsection, I have supplied more detail than in others for several reasons. For one, I was closely associated with the streptococcal research and recall it better. For another, the account serves to emphasize the contributions of Research Associates and other young investigators. And finally, it exemplifies the type of basic bacteriology that is essential as a continuing background for more targeted investigations when indicated.

Some Personal Notes

On first arriving at Bethesda, I was assigned to the National Microbiological Institute (NMI), which had been created the year before (1948) from the old Division of Infectious Diseases (DID). The Director was VICTOR HAAS, and his responsibilities included not only the Bethesda operations but also those of the Rocky Mountain Laboratory (RML), which had been a field station of NIH since 1931 and a part of DID since 1937. At Bethesda, bacteriologic and mycologic research in NMI was carried out both in the Laboratory of Infectious Diseases (LID), then headed by Karl Habel (later by Dorland Davis), and in the Laboratory of Biologics Control (LBC), headed by William Workman. NMI occupied Buildings 5 and 7.

Within LID the research was organized by units that primarily, but not exclusively, focused on given disease entities or related microorganisms. I can recall groups working on brucellosis (Birdsall Carle, Bill Hoyer), tuberculosis (Byron Olson), rheumatic fever and streptococci (Mark Schultz), enteric bacteria (Elizabeth Verder), mycology (Chester Emmons, SAMUEL SALVIN), and antigens of *Pasteurella* and *Brucella* (Carl Larson). There was a Section on Experimental Therapeutics (Harry Eagle, ARTHUR SAZ, Harry Steinman) investigating treponeme nutrition and the mode of action of penicillin, and one on Epidemiology (Joseph Bell), in which I worked for several years. Robert Huebner and members of his group were studying both viruses and rickettsia (Q fever).

In LBC, Sara Branham was investigating neisseria, Margaret Pittman haemophilus. Others present, though I don't remember all of their specific areas of research or organizational locations, were J. F. (Fritz) Bell, EDGAR RIBI, Charles Shepard, John Hornibrook, LLOYD FELTON, and Benjamin Prescott. In 1951 J. F. Bell, Hoyer, Salvin, Shepard, and Ribi moved to RML, where Larson had gone late in 1949 to succeed R. R. Parker as Director.

NIH in 1949 was small relative to today, and there was more interchange among personnel and more awareness of the scope of activities. The Health Unit, in which many of us served periods of temporary duty, was in Building 1, as was the Dental Unit. These provided both dental and medical care (emergencies, acute infections, immunizations, etc.) for commissioned officers, their dependents, and civilian employees during duty hours. The Credit Union, a one-person operation in a small room, was also in Building 1.

Each spring the senior officers attended (and picked up the tab for) the junior officers' annual picnic, which was held in and around a house called Top Cottage. It was located on the present site of Building 31, to which it had been moved from the hill that was excavated to build the Clinical Center. The picnic provided an opportunity for the members of a small community (in reality, a military post) to associate informally with one another. Nowadays few junior officers can say that they have played baseball, horseshoes, volleyball, or poker with the NIH and Institute Directors!

At that time the quarters off Cedar Lane were run in military fashion—that is, assigned to officers, as incumbents left, via a priority list in order of arrival on the post. I

never reached the top of the list before the system degenerated into the current politicized one.

All things changed as NIH grew. From a total of 2937
employees and a budget of $37.7 million in 1949, NIH expan-
ded to about 14,000 persons (including 10,500 full-time permanent) and a $4 billion budget in 1983. Intramurally, NIAID's
staff at Bethesda in 1956 had 138 persons, of whom 35 were researchers, and a budget of $920,000. The travel budget for in-
tramural operations in 1958 was $11,540, per diem was $12, and
the round-trip air fare to New York was $30.40. In 1975-1976
(when, as Acting Scientific Director, I last had an opportunity for close examination), the NIAID appropriation for intramural activities was approximately $27 million.

Organizational changes occurred, too. When NMI became
NIAID in 1955, LBC became the nucleus of a separate Division
of Biologics Standards in reaction to problems arising from
the production and use of the Salk polio vaccine. Dorland
Davis was made the first Scientific Director of NIAID, and
Huebner replaced him as Chief of LID. In 1957 LID had sections on medical mycology (Emmons), epidemiology (J. A. Bell),
and virus and rickettsial diseases (Huebner). The latter included units on influenza, respiratory viruses, infectious
hepatitis, and rickettsia. In addition, studies on poliomyelitis, rabies, and physical microbiology were carried out
in a Section on Basic Studies (Habel).

Bacteriology—which included units on bacterial metabolism (Saz), streptococci (Cole, replacing Schultz after his
death in 1952), and diarrheal diseases (Verder)—was incorporated into a new Section on Medical and Physiological Bacteriology (MPB) headed by Saz. After Eagle left, the Section
on Experimental Therapeutics was disestablished. A Laboratory
of Bacterial Diseases headed by Norman McCullough was established in 1958.

I succeeded Saz as Head of the MPB Section in 1964. Dorland Davis succeeded JUSTIN ANDREWS that year as Director,
NIAID, and JOHN SEAL arrived from the directorship of the
Naval Medical Research Institute to become our Scientific Director. With the support of Huebner, Seal, and Davis, we
eventually succeeded in gaining a long-sought consolidation
and laboratory status for the bacteriologic and mycologic activities.

In 1967 the pertinent sections were incorporated into a
new Laboratory of Microbiology (LM), of which I became Chief.
When McCullough retired in 1968, the remainder of his Laboratory became the Mycoplasma Section of LM. The Laboratory,
with a staff of 44, then consisted of Sections on Bacterial
Structure and Function (Cole), Mycoplasmas (Joseph Tully),

Immunology (SANFORD STONE), and Medical Mycology (Herbert Hasenclever).

In 1973, purportedly because of needs engendered by over-all budget and personnel restrictions, LM was disbanded. Mycology was reassigned to LCI, Mycoplasmology to the reorganized LID, and Immunology to the Office of the Scientific Director. Many employees found positions elsewhere and some retired. The remainder, which was in effect the bacterial structure and function section, became the new 15-person Laboratory of Streptococcal Diseases (LSD), and I was named Chief. We continued studies of bacterial ultrastructure, walls, membranes, and organelles; bacteriophages; and streptococcal genetics, antigens, and extracellular products until I retired in 1981—when LSD, too, was disbanded.

Epilogue

NIH contributions to bacteriologic knowledge are much more extensive than I have noted here. Not all were made in NIAID or its predecessor organizations, though this Institute has been the traditional locus of microbial research. Significant findings on the nature and roles of streptococci and other bacteria in dental caries continue to be made in NIDR's Laboratory of Microbiology and Immunology. The processes of differentiation, as exemplified in the sporulation of bacilli, have been elucidated in the Laboratory of Molecular Biology of NINCDS. Extensive investigations of pertussis, mycoplasmas, mycobacteria, fungi, and bacterial polysaccharides and toxins —once activities of NIAID in relation to biologics control—continue in the Division of Bacterial Products, part of FDA's National Center for Drugs and Biologics on the NIH campus. Bacterial taxonomy has been enriched by NIH intramural scientists: 53 are cited in 113 references in *Bergey's Manual of Determinative Bacteriology* (eighth edition), and 44 of the citations describe new bacterial genera, species, families, etc.

I regret that space limitations preclude a more thorough account of intramural NIH advances. Even for NIAID investigations, much has necessarily been omitted—for example, new approaches to the genetics of bacteria in the Laboratory of Molecular Microbiology at Frederick, ongoing fundamental studies of gonococci in the Laboratory of Microbial Structure and Functions at the Rocky Mountain Laboratory, and the 50-year involvement of RML in spirochetal diseases, such as the relapsing fevers and leptospirosis. In this latter field W. BURGDORFER and associates recently reported (1982) that the elusive cause of Lyme disease, a tick-borne entity, is a yet unnamed treponemalike spirochete. This is also the first discovery in many years by an intramural researcher of the etiology of a human infectious disease—which prompts me to reflect again on the changing nature of bacteriologic investigations at NIH.

When we maintained both epidemiologic expertise and broader laboratory coverage of bacteriology, the assistance of NIAID was often solicited in investigations of new or unsolved diseases of apparent infectious nature. Now disease outbreaks are primarily investigated in the extensive facilities of the Centers for Disease Control, Public Health Service, in Atlanta. Other factors in the decline of traditional bacteriologic research at NIH may be increased competition (often supported by NIH grants or contracts), a lack of ready access to populations in which new infections appear, the decreasing number of intramural bacteriologists, and inflexibility in program planning. For whatever reasons, such relatively recent infectious entities as Legionnaire's disease, neonatal tetanus, *Clostridium difficile* infections, scalded-skin and toxic-shock syndromes, infections due to *Bacteroides* and other anaerobes, enteritis caused by *Campylobacter* neonatal meningitis and septicemia due to Group B streptococci, most hospital-associated infections, and new approaches to cholera have not been subjects of intramural NIH investigations.

It seems clear that the trend of intramural bacteriology is away from etiology, that the magnitude of bacteriologic effort is decreasing because of more attention to newer virologic and immunologic problems, and that the remaining bacteriologic research is increasingly basic. This, I suppose, is a reflection of general trends in bacteriology, and its course will be clear in future histories.

Introduction

VIRAL HEPATITIS

A Persian fairy tale, "The Three Princes of Serendip" (an ancient name for Sri Lanka), tells of three gentlemen who were always discovering things they weren't seeking. To describe this phenomenon, Horace Walpole in 1754 coined the term serendipity, and nearly 200 years later Walter Cannon introduced it into the biological sciences. It has been said that BARUCH BLUMBERG's discovery of the Australia antigen, which turned out after years of study to mark the causative agent of type B hepatitis, was pure serendipity, for certainly the cause of hepatitis was not Blumberg's objective. But there is another aspect of serendipity inherent in Louis Pasteur's phrase "chance favors only the prepared mind." Blumberg's mind was prepared, as his earlier and later publications clearly show.

Hepatitis was not a novel disease. Sporadic outbreaks of inflammatory disease of the liver had frequently been seen, and during World War II both the allied and German armies suffered severely from hepatitis, particularly during the North African campaign. As Jay Hoofnagle's chapter reveals, however, it was Blumberg's "breakthrough" that initiated a wave of research largely in NIH laboratories.

In the following pages we learn that viral hepatitis is, in fact, a mixture of at least four distinct diseases and that the causative agents of types A and B have definitely been identified. Of particular interest has been the development of increasingly sensitive methods for detecting hepatitis B infectivity in blood samples. The application of these methods in blood banking has brought a dramatic reduction in the hazard of posttransfusion hepatitis.

D. S.

9

VIRAL HEPATITIS

Jay H. Hoofnagle

For many years progress in research on viral hepatitis was
hampered by the lack of a simple animal model and the inability to propagate human hepatitis viruses in cell culture. At a
time when many advances were being made in the understanding
and control of common viral illnesses such as polio, measles,
rubella, and mumps, little was being accomplished in the conquest of hepatitis. The inability to study hepatitis viruses
in vitro led to studies in the 1940s and 1950s in human volunteers inoculated with icterogenic plasma.

Studies with Human Volunteers

In 1951 RODERICK MURRAY at the Laboratory of Biologics
Control, National Microbiological Institute, began studies of
human transmission of viral hepatitis in volunteers from Federal prisons at Lewisburg, Pennsylvania, at McNeil Island,
Washington, and at Ashland, Kentucky. These studies were aimed
at finding means of inactivating hepatitis viruses in plasma.
First a large pool of infectious plasma was produced. This
pool was shown to be infectious in human volunteers in dilu-
tions of up to 10^7, with jaundice and/or symptomatic viral
hepatitis occurring in approximately half of the subjects inoculated.

The plasma pool was then subjected to various modes of
fractionation and inactivation. The virus of serum hepatitis
was shown to be resistant to heat (60°C for four hours), ultraviolet irradiation, beta propriolactone, and storage at
room temperature.

Blood products prepared from this icterogenic plasma were
studied for infectivity. Immune serum globulin (gamma globulin) did not transmit hepatitis, whereas albumin and a plasma

*JAY H. HOOFNAGLE, M.D., Senior Investigator, Liver Diseases
Section, Digestive Diseases Branch, National Institute of Arthritis, Diabetes, and Digestive and Kidney Diseases.*

protein fraction did. However, when the albumin and plasma protein fractions were heated at 60° for 10 hours, they no longer transmitted clinically apparent viral hepatitis. These findings established the safety of the three plasma products (made by the Cohn cold ethanol technique) but provided no new means of inactivating virus in plasma.

In further studies Murray and colleagues documented a chronic asymptomatic carrier state of serum hepatitis. Small volumes of plasma from five of six blood donors who had been implicated in cases of posttransfusion hepatitis were shown to be infectious to volunteers.

The studies by Murray and colleagues involved the inoculation of more than 300 male volunteers aged 21-35. The occurrence of chronic liver disease and three fatalities from acute, fulminant viral hepatitis led to the termination of these trials and of volunteer inoculation studies of serum hepatitis in adults.

The Australia Antigen

Unquestionably the major breakthrough in research into viral hepatitis resulted from the discovery and characterization of the Australia antigen by BARUCH BLUMBERG and his co-workers in the early and mid 1960s. Blumberg had been investigating genetic polymorphisms that occurred in various isolated populations of the world. In 1961 Allison and Blumberg had shown that repeatedly transfused individuals developed isoprecipitins,* detectable by agar gel diffusion, against proteins found in many normal human sera.

At the National Institute of Arthritis and Metabolic Diseases, Blumberg used this approach to characterize a system of genetically determined beta lipoproteins. During the investigation a precipitin line was detected that had different staining characteristics (staining more with the red protein counterstain than with the blue-black lipid stain). This unique reaction occurred between the serum of a patient with hemophilia and that of an Australian aborigine. Thus the "red antigen" came to be known as the Australia antigen. This discovery was the cornerstone of modern studies and understanding of viral hepatitis.

The Australia antigen was first described by Blumberg in collaboration with HARVEY ALTER at the NIH Clinical Center Blood Bank in 1965. They first suggested that it was another inherited protein polymorphism. It proved, however, to have

---

*Antibodies that precipitate soluble antigenic material from some members of the same species.

interesting clinical associations, being found frequently in children with leukemia or Down's syndrome. Subsequently Blumberg left NIH to pursue his research on genetic polymorphisms at the Fox Chase Institute for Cancer Research in Philadelphia. It was there, in 1967, that Australia antigen was first linked to viral hepatitis.

This association led to a surge of research. Several investigators confirmed that the antigen was intimately related to viral hepatitis and more specifically to type B (serum) hepatitis. This link established the Australia antigen as a specific serum marker of type B hepatitis and paved the way for laboratory and clinical investigation of this important disease.

For his discovery Blumberg received the Nobel Prize for medicine in 1976. It has been said that his observation was serendipitous and not the result of actual investigation of viral hepatitis. Nevertheless, it was Blumberg's persistence and deliberate pursuit of the meaning of the Australia antigen in respect to viral hepatitis that finally led to the realization of its importance.

The Hepatitis B Surface Antigen

The infectivity of plasma positive for Australia antigen was first reported by Alfred Prince in New York and Okochi in Japan. The finding was confirmed and extended by LEWELLYS BARKER and Roderick Murray of the NIH Division of Biologics Standards (DBS) in a reanalysis of the human volunteer studies conducted in the 1950s. Both the human plasma pool and the serum of chronic carriers who transmitted type B hepatitis proved to be reactive for Australia antigen. The DBS investigators showed that this infectious plasma pool when diluted far beyond the detectability of the Australia antigen could still induce hepatitis in inoculated volunteers. Furthermore, patients who contracted serum hepatitis also developed Australia antigen in their serum.

These studies documented the infectivity of human blood and blood products containing the Australia antigen and demonstrated the insensitivity of test methods for detecting the virus. On the basis of data such as these, the first attempts at prevention of type B hepatitis were instituted: the screening of blood donations for Australia antigen and the exclusion of positive units.

The initial studies of the antigen employed agar gel diffusion as a detection method. Several investigators, including Alter, HOLLAND, and PURCELL at NIH, adapted the technique of counterelectrophoresis. This soon became the standard method used by blood banks for donor screening.

SHULMAN and Barker at DBS as well as Robert Purcell and his co-workers at the National Institute of Allergy and Infectious Diseases (NIAID) developed complement fixation tests for Australia antigen that were considerably more sensitive than agar gel diffusion. Subsequently JOHN WALSH from NIH, working in collaboration with Yalow and Berson in New York, developed a more sensitive solid-phase radioimmunoassay for the antigen that has become the standard of sensitivity for detection. Also important were tests for antibody to Australia antigen, including radioimmunoassay developed by PETERSON, Barker, and co-workers, radioimmunoprecipitation by Purcell and colleagues, and passive hemagglutination by VYAS and Shulman, all in NIH laboratories.

Using electron microscopy, Blumberg's group at the Fox Chase Institute for Cancer Research had detected small (20-nanometer) spherical and tubular particles in the serum of patients with Australia antigen. Dane and co-workers in England subsequently described an associated double-shelled viruslike particle (the Dane particle), which has since been established as the intact hepatitis B virus. Almeida and colleagues, also in England, demonstrated by immune electron microscopy that the Australia antigen was the outer, surface component of the hepatitis B virus and that there was a second, antigenically distinct nucleocapsid core antigen.

These findings led to a change in the nomenclature for the Australia antigen, first to hepatitis-associated antigen (HAA) and later to hepatitis B surface antigen (HBsAg). The core component of the virus was later named the hepatitis B core antigen (HBcAg).

Biophysical characterization of Australia antigen is largely attributable to NIH investigators. Early work was conducted by Alter and Blumberg, and more detailed work by Barker and co-workers and GERIN and Purcell. The techniques of ultracentrifugation for HBsAg purification, developed in their laboratories, laid the basis for ultimate production of large amounts of HBsAg for use in serological tests and in the preparation of an inactivated-virus vaccine.

By similar means, HBcAg was purified from liver by HOOF-NAGLE, GERETY, and Barker and from plasma by Purcell and co-workers. It was used to develop serological assays for antibody to the core antigen (anti-HBc). This antibody response was found to be a reliable and specific marker for infection with hepatitis B virus.

In collaboration with Gerin and Purcell at NIH, Paul Kaplan and William Robinson from Stanford University demonstrated that the hepatitis B virus is endowed with an enzyme for replication, an endogenous DNA polymerase. Using the DNA polymerase reaction, Robinson later isolated and characterized the nucleic acid of the virus as a small, double-stranded DNA molecule.

Hepatitis B Virus Vaccines

Although a marker for hepatitis B virus was now available, attempts to propagate the virus in tissue culture remained frustratingly unsuccessful. Testing for HBsAg, however, revealed a susceptibility to the viral infection in several primate species. Barker's laboratory at the Bureau of Biologics, Purcell's at NIAID, and Maynard's at the Center for Disease Control (Phoenix) demonstrated that the chimpanzee was a reliable model for hepatitis B virus infection. This has permitted a more complete characterization of the virus and an evaluation of the safety of the vaccines.

Initial attempts at developing a vaccine for type B hepatitis centered upon the purification of Australia antigen from serum and then its inactivation by physicochemical means. Krugman and Giles at the Willowbrook State School in New York found that heating serum positive for Australia antigen at 100°C for one minute left the plasma noninfectious but still immunogenic. Children inoculated with this heat-inactivated plasma were shown to develop anti-HBs and to be immune to further challenge with infectious inocula. These studies provided the cornerstone for attempts to develop a hepatitis B virus vaccine, showing that HBsAg could be isolated from plasma and made noninfectious and that anti-HBs induced by this antigen was protective against subsequent challenge.

Purcell and Gerin at NIH and Provost and Hilleman at the Merck Institute of Therapeutic Research independently developed inactivated hepatitis B virus vaccines that were shown to be safe (noninfectious) as well as immunogenic (inducing anti-HBs) in both chimpanzees and man. Recently Szmuness and co-workers showed these vaccines to be safe and effective in multiple controlled clinical trials in high-risk, susceptible populations. The development of a reliable vaccine against type B hepatitis has been a capstone to the years of research into this common and important disease.

Molecular Biology of the Hepatitis B Virus

Current research on type B hepatitis has been directed largely toward understanding the pathogenesis of the disease and its complications and toward developing more practical

and safe vaccines. The modern techniques of molecular hybridization and monoclonal antibodies have provided means for
more intensive investigation of the virus and the disease it
causes. The genome of the hepatitis B virus (HBV-DNA) has been
cloned in bacterial systems by several groups of investigators, including the laboratories of William Robinson at Stanford University, William Rutter from the University of California (San Francisco), Pierre Tiollais from the Institut Pasteur, and HOYER, Gerin, and Purcell at NIH. Using cloned genome, HBV-DNA has been detected in serum and liver from
patients with acute and chronic type B hepatitis.

The finding of integrated sequences of HBV-DNA in the
livers of HBsAg-positive patients with hepatocellular carcinoma has tightened a link made earlier between chronic infection with hepatitis B virus (the chronic HBsAg carrier state)
and development of liver cancer.

The techniques of monoclonal antibodies and molecular biology have also aided in the development of potentially effective hepatitis B virus vaccines. Monoclonal antibodies to
HBsAg can be used to purify this antigen from serum. Furthermore, HBsAg can be produced in vitro by insertion of cloned
HBV-DNA into vectors such as *Escherichia coli*, yeast, and tissue culture cell lines. Antigen so produced could provide a
"second-generation" vaccine to replace current vaccines, which
are made from HBsAg purified from plasma.

Another approach to vaccine development has been suggested
by the amino acid sequence of HBsAg, which was determined by
cloning HBV-DNA and sequencing its nucleotides. Polypeptides
can be produced that may represent the immunogenic portions of
the surface antigen. Using the chimpanzee model, Purcell and
Gerin have evaluated the potentials of these second-generation
vaccines. HBsAg produced in vitro and short polypeptides of
the antigen have been shown to induce anti-HBs in chimpanzees
and to provide partial protection against subsequent challenge
with live virus.

More recently MOSS and colleagues in NIAID have provided a
unique and exciting approach to the development of a hepatitis
B virus vaccine that has wide-ranging implications. They inserted the HBsAg gene into a vaccinia virus DNA so as to
create a hybrid virus. Infection of laboratory animals with
this virus causes a mild vaccinia infection and a potent antibody response to HBsAg. Such hybrid viruses may provide
"third-generation" vaccines for type B hepatitis and stand as
a model approach for the development of viral vaccines of the
next century.

Type A Hepatitis

The many advances in understanding type B hepatitis led to a renewed interest in attempts to isolate and characterize the hepatitis A virus. Studies in the 1960s had suggested that marmosets might be susceptible to the latter disease. Nevertheless, the causative agent remained unknown. In 1973 STEPHEN FEINSTONE, ALBERT KAPIKIAN, and Robert Purcell in NIAID discovered a viruslike agent in the stools of human volunteers who had been inoculated with hepatitis A virus. Using immune electron microscopy, they found a 27-nm spherical particle in stools taken during the late incubation period. Convalescence serum from the same patients agglutinated and coated these viruslike particles. Subsequent studies have confirmed that the isolated particle was indeed the hepatitis A virus.

Again using immune electron microscopy, these investigators clarified much of the epidemiology and clinical course of type A hepatitis and confirmed the susceptibility of both marmosets and chimpanzees to this infection. Investigators at the Bureau of Biologics also demonstrated the hepatitis A virus in liver and bile of infected chimpanzees by means of electron microscopy.

Shortly after the description of the hepatitis A virus by Feinstone and co-workers, Provost and Hilleman of the Merck Institute described the isolation of hepatitis A virus from liver tissue of marmosets and the development of complement fixation and immune adherence hemagglutination tests for hepatitis A antigen and antibody. These assays allowed for a more extensive analysis of antibody responses and incidence in populations. Subsequently Purcell and co-workers developed a radioimmunossay for hepatitis A antigen and antibody, using viral antigen extracted from feces. Radioimmunoassay has become the standard test for this viral antibody, and specific IgM* tests have been developed for serological diagnosis of acute type A hepatitis. This group of investigators also developed an immunofluorescence microscopy assay for hepatitis A antigen in tissue, demonstrating its presence during the course of the disease.

The availability of assays for the antigen has permitted a more complete analysis of hepatitis A virus. Siegl and co-workers in Switzerland showed it to be a picornavirus containing a single-stranded molecule of RNA. The physicochemical characteristics are much like those of poliovirus, with which it shares many epidemiological features.

Techniques of molecular biology have been applied to the

---

*IgM: immunoglobulin-M (from *mu*). See Paul-Waldmann chapter, Section II.

study of type A hepatitis. Recently TICEHURST and co-workers in Purcell's laboratory at NIH reported the cloning of hepatitis A virus and partial nucleotide sequencing.

The development of a vaccine for type A hepatitis received a major impetus when Provost and Hilleman from the Merck Institute reported the propagation of the virus in tissue culture. It was found to be noncytopathic, explaining the failure of previous tissue culture studies as due to inability to detect its growth. Provost and Hilleman's discovery was thus dependent upon detection of hepatitis A antigen in the cell culture by means of immunofluorescence microscopy, a technique developed in Purcell's laboratory. The growth of hepatitis A virus in several cell culture systems was subsequently confirmed by Purcell and co-workers at NIH. Propagation of this virus in cell culture has already led to the development of experimental hepatitis A vaccines, which are currently being tested in chimpanzees and man.

Non–A, Non–B Hepatitis

Until very recently it was believed that viral hepatitis represented two diseases, infectious (type A) hepatitis and serum (type B) hepatitis. On the basis of epidemiological and clinical features, Prince and his co-workers in New York first suggested that there was a third form of viral hepatitis, which they termed type C. In 1974 Feinstone and colleagues at NIH proved this serologically in revealing cases of posttransfusion hepatitis that were due to neither hepatitis B nor hepatitis A virus infection. They referred to the disease as "non-A, non-B" hepatitis in order to stress that the causative agent(s) had yet to be identified and that non-A, non-B is a diagnosis of exclusion.

In the decade since non-A, non-B hepatitis was first described, the term has remained appropriate: the causative virus has yet to be identified, and there are still no specific serological markers. Progress in research during the 1970s and 1980s has been as slow and frustrating as progress against types A and B was during the previous two decades. An innovative breakthrough in identification of the causative agent is needed.

In 1978 several groups of investigators, including Alter and co-workers from the NIH Clinical Center Blood Bank and TABOR and co-workers from the Bureau of Biologics, demonstrated that non-A, non-B hepatitis could be transmitted to chimpanzees. The disease appears to be due to one or more transmissible agents that are probably viruses, for serum passed through a 220-nm filter is infectious and the strains that

have been studied are readily inactivated by heat (60°C for
10 hours), formalin (1:2000 dilution for 36 hours), and chloroform. Recently Feinstone and colleagues at NIH showed that
the marmoset is also susceptible to non-A, non-B hepatitis.
It is hoped that these animal models will ultimately provide
a means of isolating and identifying the causative agent.

Clinical features of non-A, non-B hepatitis were described
by DIENSTAG and others in NIAID and Hoofnagle and others in
the Bureau of Biologics. The clinical course of chronic non-A,
non-B hepatitis has been characterized by Alter and co-workers
in the Liver Diseases Section of the National Institute of
Arthritis, Metabolism and Digestive Diseases. At the present
time, this disease is the most common form of posttransfusion
hepatitis. Aach and co-workers with the Transfusion-Transmit-
ted Viruses Study Group and Alter and co-workers from the
Clinical Center Blood Bank have shown that posttransfusion
non-A, non-B hepatitis occurs in 5 to 8 percent of persons
receiving transfusions from volunteer blood donors. These
authors, in the absence of serological tests to specifically
detect the agent, have investigated the use of serum aminotransferase levels (alanine aminotransferase: ALT) as a means
of reducing the incidence of posttransfusion hepatitis. Their
studies have shown that 30 to 40 percent of cases might be
prevented if all donor blood were tested for ALT and all units
with raised levels were excluded from use. However, the problems inherent in such donor screening are many. Trials of
ALT screening of donor blood are now under way at NIH.

Non-A, non-B hepatitis has been closely linked with the
parenteral route of exposure. But epidemics have been reported. Khuroo from India and WONG and co-workers from NIAID
described large outbreaks of hepatitis that were initially
believed to be type A but that appeared on serological testing
to be non-A, non-B. Recently Balayan and co-workers from the
Moscow Institute of Virology reported the transmission of this
"epidemic" form of non-A, non-B hepatitis to a human volunteer
(Balayan himself) and to laboratory animals.

Delta Hepatitis

In 1977 RIZZETTO and co-workers from Turin, Italy, described a new antigen reactivity in the nuclei of hepatocytes
from patients with chronic type B hepatitis. This new antigen,
called delta, was none of the known hepatitis B viral antigens, such as HBsAg, HBcAg, or HBeAg. However, it was only
found in patients who had HBsAg in their serum. Delta antigen
was found in the hepatocytes; antibody to delta (anti-delta),
in the serum. The nature of this reactivity remained obscure,

and other investigators were unable to detect delta antigen reactivity in liver tissue samples from other areas of the world.

In order to further characterize the delta antigen, Rizzetto came to NIH in 1979 to work in the laboratories of John Gerin and Robert Purcell. The nature and significance of the antigen soon became apparent. In collaboration with Gerin, Rizzetto developed a solid-phase radioimmunossay for delta antigen and antibody and applied this to seroepidemiologic and virologic studies. Simultaneously Rizzetto and Purcell demonstrated that delta infection could be transmitted to chimpanzees positive for HBsAg. Chimpanzees without HBsAg in their serum did not develop delta infection. The serum of a chimpanzee in the acute phase of infection yielded a viruslike particle with an internal component of delta antigen and a surface component of HBsAg. Associated with this virus particle was a small molecule of single-stranded RNA that demonstrated no homology with HBV-DNA. These data indicated that the delta agent was a unique virus that was encapsidated (coated) by HBsAg and required hepatitis B virus for its replication.

The radioimmunoassay for delta antigen and antibody has since been used extensively to clarify the epidemiology and clinical course of delta hepatitis. This disease has a worldwide distribution but is most prevalent in the Middle East and the Mediterranean area. It is an important cause of acute and chronic liver disease. In the United States, delta infection occurs most commonly in drug addicts and in repeatedly transfused persons, such as hemophiliacs.

In recent years it has become clear that the delta agent often occurs in epidemics, a particularly severe example of which attacked Yupca Indians of Venezuela in the late 1970s. A similar severe outbreak was recently shown to have occurred at the NIH Clinical Center among children treated for leukemia in the early 1970s. The delta agent has proved to be unique among biologic agents. It is an intriguing possibility that other deltalike agents may be responsible for some little-understood diseases in man.

Three Decades of Research Into Viral Hepatitis

The last three decades have witnessed remarkable advances in the understanding of viral hepatitis. Thirty years ago this was a poorly understood disease, the diagnosis of which was unreliable and the cause unknown. Today the term viral hepatitis encompasses at least four diseases caused by different and distinct agents. The major forms can be easily diagnosed, and each has been well characterized. Further, a means of preventing the most severe and common form, type B hepatitis, is now at hand; and a vaccine for type A hepatitis should soon be available.

Many of the significant advances in the understanding of viral hepatitis have been made at the National Institutes of Health. Indeed, two of three agents known to cause viral hepatitis (the A and B viruses) were first identified at NIH, and much of what is known concerning the other agents is a result of work at this institution.

Selected References

Barker, L.F., et al. Transmission of type B hepatitis to chimpanzees. J Infect Dis 127:648-662, 1973.

Blumberg, B.S., H.J. Alter, and S. Visnich. A "new" antigen in leukemia sera. JAMA 191:541-546, 1965.

Dienstag, J.L., et al. Hepatitis A virus infection. New insights from seroepidemiologic studies. J Infec Dis 137: 328-340, 1978.

Feinstone, S.M., A.Z. Kapikian, and R.H. Purcell. Hepatitis A. Detection by immune electron microscopy of a virus-like antigen associated with acute illness. Science 182: 1026-1029, 1973.

Feinstone, S.M., et al. Transfusion-associated hepatitis not due to viral hepatitis type A or B. N Engl J Med 292:767-770, 1975.

Gerin, J.L., et al. Chemically synthesized peptides of hepatitis B surface antigen duplicate the d/y specificities and induce subtype-specific antibodies in chimpanzees. Proc Natl Acad Sci USA 80:2365-2369, 1983.

Kaplan, P.M., et al. DNA polymerase associated with human hepatitis B antigen. J Virol 12:995-1005, 1973.

Krugman, S., J.P. Giles, and J. Hammond. Viral hepatitis, type B (MS-2 strain). Studies on active immunization. JAMA 271:41-45, 1971.

Murray, R. Viral hepatitis. Bull NY Acad Med 31:341-358, 1955.

Prince, A.M. An antigen detected in the blood during the incubation period of serum hepatitis. Proc Natl Acad Sci USA 60:814-821, 1968.

Rizzetto, M. The delta agent. Hepatology 3:729-737, 1983.

Robinson, W.S., D.A. Clayton, and R.L. Greenman. DNA of human hepatitis B virus candidate. J Virol 14:384-391, 1974.

Smith, G.L., M. Mackett, and B. Moss. Infectious vaccinia
    virus recombinants that express HBV surface antigen.
    Nature 302:490-495, 1983.
Szmuness, W. Hepatocellular carcinoma and the hepatitis B
    virus. Evidence for a causal association. Prog Med Virol
    24:40-69, 1978.
Szmuness, W., et al. Hepatitis B vaccine. Demonstration of
    efficacy in a controlled clinical trial in a high-risk
    population in the United States. N Engl J Med 303:833-
    841, 1980.
Ticehurst, J.R., et al. Molecular cloning and characteriza-
    tion of hepatitis A virus cDNA. Proc Natl Acad Sci USA
    80:5885-5889, 1983.

IMMUNOLOGY—BASIC AND CLINICAL

White blood cells of the kind called lymphocytes are so uniform under the microscope that their subdivision into many different classes was long delayed. It is now known that some of these cells receive their graduate training in the thymus (T cells), while others, at least in the chicken, receive theirs in the bursa of Fabricius (B cells). B cells are the source of the soluble antibodies that circulate in the blood and interact with antigens, frequently macromolecules derived from bacterial or viral invaders. The T cells have been subdivided and designated by various descriptive adjectives, such as "helper," "killer," "suppressor." They are related to the phenomenon of fixed-tissue immunity, and their mechanisms of action are imperfectly understood at this time.

Indeed, the recent explosion in our understanding of the lymphocytes and their relationship to the immune reaction leaves immunology today one of the most confusing fields of biomedical science. For many readers, however, the following chapter should be rewarding if difficult.

It is characteristic of the immune system to differentiate between endogenous substances—those arising within the host— and exogenous agents arising outside. Thus the immune response is the principal defense against invasion by foreign organisms. Most immune reactions are directed against foreign agents. On occasion, however, immune reactions are evoked against host macromolecules, and a so-called autoimmune disease results.

Again, an immunologic response, even to a foreign agent, can be injurious if excessive, as in the allergic diseases.

Failures of the immune response also occur. These may be deliberately brought about, as by the surgeon preparing to transplant an organ or tissue from one person to another. Under these circumstances immunosuppressive agents enable the host to tolerate the foreign substance. Similarly, the immune system may fail to react adequately to foreign substances, leading to lethal infections and, in an extreme case, to the acquired immune deficiency syndrome (AIDS). Here the immune system breaks down completely and the host becomes susceptible to a variety of intruders.

The immunologist has extended his interest to a wide range of diseases that were formerly not regarded as immunologic problems. Among these are diabetes and cancer. And there appears to be no limit to the growth of clinical immunology. For all these reasons, immunology has been extraordinarily active over the past decade and promises to continue to grow and develop in the years ahead. The physician now has at his command a battery of means both to enhance and to suppress the immune response, and a considerable part of his therapy is devoted to one or the other of these activities. Each has its uses, each its hazards.

The following chapter views this field at a moment when the science is growing rapidly. Much can be written about work in progress, little as yet about final conclusions.

D. S.

10

IMMUNOLOGY—BASIC AND CLINICAL

I. Introduction

William E. Paul

Thomas A. Waldmann

Immunology is in the midst of a revolution. From a largely phenomenological science based principally upon whole-animal experimentation, it is being transformed into a deeply analytical and highly technological discipline. This change reflects the introduction of a series of powerful in vitro techniques coupled with an ever-increasing appreciation of the range of clinical situations in which immune reactions are critically involved. Now available to the immunologist are monoclonal antibodies, modern molecular and somatic-cell genetics, flow microfluorometry, and electronic cell-sorting. Perhaps the most important innovations are the recently developed techniques for propagating normal T and B lymphocytes in long-term culture and for cloning these cells.

The critical role of immunological phenomena in a variety of disease states has long provided one of the key driving forces to the pursuit of basic and clinical immunology. Moreover, the actual or potential involvement of those phenomena in a broad range of disorders, from a predominant role in infectious diseases to a still poorly understood role in malignancies, multiple sclerosis, and diabetes mellitus, manifests the centrality of these bodily defense mechanisms. The recent emergence of the profound disorder known as acquired immune deficiency syndrome (AIDS) serves to reemphasize the critical functions of the immune system.

The explosive development of immunology over the last 15 to 20 years has both served and drawn upon comparable develop-

WILLIAM E. PAUL, M.D., Chief, Laboratory of Immunology, National Institute of Allergy and Infectious Diseases. THOMAS A. WALDMANN, M.D., Chief, Metabolism Branch, Division of Cancer Biology and Diagnosis, National Cancer Institute.

ments in the intramural programs of the National Institutes
of Health. Today the immunological community at NIH includes
several large laboratories in the National Institute of Allergy and Infectious Diseases and the National Cancer Institute. It also comprises smaller but still considerable programs in the National Institute of Arthritis, Diabetes, and
Digestive and Kidney Diseases, the National Institute of Dental Research, the National Institute of Neurological and Communicative Disorders and Stroke, the National Eye Institute,
the National Institute on Aging, and the National Institute
of Child Health and Human Development.

NIH scientists are clearly among the leaders in immunology. Of 105 American immunologists listed among the 1000 contemporary scientists most cited between 1965 and 1978, 32 are
current or former NIH staff members. Among immunologists of
the National Academy of Sciences, six are now or were employed
at NIH. A former NIH laboratory chief, BARUJ BENACERRAF, received the Nobel Prize in 1981 for his immunological studies.
The NIH immunological community has made impressive contributions to the current progress and is proud of its record of
accomplishment. It would be of great value to gain insight
into what has been responsible for the flourishing of immunology at NIH, with a view to perpetuating this success and
guiding other institutions.

We do not propose, however, to attempt the type of historical presentation that would truly be required for such
analysis, both because of space limitations and because, as
participants in the process, we lack the detachment necessary
for an objective treatment. Rather, we wish to give a personal view of the development of selected aspects of immunology at NIH during a period beginning in the early 1960s in
the hope that it may later contribute to a more complete examination.

We have chosen four areas for presentation in this joint
chapter. They are immunoglobulin chemistry and genetics;
genetic control of cellular interaction and specific immune-
response genes; lymphokines; and clinical immunology. These
are aspects of immunology to which NIH scientists have made
exceptional contributions and in which the authors have been
deeply involved. We will also include brief material on our
own experiences in NIH laboratories and clinics.

IMMUNOLOGY—BASIC AND CLINICAL

II. Immunoglobulin Structure and Genetics

Thomas A. Waldmann

The immune system of vertebrates can generate millions of different types of antibody molecules that recognize and bind to potential antigens, or "nonself molecules." This extraordinary diversification despite a limited number of genes has been a major paradox stimulating immunologists and molecular geneticists for more than two decades. The solution is now emerging.

The picture as developed so far reveals that each immunoglobulin* is made up of two kinds of protein chains, designated as light and heavy. Each chain is bifunctional and has a constant and a variable region. The sequence of amino acid components is the same for the constant regions of different immunoglobulins of a given type. In contrast, the variable region of each chain has an amino acid sequence that is quite different from one antibody to another. Normally, the immunoglobulin chains are folded so that areas of extreme diversity between different molecules (termed hypervariable regions) present highly specific antigen-combining sites. In their genetic origin, immunoglobulin chains are encoded by segments of DNA that are rearranged and joined in various ways as the cells of the immune system develop. This process can generate information specifying millions of different antibodies.

Immunoglobulin molecules not only have immense variation in the amino acid sequence of their variable regions but also show great heterogeneity when one class of heavy or light chains is compared with another. Specifically, there are two

---

*One of a class of proteins present in blood serum and other body fluids and tissues, synthesized by lymphocytes and plasma cells and endowed with immunological activity. Antibodies are immunoglobulins, and all immunoglobulins probably act as antibodies.

major classes of light chains and five major classes of heavy
chains with different constant-region structures.

Monoclonal Antibodies

Critical early insights into the mystery of immunoglobulin
heterogeneity included the discovery that antibodies are immunoglobulin molecules produced by plasma cells and that malignant plasma cells produce homogeneous immunoglobulins. In 1955
Frank Putnam in his NIH lecture indicated that myeloma proteins produced by a given patient were homogeneous, but that
those of all individuals differed. Since these malignancies
came from a genetically heterogeneous human population, the
biologic basis of the differences could not be easily determined. However, MICHAEL POTTER in the pathology department of
the National Cancer Institute (NCI) reasoned that the differences between myeloma proteins from plasma cell tumors in
an inbred strain of mice, where the individuals were genetically identical, should be revealing. He therefore decided to
look for myeloma serum proteins in mice bearing transplantable
tumors that might be related to plasma cells.

THELMA DUNN, an NCI pathologist who first described plasma
cell tumors in mice, gave Potter two mice with plasmacytomas
that had been referred to her for diagnosis. Then Potter and
JOHN FAHEY of the Metabolism Branch, NCI, using paper electrophoresis, demonstrated that the serum of both mice contained
gamma globulin myeloma protein in massive quantities. Furthermore, the myeloma proteins of the mice were different.

These plasmacytoma tumors occurred so rarely in mice that
only one a year became available for study. Then, as so often
happens in science, chance presented a remarkable opportunity.
RUTH MERWIN and GLENN ALGIRE of NCI, studying the role of lymphocytes in allograft rejection, had implanted small plastic
chambers containing antigenic materials in the abdominal cavity of mice. Dunn discovered that some of these mice, of the
inbred strain called BALB/c, bore plasma cell tumors, and Potter thought that this strain might be genetically predisposed
to develop them.

Potter and CHARLOTTE ROBERTSON BOYCE of NCI found that
plasmacytomas could be induced with mineral oil. This gave
Potter an easy way to produce the tumors and of course an
abundance of myeloma proteins, all directed by the genes of
a single mouse strain. Plasmacytomas became very useful and
popular items for immunologists, and Potter sent them around
the world. Their uniformity and large supply enabled scientists to crystallize the pure antibody proteins and to disclose their molecular structure with X-rays.

Plasma cell tumors also provided investigators with large amounts of the RNA and DNA that encoded each antibody. Melvin Cohn of the Salk Institute and Potter, studying mouse myeloma proteins, and Henry Kunkel and Hugh Fudenberg of The Rockefeller University, studying human myeloma proteins, showed that they were in fact indistinguishable from natural mouse and human antibodies to environmental antigens. These were the first monoclonal antibodies.

The Hybridoma

But monoclonal antibodies specific for particular antigens were not easily obtained. Then, in 1975, immunologists George Kohler and César Milstein at the Medical Research Council's Laboratory of Molecular Biology in Cambridge, England, fused mouse plasmacytoma cells obtained from Potter to normal antibody-producing mouse spleen cells. The resulting "hybridomas" were nonstop factories for monoclonal antibodies. The availability of such uniform antibodies for a virtually unending series of antigens has revolutionized the approach to basic biological questions, to medical diagnosis in humans, and to the treatment of cancer and other diseases.

Structure of Immunoglobulins

The recognition that myeloma proteins of mice and humans produce homogeneous immunoglobulin antibodies, together with the development of new techniques for separating proteins and analyzing antibody molecules, led rapidly to the discovery that different kinds of polypeptide chains combine to produce antibodies. Initially, the pentameric IgM (five-part immunoglobulin-mu) class of molecules, made of five sets of four chains with a molecular weight of 900,000, was distinguished from the smaller monomeric immunoglobulin molecules that have a molecular weight of approximately 150,000-180,000. Subsequently, P. Grabar and J. F. Heremans, using immunoelectrophoresis, distinguished the IgA (immunoglobulin alpha) class from other classes.

Through the work of Kunkel and associates at The Rockefeller University and of Fahey, HOWARD C. GOODMAN, WILLIAM D. TERRY, DAVID S. ROWE, and Potter at NCI, the two types of light chains, lambda and kappa, were identified, and the four subclasses of IgG (immunoglobulin gamma) molecules were recognized and defined in both humans and mice.

Discovery of a New Class of Immunoglobulin, IgD

Subsequently, Rowe and Fahey, studying patients with multiple myeloma, defined a new class of immunoglobulins. They
identified two proteins that were atypical: their fast fragment in electrophoresis was exceptionally rapid, and the metabolic properties were unusual. ALAN SOLOMON, Fahey, and I had
observed that an elevated concentration of IgG protein always
led to accelerated in vivo catabolism of intravenously administered normal IgG molecules (radioisotope-labeled), but the
two myeloma proteins did not induce this effect.

Rowe and Fahey, examining the new proteins more extensively, demonstrated that they reacted with antibodies directed against known classes of light-chain antigenic determinants but not with those against heavy-chain determinants.
The myeloma protein and its heavy chains, however, did possess
specific antigenic determinants that characterized them. Subsequent studies have shown that this new class of molecules,
termed IgD (immunoglobulin delta) by Rowe and Fahey, is present only in very low concentration in serum but, as shown
by JOHN VAN BOXEL, WILLIAM E. PAUL, Terry, and IRA GREEN, is
a specific surface membrane receptor on B-lymphocytes. This
receptor may play a critical role in regulating the maturation
of B cells into antibody producers on interaction with foreign
antigens.

Further Characterization of Immunoglobulins

After the discovery of monoclonal molecules with antibody
activity, significant results derived rapidly from a variety
of novel approaches. Enzymatic cleavage of antibodies, determination of the amino acid sequence of homogeneous immunoglobulin molecules, computer analysis of these data, crosslinking
studies, and definition of the three-dimensional structure of
antibodies by X-ray crystallography led to a better understanding of the structure-function relationships of antibody
molecules and to definition of the sites thereon that combine
with antigens.

Turning back to 1959, Rodney Porter at the National Institute for Medical Research, Mill Hill, England, showed that pa-
pain digestion of IgG antibody produced two interesting sets
of fragments, Fab and Fc. Fab did not crystallize spontaneously, but bound antigen, whereas Fc crystallized spontaneously, but did not bind antigen.

Edelman and Gally of The Rockefeller University then
showed that myeloma proteins, reduced and alkylated, gave two
bands on electrophoresis in starch gel. They identified the

faster band as Bence Jones protein* and termed the two bands
of immunoglobulin chains *light* and *heavy*. These developments
and subsequent studies have led to our present understanding
of immunoglobulin molecules as comprising pairs of light
chains of either kappa or lambda type and pairs of heavy
chains of the mu, delta, gamma, alpha, or epsilon variety.

Hilschmann and Craig of The Rockefeller University determined the amino acid sequences of two kappa Bence Jones proteins. The sequences differed strikingly in the N-terminal**
half of the molecule (residues 1-107), whereas they were essentially identical in the C-terminal*** half (residues 108-
218). These areas were termed the variable and constant do-
mains. As the amino acid sequences of more immunoglobulin
chains became available, the variable regions of both the
light and heavy chains were shown to contain three hypervariable segments in which the amino acid residues varied markedly
from one chain to another.

Advances in this field were much accelerated by the
efforts of ELVIN KABAT, who had joined NIH initially as a Fogarty scholar. Kabat and his co-workers T. T. WU and Bilofsky,
using the PROPHET computer system of the NIH Division of Research Resources, tabulated the sequences of the variable regions that were available. Starting in 1976, publications of
sequences of immunological interest have aided greatly in the
development of theories about the structure and genetic basis
for diversity of such molecules. Kabat hypothesized that the
three hypervariable regions folded to form the antigen-combining site, with the amino acid residues determining complemen-
tarity. Various groups, including that of HENRY METZGER of
the National Institute of Arthritis and Metabolic Diseases,
indeed showed that radiolabeled antigens bind to these residues in the hypervariable segments.

In addition, the three-dimensional structure of antibody
molecules has been established by X-ray crystallography at
high resolution by Poljak, Saul, Epp, and Edmonston and by
DAVID SEGAL, EDUARDO PADLAN, and DAVID DAVIES at the Arthritis Institute. These latter studies, utilizing a myeloma
protein (MPC-603) that binds the antigen phosphorylcholine,
revealed at one end of the Fab fragment a large cavity with
walls formed exclusively by hypervariable residues. The antigen binds to this cavity and thus to the complementarity-
determining segments that had been predicted from the amino
acid sequence.

---

*A urinary protein seen in multiple myeloma.
**The amino (NH$_2$) end of a polypeptide chain.
***The end of the polypeptide chain bearing the free alpha
carboxyl group of the last amino acid.

The Mechanism of Antibody Diversity

Over the past few years, major insights concerning the molecular mechanisms leading to antibody diversity have been gained through molecular biology. New techniques have been used to study the arrangement of immunoglobulin genes and the rearrangements they undergo as a pluripotent stem cell matures into a plasma cell committed to produce a specific antibody molecule. The structural features of antibodies discussed above provided the first clue to the genetic source of their diversity. Hilschmann and Craig had shown that the amino acid sequences of peptide chains from different antibodies differed from one another but that the differences were confined to the N-terminal part. The amino acid sequences of the remainder of each chain were essentially the same for all antibodies of a given type.

This demonstration—that each chain has a variable region (about one-half of a light chain and one-fourth of a heavy chain) and a constant region—led WILLIAM DREYER and CLAUDE BENNETT, who had left NIH and were continuing their studies at the California Institute of Technology, to develop a radical hypothesis that turned out to be substantially correct. They proposed that the light chain is encoded by two discontinuous stretches of DNA, one for the variable and one for the constant region. Furthermore, there were hundreds or thousands of separate variable-region genes, but only one constant-region gene. This arrangement implied that a single constant-region gene must be attachable to any one of the variable-region genes. They therefore contended that immunologically competent B cells are capable of genetic behavior radically different from anything previously found in molecular genetics. The genetic material must undergo a "scrambling" process.

One of the first studies providing proof for the Dreyer-Bennett hypothesis was reported by PHILIP LEDER and DAVID SWAN of the National Institute of Child Health and Human Development. These investigators used newly developed hybridization kinetic analysis to confirm the model's prediction of only one or, at most, very few copies of the constant-region gene.

The discovery of restriction endonucleases* and their application to the mapping of gene sequences allowed Nobunichi Hozumi and Susumi Tonegawa of the Basel Institute for Immunology to test the Dryer-Bennett model in a more direct fashion. This group utilized mouse myeloma tumors, most of which were

---

*Restriction endonucleases are enzymes that cleave DNA molecules at certain sites into specific fragments of four to six nucleotides.

prepared by Potter. These tumors provide large quantities of a particular antibody and of the DNA and RNA that encode it, enabling the investigators to show that activation of the immunoglobulin genes during the maturation of B-type plasma cells is accompanied by somatic recombination. That is, the genes are indeed rearranged, or shuffled.

In further studies, Tonegawa and co-workers, examining light-chain genes of mice, and Leder, JONATHAN SEIDMAN, EDWARD MAX, PHILIP HIETER, GREGORY HOLLIS, STANLEY KORSMEYER and I at NIH, studying the kappa genes of mice and the immunoglobulin light-chain genes of humans, showed that the variable and constant regions of light chains are separately encoded but that two distinct gene segments, not just one, are needed to produce the variable region. One segment (designated V) encodes the first 95 amino acids of the variable region, and a second (designated J, or joining, because its product joins the constant and variable regions) encodes the remaining 13 amino acids of the variable region. Thus, the variable region of a light immunoglobulin chain is encoded by both a variable- and a joining-region gene segment.

As a stem cell matures into a B cell, the DNA is rearranged so that one of the 50-300 variable-region genes for a particular light chain is brought into contact with one of the 4 or 5 active joining-region genes. The constant region of the light chain is encoded by a single constant-region gene segment located on the same chromosome. Thus the noninformational DNA (intervening sequence) occupying the area between the variable and the constant region is incorporated into the precursor RNA as it is formed to transmit the code for polypeptide synthesis. The precursor RNA is programmed to remove this intervening sequence and, by a process known as RNA splicing, is rejoined so that the structural sequence forms an intact light-chain message.

LEE HOOD at the California Institute of Technology, Tonegawa at the Basel Institute, and Leder, ULRICH SIEBENLIST, JEFFREY RAVETCH, and their co-workers at NIH showed that the heavy-chain variable region was also encoded by separate pieces of genetic material. Three pieces were required to generate the region: V_H, a heavy-chain variable-segment gene; D, or diversity-segment gene; and J_H, or joining-segment gene.

When the first J segments were determined and compared with known amino acid sequences in the corresponding light-chain region, amino acid position 96 was often found to be at variance with the codons in position 96 in the germline J sequence. This suggested to Leder and co-workers that V and J segments must be capable of joining at one of several crossover points, a notion that was confirmed by cloning and determining the nucleotide sequences of several rearranged kappa light-chain genes. The region immediately surrounding position 96 formed one of the three regions of the light chains that had earlier been designated by Kabat as hypervariable and that formed the antigen-antibody combining site.

Another sort of diversity is provided by point mutations.* These have been shown to occur in the variable region by MATTHEW SCHARFF of the Albert Einstein College of Medicine, Patricia Gearhart of the Carnegie Institution of Washington, Lee Hood of the California Institute of Technology, and David Baltimore of the Massachusetts Institute of Technology.

Thus the total repertoire of unique antibody specificities is attributable to at least four genetic mechanisms: (a) a large number of germline gene segments that encode portions of the final variable-region peptide; (b) random recombination of these variable-gene segments to create multiple variable assortments, and enrichment of diversity through combination of different light chains and heavy chains; (c) flexibility at the recombination sites (variability of crossover point), which adds to the diversity; and finally (d) the occurrence of point mutations that result in changes in amino acids within the variable-region protein. Theoretically, the first three mechanisms for generating antibody diversity could alone generate at least 1 billion different antibody molecules from a few hundred different genetic segments in the embryonic DNA.

In summary, one of the most critical questions of modern biology has been resolved with the definition of the structure of antibodies and the discovery of the molecular mechanisms involved in their generation, with virtual unlimited diversity in their capacity to bind antigens in our environment.

Selected References

Dreyer, W.J., and J.C. Bennett. The molecular basis of antibody formation: a paradox. Proc Natl Acad Sci USA 54:864-868, 1965.

Köhler, G., and C. Milstein. Continuous cultures of fused cells secreting antibody of predefined specificity. Nature 256:495-497, 1975.

Korsmeyer, S.J., et al. The rearrangement of immunoglobulin genes and cell surface antigen expression of acute lymphocytic leukemias of T-cell and B-cell precursor origin. J Clin Invest 71:301-313, 1983.

---

*A mutation resulting from a change in a single base pair in the DNA molecule.

Leder, P. The genetics of antibody diversity. Sci Amer 246: 102-115, 1982.

Potter, M. Immunoglobulin-producing tumors and myeloma proteins of mice. Physiol Rev 52:631-719, 1972.

Rowe, D.S., and J.K. Fahey. A new class of human immunoglobulins. I. A unique myeloma protein. J Exp Med 121:171-183, 1965.

Seidman, J.G., and P. Leder. The arrangement and rearrangement of antibody genes. Nature 276:790-795, 1978.

IMMUNOLOGY—BASIC AND CLINICAL

III. Genetic Control of Cellular Interactions and Specific Immune Response Genes

William E. Paul

Background

My description of NIH research on cellular interactions, immune-response genes, and lymphokines* dates largely from 1968. I have chosen this year as a starting point partly for the quite personal reason that it was then that BARUJ BENACERRAF, IRA GREEN, and I came to the National Institutes of Health. Benacerraf had been one of the major figures in the remarkable flowering of immunology at New York University during the previous decade under the leadership of Lewis Thomas and Chandler Stetson. JOHN SEAL, then Scientific Director of the National Institute of Allergy and Infectious Diseases, recognized that the Laboratory of Immunology, originally established under JULES FREUND's direction, needed strong scientific leadership if NIAID's immunology research was to achieve the stature implicit in its initial promise. He succeeded in convincing Benacerraf that NIH could provide the proper setting for his developing research program. Seal proved to be a scientific director of great acumen. Among the distinguished laboratory chiefs he appointed were WALLACE ROWE, SHELDON WOLFF, ROBERT CHANOCK, NORMAN SALZMAN, FRANKLIN NEVA, and RICHARD ASOFSKY.

Benacerraf, Green, and I arrived during a period of change for three units that were to become the largest and most productive immunological research laboratories at NIH: the Metabolism and Immunology Branches of the National Cancer Institute, and the Laboratory of Immunology, NIAID. THOMAS WALD-

---

*From Latin *lympha,* water + Greek *kinesis,* movement. A class of soluble proteins released by sensitized lymphocytes on contact with antigens. They play a role in lymphocyte transformation and cell-mediated immunity.

MANN succeeded NATHANIEL BERLIN as Chief of NCI's Metabolism Branch. Under Waldmann's leadership, this has become one of the preeminent clinical immunology laboratories in the world. WILLIAM TERRY succeeded JOHN FAHEY as Chief of NCI's Immunology Branch. He recruited an exceptional group of young scientists, including DAVID SACHS, GENE SHEARER, HOWARD DICKLER, RICHARD HODES, and ALFRED SINGER. Terry's efforts resulted in the development of an outstanding cellular immunology-immunogenetics center. Benacerraf reorganized NIAID's Laboratory of Immunology. Although he left NIH only two years later to become a department chairman at Harvard Medical School, his impact on the NIAID research program in immunology was immense.

Green and I had come with Benacerraf as senior investigators, and our work prospered. Indeed, I was asked to succeed Benacerraf as Chief of the Laboratory in 1970. ROSE MAGE, ROSE LIEBERMAN, and JOHN INMAN, members of the Laboratory before the arrival of "the NYU mafia" (Green, Benacerraf, and I), developed important research programs in the genetics, chemistry, and antigen-binding capacity of immunoglobulins. Others who joined the Laboratory subsequently were ETHAN SHEVACH, MYRON WAXDAL, RONALD SCHWARTZ, DONALD MOSIER, and RONALD GERMAIN. All made major contributions.

On a personal note I must mention a group of Bethesda colleagues, outside the Laboratory of Immunology, with whom I have had exceptionally useful collaborations: Irwin Scher, formerly of the Naval Medical Research Institute; ALAN ROSENTHAL, now at Merck Research Laboratories; and Asofsky, of the Laboratory of Microbial Immunity, NIAID. In addition, it has been my special good fortune to work with an outstanding group of postdoctoral fellows, including JOSEPH DAVIE, DAVID KATZ, JACK STOBO, Shevach, CHARLES JANEWAY, Jr., FRED FINKELMAN, JAMES MOND, BENJAMIN SCHWARTZ, and Ronald Schwartz. They and my most recent postdoctoral fellows have been a key to the success of our research program.

In closing this short introduction, several important points should be made which, in my opinion, describe some of the attributes that have been critical to the development of NIH as a highly productive immunological research center. The Institutes have appointed young people to positions of research independence and have supported them in a way that has allowed the emergence of true creativity. Interaction among research groups has been a hallmark of the NIH immunology community, with divisive competitiveness held to a minimum. We have had the good fortune to work with outstanding postdoctoral fellows, both M.D.'s and Ph.D.'s, who have in a real sense provided much of the spark that has made the NIH research engine run. Finally, NIH has offered opportunities for truly independent, creative individuals to work on important problems freed of some of the constraints and uncertainties of short-term funding that have often had inhibiting effects in extramural research settings.

Cellular Interactions and Immune–Response Genes

T-lymphocytes are the principal regulatory cells of the immune system and are responsible for cellular immune responses. These critical functions are mediated by sets of distinct T cell subpopulations. Among these are the T cells that help B cells differentiate into antibody secretors; those that produce interleukin 2, a lymphokine critical to cytotoxic T cell proliferation and differentiation; those that suppress immune responses; those that cause the activation of macrophages to destroy intracellular parasites; and those that are directly cytotoxic to cells bearing viral, tumor, or foreign cellular antigens.

Virtually all the responses of T cells, in contrast to those of B cells, are mediated through their interactions with other cell types. Thus, the study of T cell function and physiology has principally involved the study of interactions of T cells with other cells, including macrophages, B cells, other T cells, and "target" cells that are lysed by cytotoxic cells. Such interactions have been fascinating and highly instructive. Their study has led to the observation that T cells express receptors with complex antigen-recognition properties that virtually force them to "see" antigen on cell surfaces, and has provided an explanation of how certain genes regulate the specificity and degree of immune responses.

In turn, this information has provided a potential key to clarifying the association between histocompatibility (tissue type) and susceptibility to a group of diseases. Moreover, it should provide a rational basis for attempts to deal with the disordered T cell responses and abnormal immunoregulation that characterize many important acute and chronic disorders.

A substantial part of our understanding of the recognition events determining interactions of T cells with other cell types and the nature of immune-response genes has been due to the work of NIH intramural scientists. Benacerraf and colleagues, while at New York University School of Medicine, had discovered that a set of genes, designated immune-response (Ir) genes, determined the responses of guinea pigs to simple antigens. Moreover, they had shown that allelic genes* controlled the ability of guinea pigs to respond to distinct

---

*One of a pair on homologous chromosomes.

antigens, implying that these Ir genes acted specifically.
Then Hugh McDevitt and his group at Stanford demonstrated
that, in mice, Ir genes were linked to the major histocompatibility complex (MHC) of that species. In NIAID LEONARD
ELLMAN, JOHN MARTIN, Green, and Benacerraf showed that guinea
pig Ir genes were also linked to the MHC.

Several scientists at NIH then undertook an exploration
of the mechanisms through which Ir genes act. Green, Benacerraf, and I, working at NYU, had demonstrated a genetic
limitation to the ability of T cells to convey responsiveness to antigens. More specifically, we had shown that T
cells from animals with an Ir gene allowing them to respond
to the dinitrophenyl conjugate of poly(L-glutamic acid, L-
lysine), or DNP-GL, could not transfer such responsiveness
to a recipient that was not a genetic responder. Only if cellular constituents of the recipient animal were of a responder
genotype would a response ensue. What the nature of these
cellular constituents might be was derived from studies initiated by JOOST OPPENHEIM, then in the National Institute of
Dental Research and now in NCI, and carried to fruition by
Rosenthal in NIAID.

Both scientists were interested in the potential role of
macrophages* in the capacity of T-lymphocytes to be activated
by antigen. Oppenheim and Rosenthal demonstrated that a primed
T cell population from which macrophages had been removed
did not respond to antigen. Rosenthal then showed that the
role of macrophages was to take up and present antigen to T
cells. This raised the possibility that the defect in Ir gene-
controlled responsiveness to individual antigens might revolve
about some abnormality in the way the macrophages "handled"
antigen or in the macrophage/T cell interaction.

Shevach and Rosenthal then demonstrated that antigen presented by macrophages from a responder-type (R) guinea pig
could activate proliferation of primed T cells from the F_1
hybrid of R and nonresponder-type (NR) parents, but that activation did not occur when the presenting macrophages were
from the NR parent. This indicated that some aspect of the
antigen-presenting function was associated with the responder
phenotype (overall genetic product). Ronald Schwartz and I
extended these findings, using mice, to demonstrate that the
genes essential to the macrophage capability resided in the
I region of the MHC. Since this was precisely the region to
which the Ir genes had been mapped, our result strongly sug-

---

*Large, mononuclear, phagocytic cells occurring in the
walls of blood vessels and in connective tissue. Some, when
stimulated by inflammation, become mobile and act in the
body's defense against invaders.

gested that Ir genes or their products determine the capacity
of macrophages to present antigen to primed T cells.

In 1970 Shevach, Green, and I began to investigate how the
I region MHC genes expressed in macrophages might be involved
in Ir gene-determined responsiveness. We showed that the
response of T cells from an (R x NR)F_1 guinea pig to antigen
in the presence of (R x NR)F_1 macrophages could be inhibited
by appropriate antisera—that is, antisera to histocompatibility antigens of the responder parent but not to those of the
nonresponder parent.

The inhibiting antisera were later shown by Benjamin
Schwartz, Shevach, and colleagues in NIAID to recognize class
II MHC antigens expressed on guinea pig macrophages and B
cells. At about the same time, several groups in the United
States, including that of Sachs in NCI, described the class II
MHC antigens of mice, showed that they were principally expressed on B cells (later, also on macrophages), and demonstrated that the genes coding for them were found in the I
region of the MHC. Then Ronald Schwartz, Sachs, C. S. David,
and I demonstrated that antibodies to class II molecules inhibited Ir gene-controlled T cell proliferative responses of
mice, just as comparable antibodies had inhibited macrophage-
dependent responses of guinea pigs.

This led to the concept that Ir genes actually encode
class II molecules and that the polymorphic form of a class
II molecule expressed on a macrophage somehow determines the
immune-response phenotype of an animal. The most decisive confirmation of this work came from studies in Ronald Schwartz's
laboratory indicating that monoclonal anti-class II antibodies inhibit Ir gene-controlled interactions of antigen-
pulsed macrophages with members of a cloned T cell line.

How the class II molecules might determine responsiveness
became appreciated through a parallel set of studies, some of
which had their beginnings in the NIH intramural program. Rosenthal and Shevach showed that macrophages could only present
antigen to primed T cells if the donors of both shared histocompatibility antigens. Simultaneously, Katz and Benacerraf,
then at Harvard Medical School, discovered that T cell/B cell
collaboration occurred only if the donors of both cell types
possessed I region genes of the same type. These observations
led to the concept of "genetic restriction of cellular interactions," implying that T cells only interact with macrophages
and B cells when all are of homologous MHC types.

Progress in understanding the significance of this MHC restriction derived from the finding of a similar restriction
in the capacity of cytotoxic T cells to lyse target cells. In
landmark studies, Shearer in NCI's Immunology Branch and Peter
Doherty and Rolf Zinkernagel at the Australian National Uni-

versity in Canberra showed simultaneously that cytotoxic T
cells, nominally specific for a hapten (partial antigen) or
a virus, could lyse cells bearing this target only if they
were derived from an animal of the same MHC type as the T cell
donor. The Australian group and Shearer went on to demonstrate that the gene necessarily common to this system specified a class I (rather than class II) MHC molecule.

This histocompatibility restriction of the action of cytotoxic T cells proved to be much more amenable to detailed
analysis than the in vitro proliferation systems. Using this
technique, Shearer and others rapidly provided evidence implying that the T cell bore receptors by which it recognized both
the antigen (virus or hapten) on the target cell and the particular polymorphic form of class I MHC molecule that the target cell expressed. It now seems clear that the receptor of
the cytotoxic T cell "corecognizes" an antigenic determinant
and a class I MHC gene product, often termed a restriction
element.

The insights obtained from the study of the MHC restriction of cytotoxic T cells were rapidly shown to apply with
equal force to the antigen-recognition process implicit in
macrophage/T cell and B cell/T cell interactions. In these
systems it became apparent that T cells possess receptors that
recognize both antigen and a restriction element on a class
II MHC molecule. Among the NIH groups that contributed to
this understanding were my own and those of Ronald Schwartz,
Shevach, JAY BERZOFSKY and Sachs, and Singer and Hodes.

Singer and Hodes, working in NCI, then went on to solve a
particularly perplexing problem in T cell/B cell interactions.
Although Katz and Benacerraf had reported that helper T cell
interactions with B cells were MHC-restricted, considerable
uncertainty had grown on this point over the years because
in most experiments the B cell population was the source of
the antigen-presenting macrophages as well as the responding
B cells. Thus, the apparent T cell/B cell MHC restriction
might actually represent a macrophage-restricted T cell activation, with subsequent production of nonspecific helper
factors capable of recruiting both syngeneic* and allogeneic**
B cells.

Singer and Hodes demonstrated that this did indeed occur
and was the explanation for the mechanism of cellular interactions between T cells and one of the two principal B cell
classes (Lyb5+ B cells), which Mosier and I, working with
Irwin Scher and Aftab Ahmed of the Naval Medical Research
Institute, had identified through our studies of the immune

---

*Having cell types that are antigenically identical and
**antigenically distinct but of the same species.

defects of mice bearing the mutant X chromosomal gene *xid*. However, the interactions of T cells with the other major B cell class (Lyb5⁻ B cells) were subject to precisely the type of MHC restriction envisaged in the initial reports of Katz and Benacerraf.

The concept that has emerged, based on a large body of work by both NIH and non-NIH scientists, is that T cells bear receptors capable of corecognizing an MHC gene product (either a class I or a class II MHC molecule) and an antigen. As already noted, the corecognized MHC gene product has been designated the restriction element. It is not surprising that primed T cells from a mouse of one MHC type fail to respond to an antigen presented by macrophages of a different MHC type, for the primed T cells will have been selected by their ability to recognize antigen plus self-MHC restriction elements on autologous macrophages. Only such "self cospecific" T cells will have been primed.

Ir gene-controlled unresponsiveness is interpreted in this light as the failure of T cells to corecognize the "pair" consisting of a given antigen and a given restriction element. This theory implies that examining the structures of the antigen and the restriction elements will be critical to an understanding of how Ir genes function. Structures of protein antigens critical to T cell activation have been examined by Rosenthal and his colleagues for insulin, by Ronald Schwartz and others for cytochrome *c*, and by Berzofsky for myoglobin. These have yielded important insights into the antigenic structures involved in the recognition by T cells and have delineated sequences that may be the sites of interaction of antigens with class II MHC molecules.

Similarly, chemical analysis of the primary structure of MHC-encoded class I and II molecules has been carried out by JOHN COLIGAN and THOMAS KINDT, NIAID, in collaboration with Stanley Nathenson at Albert Einstein College of Medicine; while JONATHAN SEIDMAN and his colleagues, then at the National Institute of Child Health and Human Development, were among the first to obtain nucleic acid clones for the constituent polypeptide chains of both class I and class II molecules.

A final and very exciting development at the time of this writing is that the structure of the T cell receptor for antigen may soon be established. The nature of the molecules that mediate recognition of antigen and restriction elements has been one of the major unsolved problems of contemporary immunology. Recently monoclonal antibodies have been prepared that bind to and specifically inhibit activation of the antigen-specific T cell hybridoma against which they were prepared, but do not interact with T cell hybridomas of dis-

174 WILLIAM E. PAUL

tinct antigen reactivity. Such monoclonal antibodies appear
to be specific for idiotypic determinants on T cell receptors.
Several groups in this country have prepared such antibodies,
including that of Ronald Schwartz in NIAID. LAWRENCE SAMELSON
and Ronald Schwartz have shown that the T cell molecule identified by the antibody is a disulfide-linked heterodimer consisting of chains of 48,000 and 42,000 daltons. The chemical
characterization of this "receptor" and the molecular cloning
of its gene should provide information critical to explaining how T cells recognize and respond to both antigen and MHC
restriction elements on the surface of antigen-presenting
cells. STEPHEN HEDRICK, DAVID COHEN, and MARK DAVIS of NIAID
have recently obtained cDNA clones that appear to specify one
of the two constituent chains of the T cell receptor.

The rapid advances now being made toward an understanding
of the function of restriction elements and of the nature of
the T cell receptor indicate that a climax may be at hand in
the endeavor, begun in the 1960s, to explain Ir gene function.
NIH intramural scientists in at least four Institutes have
contributed importantly to this fascinating trail of research.
Although considerable progress might have been made without
their efforts, the pathways followed would certainly have been
different and perhaps less exciting and illuminating.

Selected References

Coligan, J.E., et al. Primary structure of a murine transplantation antigen. Nature 291:35, 1981.

Margulies, D.H., et al. H-2-like genes in the Tla region of
mouse chromosome 17. Nature 295:168, 1982.

Paul, W.E., et al. Independent population of primed F_1 guinea
pig T lymphocytes respond to antigen-pulsed parental peritoneal exudate cells. J Exp Med 145:618, 1977.

Rosenthal, A.S., and E.M. Shevach. Function of macrophages
in antigen recognition by guinea pig T lymphocytes. I.
Requirement for histocompatible macrophages and lymphocytes. J Exp Med 138:1194, 1973.

Sachs, D.H., and J.L. Cone. A mouse B cell alloantigen determined by gene(s) linked to the major histocompatibility
complex. J Exp Med 138:1289, 1973.

Shearer, G.M., T.G. Rehn, and C.A. Garbarino. Cell-mediated
lympholysis of trinitrophenyl-modified autologous lymphocytes. Effector cell specificity to modified cell surface
components controlled by the H-2K and H-2D serological regions of the murine major histocompatibility complex. J
Exp Med 141:1348, 1975.

Shevach, E.M., W.E. Paul, and I. Green. Histocompatibility-linked immune response gene function in guinea pigs: Specific inhibition of antigen-induced lymphocyte proliferation by allo-antisera. J Exp Med 136:1207, 1972.
Shevach, E.M., and A.S. Rosenthal. Function of macrophages in antigen recognition by guinea pig T lymphocytes. II. Role of the macrophage in the regulation of genetic control of the immune response. J Exp Med 138:1213, 1973.

IMMUNOLOGY—BASIC AND CLINICAL

IV. Lymphokines

William E. Paul

The immune system consists of many distinct cell types whose activities are mutually regulated in the course of immune responses. One of the principal agents of the cellular communications necessary for this regulation is a family of extremely potent proteins made by cells of the immune system and designated as lymphokines (more properly, cytokines, since some are products of macrophages and others of lymphocytes). We now recognize that these communication molecules act on their target cells very much as hormones do and that the insights obtained from studies of hormone/receptor interactions are applicable here.

Work from many laboratories throughout the world had established the existence of soluble factors with important immunological effects. Among these are T-lymphocyte products, first described in the 1960s: a migration inhibition factor (MIF), that inhibits macrophage migration; a macrophage activation factor; lymphotoxin, a factor that kills or limits the growth of certain cell lines; and a blastogenic factor, that causes the proliferation of lymphoid cells.

Although immunologists recognized that such factors might be of great physiologic and pathophysiologic significance, progress in purifying them and understanding their mechanism of action was quite slow, partly because of the low concentrations in which they were produced and partly because some of the initial assays were not sufficiently sensitive or quantitative. During the 1970s, however, several developments led to an enormous increase in immunologists' attention to lymphokines.

One of the seminal findings was made in 1976 by ROBERT GALLO and his colleagues in NCI. They reported that they could propagate in long-term culture T-lymphocytes from human peripheral blood in the presence of a soluble factor that had been produced by human peripheral blood cells stimulated

by phytohemagglutinin.*   The soluble material was initially
designated T cell growth factor (TCGF), but is now generally
referred to as interleukin 2 (IL-2).

This discovery has had wide significance. The recognition
that T cells might be propagated in culture in the presence of
IL-2 led to the development of a technology to create, maintain, and clone long-term lines of specific T cells of most of
the recognized functional types. Much of the work that allowed
T cell cloning to become a major technology for modern cellular immunology was done outside NIH, but STEVEN ROSENBERG and
his group in NCI and BENJAMIN SREDNI and RONALD SCHWARTZ of
NIAID were responsible for several important technical innovations. Schwartz and his colleagues made imaginative use
of cloned T cell lines to establish unambiguously that individual histocompatibility-restricted T cells corecognized
class II MHC (major histocompatibility complex) molecules and
antigen. Furthermore, they showed that cloned T cells specific for a given antigen and a self-class II MHC molecule
often recognize and react to macrophages bearing specific
foreign class II MHC molecules. This implies that the high
frequency of T cells specific for foreign histocompatibility
antigens and responsible for the prompt rejection of foreign
transplanted tissue is due to the fact that they are actually
T cells specific for conventional antigens and self-MHC molecules that crossreact with the foreign molecules.

IL-2 was also seen to play an important role in the proliferation of T cells in response to physiologic stimulants.
It is probably an essential factor in their clonal expansion.
Among the several groups responsible for major progress in
elucidating the chemistry and function of IL-2 was JOHN FAR-
RAR's in the National Institute of Dental Research (NIDR).
Farrar developed a mouse T cell line that secretes large
amounts of IL-2 in the presence of phorbol esters. Purification of this potent mediator could then be undertaken. Farrar
and his colleagues showed that mouse IL-2 is a glycoprotein
with a molecular weight of approximately 21,000, existing in
several charged forms with pIs** between 4.5 and 4.9.

An equally important element in understanding responsiveness to IL-2 was the recent development by NIH scientists of
reagents that recognize IL-2-binding receptors on human T

---

*A lectin from kidney beans (hence *phyto-* , plant) that
is both a mitogen (mitosis-inducer) and a hemagglutinin (red
blood cell agglutinant), more stimulating to T- than to B-
lymphocytes.

**For a given solution, the acidity-alkalinity value (pH)
at which a charged molecule does not migrate in an electrical
field (isoelectric point).

cells. TAKASHI UCHIYAMA, SAMUEL BRODER, and THOMAS WALDMANN in NCI identified a monoclonal antibody, anti-Tac, that appears specific for the IL-2 receptor. Indeed, WARREN LEONARD, WARNER GREENE, Waldmann, and their colleagues in NCI have shown that anti-Tac blocks the activation of T cells by IL-2 and prevents it from binding to them. Furthermore, in cross-linking studies, they demonstrated that IL-2 associates with the antigen recognized by anti-Tac, strongly supporting the concept that anti-Tac binds to the IL-2 receptor. The IL-2 receptor is not expressed on resting T lymphocytes but is induced as a result of T cell activation. It is a molecule of about 55,000 daltons. THOMAS MALEK and ETHAN SHEVACH in NIAID have recently prepared monoclonal antibodies against the mouse IL-2 receptor. Their results entirely parallel those obtained with the antibody to the corresponding human receptor.

The process of T cell activation and the expression of receptors specific for IL-2 appear to depend on prior stimulants acting on T cells. In most cases T cell activation is a multistep process. It begins with the T cell binding either a mitogenic lectin (such as phytohemagglutinin) or a complex of antigen and an MHC molecule displayed on an antigen-presenting cell. At the same time, the T cell appears to require an interaction with the macrophage product interleukin 1 (IL-1). These events cause cells to produce and become sensitive to IL-2. Much of the work involved in establishing this picture of the cell biology of T-lymphocyte activation came from the NIDR immunology group then headed by JOOST OPPENHEIM.

The trail of research that led to these insights began with the work of IGAL GERY, then at Yale and now in the National Eye Institute. He described a macrophage product with the ability to help thymocytes* respond to concanavalin A.** This macrophage product, initially termed lymphocyte-activating factor, is now designated IL-1, as mentioned above. STEVEN MIZEL in Oppenheim's group undertook to purify the material from murine sources and made substantial progress. He has continued and expanded his work at Pennsylvania State University, where the purification is nearing completion. IL-1 is a 15,000-dalton glycoprotein now recognized to express a wide range of actions related to the inflammatory process.

Largely through the work of CHARLES DINARELLO and SHELDON WOLFF, now at Tufts University but both formerly in the Laboratory of Clinical Investigation of NIAID, this mediator is known to act as an endogenous pyrogen. The NIDR group demon-

---

*Lymphocytes arising in the thymus.
**A hemagglutinin and mitogen from the jack bean. Like the phytohemagglutinins, it stimulates T- more than B-lymphocytes.

strated that it induces an amyloid precursor protein; JOHN SCHMIDT and IRA GREEN of NIAID, that it is a stimulator of fibroblast proliferation; and others, that it initiates collagen secretion.

Proliferation and differentiation of B-lymphocytes, the precursors of antibody-secreting cells, are also influenced by lymphokines. MAUREEN HOWARD and I in NIAID and Farrar in NIDR demonstrated that IL-2-producing T cell lines also produce a soluble factor that induces proliferation of mouse B cells stimulated by anti-immunoglobulin antibodies or antigen. This material, designated B cell growth factor (BCGF), is distinct from IL-2. It has a molecular weight of 15,000 and pIs between 6.4 and 7.4. Its purification is now under way.

ANTHONY FAUCI and his colleagues in the Laboratory of Immunoregulation, NIAID, have described a factor derived from human T cells that appears to promote the growth of human B cells in a manner analogous to the action of BCGF on mouse B cells. They have prepared a BCGF-secreting hybridoma from T lymphoma and T cells that provides a source for the purification of this lymphokine.

The availability of BCGF has allowed both groups to begin an analysis of the precise mechanisms through which resting B cells are stimulated to enter the cell cycle, proliferate, and then differentiate into antibody-secreting cells. Furthermore, this emerging information promises to make feasible the long-term growth and cloning of B cell lines. Benjamin Sredni, Howard, and I in NIAID have made initial progress toward this goal.

Thus, in the large arena of studies of the cellular communication factors of the immune system, NIH scientists have played an important role. One result is a rational basis for the continued biological study of lymphocyte and macrophage activation. Through examination of the lymphokines and their receptors, a new physiologically based immunopharmacology should become available, promising an entirely new rationale for the treatment of a wide variety of diseases involving dysregulated or insufficient immune responses. It is to such ends that NIH intramural scientists and their colleagues continue to explore these powerful and fascinating substances.

Selected References

Howard, M., et al. Identification of a T-cell derived B-cell growth factor distinct from interleukin 2. J Exp Med 155: 914, 1982.

Mizel, S.B., and D. Mizel. Purification to apparent homogeneity of murine interleukin 1. J Immunol 126:834, 1981.

Morgan, D.A., F.W. Ruscetti, and R. Gallo. Selective in vitro
    growth of T lymphocytes from normal human bone marrows.
    Science 193:1007, 1976.
Samelson, L., R.N. Germain, and R.H. Schwartz. Monoclonal
    antibodies against the antigen receptor on a cloned T
    cell hybrid. Proc Natl Acad Sci USA (in press).
Uchiyama, T., S. Broder, and T.A. Waldmann. A monoclonal
    antibody (anti-Tac) reactive with activated and function-
    ally mature human T cells. I. Production of anti-Tac mono-
    clonal antibody and distribution of Tac (+) cells. J Im-
    munol 126:1393, 1981.

IMMUNOLOGY—BASIC AND CLINICAL

V. Clinical Immunology

Thomas A. Waldmann

The NIH Clinical Center has provided an environment exceptionally conducive to clinical research. Features that have been especially important and virtually unique include the proximity of patient wards to research laboratories and the access to large numbers of patients with rare yet instructive diseases, such as those due to inborn genetic errors affecting the immune response. Such patients are admitted under specific prospective research protocols. These clinical investigations in immunology have provided unique scientific problems, bases for hypothesis, and directions for basic research.

As discussed earlier, studies of patients in the Clinical Center have led to the discovery of new classes of immunoglobulin molecules and to the description of such lymphokines as interleukin 1 and 2. By applying basic insights to clinical issues, immunologists at NIH have been able to discover new diseases affecting the immune system and to define previously undescribed pathogenic mechanisms underlying immunodeficiency and autoimmune and neoplastic diseases. They have devised new methods for the diagnosis of these diseases and have established the scientific base required for the development of rational approaches to therapy.

Background

I came to NIH as a Clinical Associate in 1956, shortly after the Clinical Center opened, and joined the Metabolism Branch of the National Cancer Institute. NATHANIEL I. BERLIN, the Chief of the Branch, had gathered a series of senior investigators who focused on the physiological factors controlling biological processes and on the disorders in these processes that lead to disease. My own career was influenced

ISBN 0-12-667980-0

by other investigators in the Branch, especially Berlin, who was interested in the regulation of the synthesis and degradation of hematopoietic* cells, JOHN FAHEY, who was studying immunoglobulins, and JESSE STEINFELD, whose research concerned the metabolism of these protein molecules. When Berlin was appointed scientific director of NCI, I became Chief of the Metabolism Branch.

In subsequent years the primary focus of the Branch has become the regulation of the human immune response. WARREN STROBER, MICHAEL BLAESE, SAMUEL BRODER, DAVID NELSON, ANDREW MUCHMORE, JAY BERZOFSKY, STANLEY KORSMEYER, and WARNER GREENE joined the group. Each of these investigators has made major contributions to different facets of the study of the human immune response and its disorders. They have provided insights concerning the arrangement of immunoglobulin genes, the regulatory T cell network, cell-surface receptors of lymphocytes, genetic regulation of the immune response, the nature and action of cytotoxic cells, and the metabolism of immunoglobulins.

Immunoglobulin–Deficiency States

Originally, I was especially interested in the rates of synthesis, transport, and catabolism of albumin and the different classes of immunoglobulin molecules in normal and immunoglobulin-deficient persons. These studies led to the discovery of pathogenetic mechanisms for immunoglobulin deficiency and of hitherto unknown immunodeficiency diseases.

Strober and I showed that hypogammaglobulinemia** can be caused by hypercatabolism (excessive metabolic breakdown) of immunoglobulins as well as by the previously recognized mechanism of decreased immunoglobulin synthesis. In some cases hypercatabolism affected all immunoglobulin classes, as in familial hypercatabolic hypoproteinemia, the syndrome WILLIAM TERRY and I defined. In other cases, only a single class was involved, as in patients with myotonic dystrophy, who have a short survival of IgG. In addition, we showed that patients with selective IgA deficiency may have a short survival of IgA associated with the development of anti-IgA antibodies. Such antibodies are a major cause of blood transfusion reactions.

---

*Blood-cell producing.
**An abnormally low level of generally all classes of gamma globulin (antibody-producing protein) in the blood, resulting in immunological deficiency.

Hypoproteinemia and Immunodeficiency

The analysis of patients with an abnormally short immuno-globulin survival also led to the discovery of the phenomenon of protein-losing enteropathy, a cause of hypoproteinemia (low blood protein) and immunodeficiency associated with many disease states. This discovery of excessive loss of serum protein into the intestinal tract emerged from a study of patients who were previously diagnosed as having "idiopathic hypoproteinemia." Shortly after the Clinical Center opened, investigators from several Institutes joined in the study of such patients. FREDERICK BARTTER of the National Heart In-stitute (NHI) and Steinfeld of the Metabolism Branch, NCI, followed the fate of intravenously administered albumin and showed that the hypoproteinemia in many of these patients was due to shortened survival of protein rather than decreased synthesis.

The site of this accelerated catabolism, however, was not defined until ROBERT S. GORDON, Jr., of NHI developed radio-iodine-tagged polyvinylpyrrolidone (PVP), a macromolecule that is unaffected by mammalian enzymes and is not absorbed from the intestine. Intravenously administered PVP appearing in the feces of hypoproteinemic patients demonstrated that their hypoproteinemia was due to excessive protein loss from the gastrointestinal tract.

To quantitate such protein loss, I subsequently developed other approaches, including [51]chromium-labeled albumin and [67]copper-labeled ceruloplasmin. Various techniques for de-tecting the condition have led to its association with over a hundred diseases. Some of the gastroenteropathies (stomach/intestine diseases) that we identified as marked by protein loss were such previously undescribed syndromes as allergic gastroenteropathy and intestinal lymphangiectasia.

We used the latter term to define a disease characterized by a generalized disorder of lymphatic channel development and associated with hypoproteinemia, edema, and frequently chylous effusions. In these patients Gordon demonstrated the sus-pected disorders of small intestinal lymphatics on peroral biopsy. Subsequently, Strober and I demonstrated that these patients had an immunodeficiency state characterized by hypo-gammaglobulinemia, lymphocytopenia,* skin anergy,** and im-paired homograft rejection, due to excessive gastrointestinal loss of immunoglobulins and lymphocytes through the disordered intestinal lymphatic channels. All of the disorders could be reversed by pericardiectomy in those patients with constric-

---

*Reduction in the number of lymphocytes in the blood.
**Diminished reactivity to specific antigens.

tive pericarditis, by corticosteroids in one subset of patients, or by placing the patient on an exceedingly low-fat
diet.

Thus, studies of patients admitted to the Clinical Center
initially with the ill-defined diagnosis "idiopathic hypoproteinemia" led to the discovery of protein-losing enteropathy
as a frequent cause of hypogammaglobulinemia; to identification of diseases, such as intestinal lymphangiectasia; and to
definition of an associated immunodeficiency state, disordered
cell-mediated immunity, with a previously unrecognized pathogenetic mechanism, the loss of lymphocytes into the bowel.

The Suppressor T Cell

Although it is clear from such studies as those just discussed that hypogammaglobulinemia can be caused by diminished
survival of immunoglobulin molecules, profound hypogammaglobulinemia is usually due to decreased immunoglobulin synthesis. As part of a program to define the immunoregulatory
disorders in the latter condition, Broder, Blaese, Strober,
and I focused our attention on patients with common variable
immunodeficiency disease. This is the diagnosis applied to
a heterogeneous group of diseases characterized by hypogammaglobulinemia due to different causes.

Prior to our studies it had been assumed that decreased
immunoglobulin synthesis was always caused by intrinsic defects of B and plasma cells, the cellular sites of immunoglobulin synthesis. I was stimulated to consider an alternative pathogenetic mechanism by a seminal discovery of Richard
Gershon at Yale Medical School: a new type of lymphocyte in
mice, the suppressor T cell. This acts as a negative regulator, participating in the control of virtually all the immune
responses. Subsequently, our understanding of the role of
suppressor T cells in the regulation of the immune response
of mice was extended by the work of PHILIP BAKER of NIAID,
who studied the response of mice to polysaccharide antigens
presumed to be T cell independent, and by ALFRED STEINBERG
of NIAMD, who studied the immune response to synthetic polynucleotides.

In our own studies we considered the possibility that common variable hypogammaglobulinemia in certain patients might
be due to excessive suppressor T cell activity rather than
to a B cell/plasma cell defect. To examine this hypothesis,
we developed two procedures: an in vitro immunoglobulin biosynthesis technique to study the terminal maturation of human
B-lymphocytes and a coculture technique to evaluate suppressor T cell function. Applying these procedures to study the

pathogenesis of common variable immunodeficiency, we demonstrated that some patients had normal B cells but an excessive number of activated suppressor T cells that inhibited B cell maturation and antibody synthesis. We suggested that the hypogammaglobulinemia in this subset of patients might be caused by these suppressor cells.

Our basic observations were rapidly confirmed, but questions were raised concerning their biological significance. These questions have largely been answered. The most critical issue, however—whether abnormal activation of suppressor cells is the primary pathogenetic mechanism causing the hypogammaglobulinemia—will only be answered definitively when therapeutic techniques are developed for eliminating suppressor T cells in these patients without affecting the function of their B cells and helper T cells. Since publishing our initial study, we have demonstrated excessive suppressor T cell activity in an array of diseases, including thymoma with associated hypogammaglobulinemia, and selective IgA deficiency.

GIOVANNA TOSATO and Blaese, NCI, and BARTON HAYNES and ANTHONY FAUCI, NIAID, with their collaborators also showed that suppressor T cells play a major role as a host defense controlling the B cell activation and proliferation induced by Epstein-Barr virus in infectious mononucleosis.

Other Suppressor Cells

In other studies abnormal suppression was shown to be caused by cells of the immune system other than T-lymphocytes. For example, Broder and I showed that adherent suppressor cells, most likely monocytes, play a role in the polyclonal immunoglobulin deficiency observed in patients with multiple myeloma and increased numbers of infections. Such cells were also shown by DAVID KATZ and Fauci of NIAID to be of significance in the disorders of cell-mediated immunity in patients with sarcoidosis.

The study of suppressor T cells in common variable hypogammaglobulinemia represented the first demonstration that a disorder of suppressor T cell activity could cause human disease, thus initiating a field of research concerning the delicate balance of cell interactions in the human homeostatic immune network and the disorders that can result from their imbalance.

Autoimmune Diseases

The complex mechanisms of disordered immune regulation that lead to the development of autoimmunity in animal models and human disease have been the subject of intensive investigation at NIH. NORMAN TALAL and Steinberg initiated many of these investigations at NIADDK. Fauci, TOM CHUSED, and IRA GREEN in NIAID have also made elegant contributions to our understanding of the disorders of immune regulation in systemic lupus erythematosus.

Disorders of immunoregulation leading to autoimmune diseases, in which the immune system destroys host tissues, are very complex, and a number of underlying abnormalities have been identified. Hyperactivity of B cells is virtually universal. In addition, there is often an abnormality of the network of regulatory T cells, especially a suppressor T cell deficiency. A deficiency of suppressor T cell function is evident in systemic lupus erythematosus, and has also been shown by Strober and co-workers at NCI to be a major factor in the disordered immunity of patients with primary biliary cirrhosis. Patients with rheumatoid arthritis have a restricted defect of suppressor T cell function relating specifically to the Epstein-Barr virus, as shown by Tosato, Steinberg, and Blaese of NCI and NIAMDD using an in vitro immunoglobulin biosynthesis system with Epstein-Barr virus as the simulating agent. Indeed, failure in the regulation of B cell responses induced by Epstein-Barr virus may contribute to many of the immune abnormalities underlying rheumatoid arthritis.

Clearly, hyperactivity of B cells or helper T cells, or a deficiency of suppressor T cells has been demonstrated in many rodent models of autoimmune disease as well as in patients with such disorders.

ELIZABETH RAVETCH and Steinberg, NIADDK, demonstrated that multiple genes control responses to self-antigens and that multiple genetic defects underlie the production of autoantibodies in systemic lupus erythematosus. Family studies by Miller and Schwartz at the Tufts Medical Center support the view that the development of lupus reflects abnormalities of two functionally distinct sets of genes. That is, abnormalities of both a gene-controlled suppressor T cell function and a gene-related B cell hyperactivity may be required.

Leukemias of Immunoregulatory Lymphocytes

One of the major features of the human immune response that has hindered study is that the peripheral blood lymphocytes represent mixtures of complex populations of cells with different and at times opposing functions. This problem was circumvented and a number of important insights into the control of the human immune response were made possible by the study of neoplasms of the B cell/plasma cell and the T cell series, which represent clonal expansions of homogeneous cells. The recognition that so-called paraproteins derived from patients with multiple myeloma represent homogeneous immunoglobulins was indispensable to an understanding of the structure and function of these molecules. Clonal malignancies of T cell origin, which Broder and I have been studying, are also of great interest, as these neoplastic T cells in some cases retain immunoregulatory function.

We first focused our studies on patients with the Sézary syndrome, a serious disorder characterized by exfoliative erythroderma, generalized lymphadenopathy, and circulating malignant T-lymphocytes with a propensity to infiltrate the skin. The leukemic T-lymphocytes did not produce immunoglobulins, nor could they function as suppressor cells. We demonstrated, however, using an in vitro coculture system, that the Sézary leukemic cells originate from the subset of T cells that are dedicated to helper interactions with B cells and are required for their maturation into cells capable of synthesizing and secreting immunoglobulin.

Other types of T leukemic cells function as suppressor cells or their precursors. For example, major advances concerning the nature of immunoregulatory cells and the cause of the malignant transformation of T-lymphocytes have emerged from studies of patients with a recently defined leukemia termed adult T cell leukemia (ATL) by its discoverers, UCHIYAMA, Takatsuki, and their co-workers from the Kyoto Medical School in Japan. ATL is an aggressive malignancy of mature T cells associated with skin infiltration, hypercalcemia, and pulmonary infiltrates. The disease shows an interesting geographic clustering, with most cases occurring in southwest Japan, the Caribbean, and to a lesser extent in the southeastern United States. In contrast to Sézary leukemic T cells, those of ATL never function as helper cells. In most cases we studied, they suppressed the immunoglobulin synthesis of cocultured normal lymphocytes.

In a critically important series of studies, ROBERT GALLO and his co-workers at NCI demonstrated that ATL is caused by a unique type-C retrovirus,* which they have termed human T cell leukemia/lymphoma virus (HTLV). These studies were the

---

*Retrovirus: a virus containing reverse transcriptase, an enzyme of RNA viruses that catalyzes the transcription of RNA to DNA, which then enters the genome of the host cell and serves in replication of the virus.

first to provide credible evidence that a retrovirus might be involved in a human cancer. The first step in this discovery, as discussed in Section IV of this chapter, was the demonstration that mature human T cells can be maintained in culture containing interleukin 2 (T cell growth factor). In 1980 Gallo and his co-workers, using cultures of T cells obtained from a patient with a highly malignant form of the Sézary T cell leukemia and subsequently from ATL patients, isolated HTLV. Electron microscopy revealed typical retroviral particles budding from cell membranes, and particulate reverse transcriptase was demonstrated in the culture media.

Characterization of these HTLV strains according to nucleic acid hybridization, and immunological studies of viral transcriptase and of the viral core proteins, provided evidence that the viruses obtained from different patients with ATL were related or identical to one another. In contrast, HTLV sequences were not found in either the DNA of healthy individuals or the B cells of the ATL patients, indicating that the virus was exogenous and not transmitted in the germline. It was also shown that this retrovirus was not related to previously identified animal retroviruses. Following the initial studies, many isolates of HTLV-1 have been made from ATL patients both by Gallo's group in the United States and by Hinuma's in Japan. A separate but distantly related virus, HTLV-2, has also been identified in cell lines from a patient with a T cell-type hairy cell leukemia.

One interesting feature that Broder, Greene, Takashi Uchiyama, and I identified in collaboration with Gallo is that the leukemic T cells of ATL always react with the monoclonal antibody we prepared, anti-Tac, which identifies the inducible T cell receptor for T cell growth factor. They are thus distinguishable from normal T cells and from other types of leukemic cells that are Tac-antigen negative. In addition, the demonstration that adult T cell leukemic cells universally manifest large numbers of the inducible receptor for the growth factor may partially explain their uncontrolled growth. Finally, we are currently evaluating the efficacy of intravenously administered anti-Tac monoclonal antibody in the treatment of ATL patients, whose normal T cells are Tac-antigen negative and whose leukemic cells are Tac-antigen positive. Thus, basic studies initiated by Gallo of T cell growth factor and its receptor to explain the normal growth of T cells have aided in the discovery of the first human cancer retrovirus and are providing information valuable in the diagnosis and, conceivably, the therapy of this form of leukemia.

Research on B Cell Leukemias

Recent studies on clonal leukemias of the B cell series, using the techniques of molecular genetics, have provided insights into the normal events controlling B cell maturation and the disorders in these events associated with B cell neoplasms. As noted in Section II of this chapter, immunoglobulins are encoded by a series of genetic elements that recombine to bring together variable gene segments to create multiple different assortments. The hierarchy of these immunoglobulin gene rearrangements that occur in all cases as primitive stem cells mature into B cells has been established by Alt, Baltimore, and their co-workers at the Massachusetts Institute of Technology, analyzing lymphocytic leukemias of mice, and by Korsmeyer, PHILIP HIETER, ILAN KIRSCH, Ravetch, PHILIP LEDER, and me at NIH, studying immunoglobulin gene arrangements of human leukemias of B cells, T cells, and their precursors.

In contrast to B cells, the cells of human T cell leukemias revealed no immunoglobulin gene rearrangements affecting the light-chain genes or 90 percent of the heavy-chain genes. However, virtually all "non-T, non-B" acute lymphocytic leukemic cells of childhood had undergone immunoglobulin gene rearrangements, indicating that these cells were in the B-lymphocyte precursor series. New patterns of such rearrangement were observed in the pre-B cell leukemias and B cells of these patients, though not in mature B cells. These patterns clearly indicated that there is a hierarchy of immunoglobulin gene rearrangements as a stem cell matures into a B cell, with gene rearrangements in heavy chains preceding those of light chains and, in light chains, kappa gene rearrangements preceding lambda. In some cases of leukemia of immature clonal lymphocytes, cells had undergone aberrant rearrangements of both sets of heavy-chain genes and no longer had the genetic material needed to produce an immunoglobulin molecule. The cells were arrested in the B cell precursor state of maturation. This observation provides insight into the pathogenesis of the failed maturation of these immature leukemic cells.

Analysis of further rearrangements within the immunoglobulin gene locus observed in malignant cells from all patients with Burkitt's lymphoma has provided exciting new information concerning the nature of the malignant transformation in B-lymphocytes of this neoplasm. Burkitt recognized that the lymphoma bearing his name is associated with Epstein-Barr virus infection and is largely restricted to tropical regions of Africa where malaria is also endemic. However, the Epstein-Barr virus and malaria are both common, while Burkitt's lymphoma is relatively rare. Thus it was clear that additional events are involved in causing infected B cells that are apparently predisposed to malignant transformation to become frankly neoplastic.

In early studies, Klein demonstrated in all cases a chromosomal abnormality in the malignant tumor cells. The consistent cytogenetic hallmark of Burkitt's lymphoma is a reciprocal translocation involving the distal end of the long arm of chromosome 8 at band q24 and another chromosome. It was of interest that this translocation always involved the exact site of the immunoglobulin genes,* as defined by Kirsch, Leder, and their co-workers at NICHD.

Considerable attention has been focused on the chromosomal segment that is uniformly involved, 8q24, and on an oncogene found on this segment.** Within the past few years, a set of cancer-related genes has been identified within higher eukaryotic organisms. These so-called cellular onc genes (c-onc) represent the normal cellular homologs of the transforming principles identified in a number of retroviruses (v-onc). These c-onc genes have been highly conserved throughout evolution and are probably the source of the transforming v-onc sequences present in viruses and, in their c-onc form, presumably play important roles in normal cellular growth and differentiation as well as malignant transformation.

Rebecca Taub, Leder, and co-workers and Gallo, RICARDO DALLA-FAVERA, and their group at NCI, working with Croce at the Wistar Institute, demonstrated that one of the c-onc genes, the human c-myc gene, was located at 8q24 and that the part of chromosome 8 that was translocated contained this gene in all cases. The implication of this onc gene translocation to the site of the actively transcribed immunoglobulin genes awaits identification of the c-myc gene product and its effect on normal B cells. It is important to note, however, that mouse plasma cell tumors have a comparable translocation of the c-myc gene locus to the site of the mouse immunoglobulin genes. This onc gene is also known to be activated by the nearby integration of a virus in a bursal (B cell) lymphoma of chickens. These observations support the hypothesis that the gene translocation in these B cell/plasma cell neoplasms plays a role in the malignant transformation.

---

*Chromosome 14 band q32 for heavy-chain genes, chromosome 2p13 for kappa immunoglobulin genes, and 22q11 for lambda immunoglobulin genes.

**See chapter by Scolnick for further information on oncogenes.

Therapeutic Implications

Better understanding of pathogenetic mechanisms that underlie immunological diseases and the development of drugs
that affect the immune system have led to new and more effective therapies. For example, Fauci and SHELDON WOLFF have
shown that Wegener's granulomatosis can be effectively treated
by a combination of cyclophosphamide and a steroid. The disease is characterized by granulomatous vasculitis of the upper
and lower respiratory tracts, together with glomerulonephritis. Untreated, it usually ran a rapidly fatal course, with
90 percent of patients dying within two years, and death occurred despite corticosteroid therapy. Isolated reports of the
use of cytotoxic agents had been reported by Fahey and others.
Fauci and Wolff of NIAID then initiated a prospective clinical
trial of daily low-dose cyclophosphamide and alternate-day
prednisone. Complete remissions were induced and maintained
without life-threatening complications in 93 percent of 85
patients over the 21 years of the study, and only 6 have died
of active disease.

MICHAEL FRANK and his co-workers observed an equally
striking reversal of the clinical and biochemical abnormalities of patients with hereditary angioedema when treated
with a modified androgen. Hereditary angioedema is characterized by episodic swelling of the extremities, face, abdominal viscera, and airways, with a reported 30 percent mortality usually caused by airway obstruction. The disease
appears to be due to deficient activity of the inhibitor of
the activated first component (C1 esterase) of the series of
complement proteins. Androgens were first introduced in the
treatment of hereditary angioedema by STEPHEN SPAULDING but
produced virilizing effects. JEFFREY GELFAND, Frank, and their
co-workers at NIAID initiated a double-blind therapeutic trial
with danazol, a synthetic derivative of ethynyltestosterone
that has a markedly attenuated androgenic potential. Only one
attack occurred in 46 courses with danazol, whereas 44 of 47
patients on placebo developed attacks. Levels of C1-esterase
inhibitor increased three- to fourfold during therapy. Thus,
danazol was effective in preventing attacks in hereditary
angioedema and correcting the underlying biochemical abnormality.

It is clear from this brief review that research in the
field of immunology at NIH has led to a dazzling record of
advances, especially in our basic understanding of the immune response and its regulation by genetic and other factors.
In addition, these studies of the immune system have led to the
discovery of new clinical syndromes, to the definition of new

biological bases of human disease, and to new methods for the diagnosis and therapy of diseases affecting the immune system.

Selected References

Gallo, R.C., and F. Wong-Staal. Retroviruses as etiologic agents of some animal and human leukemias and lymphomas and as tools for elucidating the molecular mechanism of leukemogenesis. Blood 60:545–557, 1982.

Gershon, R.K. T cell control of antibody production. Contemp Top Immunobiol 3:1–40, 1974.

Taub, R., et al. Translocation of the c-myc gene into the immunoglobulin heavy chain locus in human Burkitt lymphoma and murine plasmacytoma cells. Proc Natl Acad Sci USA 79:7837–7841, 1980.

Waldmann, T.A. Protein-losing enteropathy. Gastroenterology 50:422–443, 1966.

Waldmann, T.A., and W. Strober. Metabolism of immunoglobulins. In Progress in Allergy, P. Kallo and B.H. Waksman (eds.), Vol. 13, pp. 1–110. Basel and New York: S. Karger, 1969.

Waldmann, T.A., and S. Broder. Suppressor cells in the regulation of the immune response. In Prog Clin Immunol, R. Schwartz (ed.) 3:155–199, 1977.

Introduction

ORGANIC CHEMISTRY IN A BIOMEDICAL RESEARCH ORGANIZATION

Biomedical science is firmly rooted in chemistry and continues to derive sustenance from the works of the organic chemist. Initially the primary concern was to answer the question, What? This focuses on the structure of natural products and the composition of organs and tissues of the animal and vegetable world. It is the analytical question.

Next came the endeavor to answer, How? How do the ingredients of the body fluids cross cell membranes? How do they interact with one another? How do the many biological catalysts perform their vital functions? Scientists everywhere seek to answer the mechanistic question.

Last, there are some bold investigators who ask, Why? Scientists have been cautious in doing so lest they appear to imply purpose in nature—a consideration of philosophers and theologians. Nonetheless, this has proved an interesting area of inquiry. Why is there intracellular compartmentalization? Why has an immune system evolved, or a DNA-based genetics? Why does this or that characteristic have survival value? Here one enters the realm of the teleological question. In the following pages "teleological thinking" is suggested in respect to the role of opiate receptors in the brain and to the evolution of venoms.

Eighteenth century medicine was largely organ-based. Physicians and pathologists explored the nature and functions of the liver, the stomach, the lungs. With the nineteenth century came the widespread use of the microscope, and medicine, as well as pathology, became cellular. The twentieth century may be regarded as the molecular century of biomedicine. In addition to molecular biology, there is an approach at the molecular level for each of the subspecialties of medicine —molecular pathology, pharmacology, psychiatry. Concurrent with this shift of interest and emphasis, the contributions of the organic chemist have become more prominent. Numerous examples of "molecular thinking" as applied to medical and biological problems will be found in this chapter.

D. S.

11

ORGANIC CHEMISTRY IN A BIOMEDICAL RESEARCH ORGANIZATION

Bernhard Witkop

It is easy to enumerate historical events, but much more difficult to bring to life the intellectual atmosphere and pioneering spirit of past research. For this reason the history of science is often told as a chronicle of anecdotes. The present chapter will tend to do so, though it will also recount certain significant achievements in organic chemistry. We begin in the Division of Chemistry, formally created on June 20, 1905, in the Hygienic Laboratory, predecessor of the National Institutes of Health. The Laboratory of Chemistry, successor to the Division, is now in the National Institute of Arthritis, Diabetes, and Digestive and Kidney Diseases.

Early Fundamental Research
Supported by the Government

WILLIAM MANSFIELD CLARK (1884-1964), appointed to head the Division in 1920, is remembered for his extensive studies of oxidation-reduction systems. His first 10 papers appeared in *Public Health Reports* from 1923 to 1926. Their reissuance in 1928 as *Hygienic Laboratory Bulletin No. 151* (340 pages) shows a surprising early interest in the Government's basic research.

At that time there were few voices on Capitol Hill pleading for an expanded Federal role in the health sciences. One determined advocate, however, was Senator Joseph Eugene Ransdell (1858-1954) from Louisiana. In his mind fundamental research would guide scientists to find cures for diseases. He had introduced a bill in the Senate for a National Institute of Health in 1926. After many defeats and revisions, his bill finally passed the House and Senate in 1930 and was

BERNHARD WITKOP, Ph.D., Sc.D., Chief, Laboratory of Chemistry, National Institute of Arthritis, Diabetes, and Digestive and Kidney Diseases.

signed into law by President Hoover on May 26 of that year
(Public Law 71-251)—"An Act to establish and operate a National Institute of Health, to create a system of fellowships
in said institute, and to authorize the Government to accept
donations for use in ascertaining the cause, prevention, and
cure of disease affecting human beings, and for other purposes."

Ransdell, as a former legislator, discussed "Chemistry
and the National Institute of Health" in the *Chemist*, May
1931. Thirty-five years later, evidence supporting his conviction that fundamental research would lead to medical advances
appeared in a report of the National Academy of Sciences'
Committee for the Survey of Chemistry, chaired by Frank H.
Westheimer (1). There were also instances of private support
to NIH laboratories. A donation of $100,000 from the Chemical
Foundation financed fellowships in the Laboratory of Chemistry
for more than a quarter century.

Science, according to Karl Popper, is essentially based
on tradition in a twofold manner: conservative and revolutionary. This is illustrated in the history of two substances
that much interested Clark. In extension of the classical
work of Paul Ehrlich, he determined the oxidation-reduction
potentials of methylene blue—Ehrlich's favorite neurotropic
histochemical stain—and the acid-base equilibria of arsphen-
amine solutions. Little did Clark realize that a derivative
of methylene blue, chlorpromazine, was to be the most important neuroleptic drug of the century. He knew that arsphen-
amine, Ehrlich's salvarsan, had ushered in modern chemotherapy, but it was not clear until recently that the so-called
"magic bullet" was actually magic buckshot (2). Salvarsan, or
"606" (the 606th drug that Ehrlich tested against syphilis),
was not a true compound but a mixture.

Not only was Clark, as Chief of the Division of Chemistry,
the commanding general of the oxidation-reduction troops, but
when the occasion required he performed like a first-class
soldier, even outside his immediate responsibilities. This
is illustrated by an occurrence during investigation of the
health hazard from gasoline containing tetraethyl lead. The
hazard was discussed in *Public Health Bulletin No. 163:*

Early in 1923 tetraethyl lead began to be used in
an endeavor to increase the efficiency of gasoline as
a motor fuel. The possible danger from such wide distribution of a lead compound aroused fear on the part
of those concerned with public health, and these fears
were intensified when fatal poisoning occurred in the
manufacture and mixing of the concentrated tetraethyl
lead itself in Deepwater, N.J., Dayton, Ohio, and

Bayway, N.J. As a consequence of such apprehensions, the distribution of tetraethyl lead was stopped on May 5, 1925, and the sale of gasoline containing tetraethyl lead was thereby generally discontinued.

The Division of Chemistry was directed to investigate the effects of human exposure to lead-containing fumes. Since distribution of tetraethyl lead had been stopped, the investigation was launched as rapidly as possible. The Division needed a large electric furnace to analyze samples of feces. Clark donned overalls and, starting with bricks and wire, proceeded to build a furnace and a thermocouple to control the temperature. It was then possible to complete the investigation without delay.

Clark often made complicated pieces of apparatus for members of the chemistry staff. One soon came to admire this great scientist, not only for his ability as a chemist but also for his skill as a glassblower and machinist. Clark set aside a room for use as a machine shop, providing a lathe and other equipment. ELIAS ELVOVE and other contemporaries particularly recall Clark's friendliness in working with his staff.

To the layman, acid-base concepts—delineated in terms of pH—are not easily recognizable as fundamental parameters of living systems. Clark had earlier solved a practical problem by applying his knowledge of pH: the concentration of protons (H^+) in a solution. The airplane industry needed plywood, which is manufactured with glues based on casein. At that time casein, the protein of defatted milk, was imported from Argentina because glue manufacturers rejected the American-made product as inhomogeneous. Clark knew that proteins, having basic and acidic groups, are least soluble at their isoelectric point—the point at which they carry no net charge. Supervising the precipitation of casein from skim milk in a huge vat, Clark insisted that acid be added until the pH of the whey reached the isoelectric point of casein, though the casein appeared to have already separated. Rendered insoluble, the casein aggregated into large granular curds that could be easily washed from the whey and secured. This material was entirely satisfactory for glue manufacture.

Living systems are complex: proton donors and their conjugate acceptors constitute an "acid-base continuum." Potential oxidants and reductants contribute to the complexity, building to an oxidation-reduction acid-base continuum that involves electron and proton transfers and sometimes the incorporation of oxygen. Further, the oxidant, the reductant, or both may enter into processes of coordination. Where systems of even greater complexity occur in nature, the continuum

will have many variables. The investigator then works by a
series of zigs and zags, since he must control all parameters
save the one in question. Nature, however, is under no such
restriction—and Clark put it thus in considering the degrees
of freedom open to the metabolism of the amoeba:

> I once met a lively young cell
> Whom I then proceeded to tell
>   Of pH, electrons,
>   P wiggles and protons;
> To which he replied, "Go to ----!"

Clark accepted the DeLamar Professorship of Physiological
Chemistry at The Johns Hopkins School of Medicine in 1927 and
was succeeded at NIH by CLAUDE HUDSON.

The Era of Classical Carbohydrate Chemistry

Claude Silbert Hudson (1881-1952) headed the Laboratory
until 1950. Under his strong leadership, Emil Fischer's carbohydrate legacy was broadened to a solid foundation of sugar
chemistry: mono-, di-, and polysaccharides and the dynamics
of anomers in sugar solution.

Hudson's colorful personality comes to life in fanciful
anecdotes built against a sugar background. One of these re-
fers to the property of certain compounds to exist in mirror-
image forms—the *levo* (left) and *dextro* (right) isomers—or in
a *racemic* mix (L-D) of the two. It was said that two Hudsons
dwelt in opposed mirrors from which they emerged at appropriate times. L-Hudson was the convivial one, who partook of
intoxicating beverages, was strongly drawn to beautiful women,
and was in general sinful. D-Hudson was the serious, sober,
gentlemanly scientist. On the occasion of the Organic Symposium of the American Chemical Society at Richmond, L-Hudson
was in charge. It became necessary for him to leave the auditorium, but alas, the only inconspicuous exit was a spiral
staircase that was dextrorotatory. He finally ascended this
with the help of friends, but claimed for years that he had
been racemized in the process.

Hudson was always a lone worker and a member of no school.
His early training in physics with Nernst in Göttingen (1902)
gave him an exactitude in measurement and thought. His association with the great and imaginative Van't Hoff in Berlin
(1903) (where he met Fischer) made a profound impression upon
him. Van't Hoff had published some speculations on "optical
superposition," or the possibly additive nature of optical
rotatory power. More data were required, and Hudson recog-

nized that the largest known group of optically active isomers of established configuration was at hand in the carbohydrates. These proved ideal for the further exploration of Van't Hoff's hypothesis.

Hudson's contributions are fundamental to the health sciences through their basic advancement of organic chemistry. For example, he showed that mutarotation of natural glucose in water was subject to general acid-base catalysis, and expressed this in mathematical terms.

In his "lactone rule" formulation, Hudson noted that the optical rotatory sign of an aldonic acid lactone, of significant rotation, was controlled by the configuration of the carbon bearing the hydroxyl group involved in the ring closure, whereas the rotatory sign of the amides, phenylhydrazides, and benzimidazoles of the aldonic acids was conditioned by the configuration of the center adjacent to the carboxyl function.

From *Sedum spectabile* he isolated sedoheptulose, which the enzyme transketolase evokes from two pentose 5-phosphates as the 7-phosphate (3). The 1,7-diphosphate of sedoheptulose participates in the dynamics of photosynthesis, as Melvin Calvin discovered.

From Carbohydrates to Molecular Immunology

In 1951 Hudson retired as Chief of the Laboratory and the Section on Carbohydrates, and HEWITT G. FLETCHER, Jr., became Chief of the Section. Under Fletcher, the Section embarked on a program of synthetic carbohydrate chemistry, predominantly involving ribose, deoxyribose, and deoxyacetamido sugars. Over the years some 40 postdoctoral fellows and visiting scientists at NIH have worked in this area.

After Fletcher's untimely death in 1973, his successor, CORNELIS P. J. GLAUDEMANS, emphasized the role of carbohydrates in the typing of bacterial antigens and studied the interactions of polysaccharides and antibodies. With the recent blossoming of monoclonal antibodies, the Section has become heavily involved in studying, at the molecular level, how immunoglobulins interact with invading molecules. Today the work on site-mapping of these proteins is extensive, and the Section on Carbohydrates is in the forefront of this aspect of molecular immunology.

The Story of Mottled Enamel and the Fluoridation of Drinking Water

In the early 1930s a special investigation aroused great public interest. The Division of Chemistry cooperated in a study related to chronic endemic dental fluorosis, or "mottled enamel." Experiments with rats indicated that human mottled enamel is probably caused by fluoride in drinking water. It was necessary to develop and validate a sensitive method for measuring traces of fluoride in water, accurate to 0.1 part per million. H. TRENDLEY DEAN was assigned to NIH to study the mottled enamel problem. While the research progressed in the Division of Chemistry, Dean developed a method for expressing mottled enamel on a quantitative basis. Through this collaborative effort, it became possible to determine the mottled-enamel threshold of fluoride in drinking water and eventually the optimum fluoride level for the prevention of dental caries.

[These investigations are further described in Bieri's chapter, "Nutrition Studies."]

Antimalarials

As World War II approached, the Director of NIH, ROLLA E. DYER, started to feel the "pressure of mission orientation." The Office of Scientific Research and Development (OSRD) was anxious to avoid dependence on the quinine monopoly of the Dutch East Indies and to develop an extensive antimalarial program. A well-known specialist in opium alkaloids, LYNDON F. SMALL (1897-1957), heading a Drug Addiction Laboratory at the University of Virginia, was asked to shift his interest from morphine to quinine substitutes. His decision was probably not easy. But eventually Small and a few associates moved to Washington and were attached as a unit to Hudson, then Director of NIH's Division of Chemistry.

In this new field Small and his group moved ahead energetically as part of the far-flung antimalarial program of OSRD. They synthesized hundreds of compounds. A dozen or more derived from polynuclear hydrocarbons were effective enough to replace quinine and atabrine. Many were tested intensively, both pharmacologically and clinically, in a program coordinated by JAMES A. SHANNON, later Director of NIH.

Synthetic Analgesics

But this program on antimalarials was for Small only an interlude. Because of the threat to our opium sources posed by the Korean war, he was requested in 1950 to reassemble the Drug Addiction Laboratory's personnel to undertake the synthesis of morphine and codeine replacements. The group developed several synthetic analgesics more potent than morphine or codeine, with less side-action liability. These synthetics could substitute for the natural drugs should the need arise.

As Hudson was linked to Nernst, Van't Hoff, and Fischer, Small had spent 1926 and 1927 with Heinrich Wieland (1877-1957) in Munich. There he became acquainted with the complex chemistry of the morphine alkaloids, with alpinism from Mount Etna to the Matterhorn, and with Bavarian life style. After Small's death in 1957, the tradition carried over to his successor, the present writer (4), and thus assured the continued study of natural products in the Laboratory of Chemistry. ERICH MOSETTIG (1898-1962), a collaborator and colleague of Small for many years, came from Ernst Späth's laboratory in Vienna and exemplified this tradition in his life and work (5).

Others who pursued the quest for morphine substitutes were NATHAN B. EDDY, LEWIS SARGENT, ARTHUR E. JACOBSON, and more recently ARNOLD BROSSI.

These efforts started in 1947 with methadone, a strong analgesic—more active orally than morphine—with a completely new structure. It had been developed by Gustav Ehrhart at the I. G. Farbenindustrie in 1938-1944. At NIH chemical transformations of methadone and its isomer isomethadone led to all possible isomeric reduction products: α- and β-methadols and isomethadols and their O-acetyl derivatives—24 compounds in all. These were fully characterized chemically and evaluated in mice for toxicity and analgesic activity and in monkeys for physical-dependence liability. Allo-acetyl isomers were powerful, long-acting analgesics after oral or subcutaneous administration, but they fully supported morphine dependence in monkeys. A few were tested in man. L-α-acetylmethadol (LAAM) has proved to be a good substitute for methadone—more potent and longer acting—in narcotics withdrawal regimens.

Between 1952 and 1975 two new classes of synthetic analgesics, the 6,7-benzomorphans and 5-phenylmorphans, were derived deductively by excision of various portions of levorphanol. In animal tests, both classes of compounds showed for the first time consistent separation of analgesic activity and dependence potential. A practical "fallout" was the discovery (at NIH) and the development (at the Smith, Kline & French Laboratories) of phenazocine (Prinadol, Narphen), a potent analgesic when administered orally or parenterally. It has proved to be a more than adequate substitute for morphine and codeine, fulfilling the principal goal projected in 1950.

Research in the benzomorphan series has proliferated to a national and international extent. A reportedly useful analgesic with low abuse potential, pentazocine (Talwin), was synthesized at the Sterling-Winthrop Laboratories. In addition, the firm has released several potentially life-saving narcotic antagonists, including cyclazocine, which may prove valuable in the deterrence of heroin abuse. This agent also is a strong analgesic without apparent abuse liability.

While this report is being written, the situation has changed: pentazocine in combination with another prescription drug, tripelennamine (Pyribenzamine), has become a popular heroin substitute. The results of overdoses are devastating: brain infections, strokes, seizures, and death—almost 100 fatalities in 1980. This situation points to the precarious nature of conclusions on the abuse potential of analgesics and narcotics substitutes.

EVERETTE MAY reviewed these developments in the Third Smissman Award Address (6).

The Legacy: Separation of Analgesic from Addictive Effects

The Laboratory's basic research on analgesics has stimulated similar efforts in pharmaceutical organizations. Several laboratories have apparently succeeded in synthesizing nonaddicting analgesics. Three such drugs are nalbuphine (Nubain, Endo Laboratories), butorphanol (Stadol, Bristol Laboratories) and buprenorphine (Tamgesic, Reckitt & Colman). These compounds do not sustain the dependence syndrome in rhesus monkeys or appear to cause dependence in man. They are being introduced into clinical use.

Buprenorphine is reported to be a safe and effective new pharmacotherapy for heroin dependence, offering significant advantages over naltrexone or methadone (7). Investigators note, however, that addicts "like" the drug (8). Although this would be a positive stimulus for heroin addicts in replacement therapy, the contentment and euphoria induced by the drug could possibly lead to its abuse.

Potent analgesics that do not have the dependence liability, respiratory depressant, and other side effects of morphine may of course prove useful in clinical settings. Bupre-

norphine, butorphanol, and nalbuphine are candidates. It is
also conceivable that the psychological effects of agonists/
antagonists like buprenorphine could be utilized in easing
the despair of terminal cancer patients.

Other promising agents are to be found among the *N*-[(tetrahydrofuryl)-alkyl] and *N*-(alkoxyalkyl) derivatives of (-)-
normetazocine (9). They are powerful nonmorphinelike analgesics with low toxicity, some attaining analgesic potencies
more than 100 times that of morphine. Their therapeutic ratios
range from 6000 to 27,000, comparing favorably with those of
morphine (1064) and pentazocine (169). Clinical trial may
help to discover here the elusive strong analgesics with low
toxicity and potential for abuse.

Predicting the Abuse Potential of New Drugs

For the past several decades the Medicinal Chemistry Section has been testing centrally acting analgesics. One of
the great strengths of the program has been a single technician, LOUISE ATWELL, who has personally tested nearly all
of the thousands of potential analgesics obtained since 1951.
The testing procedure, developed by Eddy in 1949, is the hot
plate assay in mice.

The assay is not completely objective—unlike, for example, the mouse tailflick. Close attention and good coordination are required in using a stopwatch to mark reaction time.
Atwell's continued improvements in the procedure make it one
of the most useful in the field. The Medicinal Chemistry
Section continues its research on analgesics, with emphasis
on the interaction between drugs of new molecular types and
the opiate receptors of brain.

In 1950 M. H. SEEVERS and Eddy, working at the University
of Michigan, found that the rhesus monkey could become physically dependent on opiates and synthetic drugs of like action,
or opioids. One disadvantage in the use of monkeys for pre-
dicting dependence liability is their high cost. And great
caution must be exercised in their care, extending of course
to drug administration. Again Eddy's hot plate assay has
proved valuable, for it permits use of the mouse in establishing a starting dose at which a drug can be safely administered to monkeys. Thus, the mouse has become a cornerstone
in the search for potent analgesics without serious side effects (10).

It is doubtful, though, that any animal assay for abuse
potential would be as effective as a test on human subjects.

Such tests were once performed at the Addiction Research Center in Lexington, Kentucky, but have been discontinued in response to human rights groups.

Practical Synthesis of Opium Alkaloids

A number of laboratories are seeking methods for the total synthesis of opiates, especially codeine. The medical importance of codeine as an analgesic and antitussive is reflected in mounting United States production and use, now exceeding 50,000 kg annually, and in worldwide production at about 190,000 kg. Economic aspects of the licit opiate market are significant. The price of codeine (1980) is about $1000 per kg and rising, and prices of more complex opium derivatives are much higher. Codeine is manufactured in the United States by O-methylation of morphine, which is obtained exclusively from opium or poppy straw purchased abroad. Since domestic cultivation of poppy for opiate production is illegal and no practical total synthesis is available, all United States supplies of opium-derived drugs depend on foreign sources. International economic and political problems complicate raw material production, exacerbating the difficulty of meeting the nation's needs.

In 1980 KENNER C. RICE of the Section on Medicinal Chemistry, headed by Brossi, succeeded in straightforward total synthesis of three opioids: ($\pm$)-dihydrothebainone, ($\pm$)-nordihydrocodeinone, and ($\pm$)-dihydrocodeinone. Overall yields of 37, 30, and 29 percent, respectively, were obtained from readily available 3-methoxyphenethylamine with isolation of only six intermediates. A practical total synthesis of thebaine, codeine, and morphine appears finally to be in hand (11).

Such syntheses also make available codeine, morphine, and the morphine antagonist naloxone with dextrorotatory antipodes not found in nature. These are useful for studies on binding with the newly discovered and defined opium receptors. Here interests in synthetic opiates and endogenous brain peptides intersect.

One might reflect anew on Thomas Sydenham's assertion "Among the remedies which it has pleased Almighty God to give man to relieve his sufferings, none is so universal and so efficacious as opium." It was a great surprise when, in 1975, John Hughes and Hans Kosterlitz of the University of Aberdeen isolated from brain tissue two peptides with opiatelike activity, now known as enkephalins. Similar brain peptides with opioid effects, the endorphins, were later isolated from the pituitary. It has also been shown that naloxone blocks the action of enkephalins and endorphins. We have crossed the threshold of a new era of neurobiology and neuropsychiatry.

Interplay Between Metabolic Problems and Developments in Instrumentation

"If you can look into the seeds of time, / And say which grain will grow and which will not. . . ." Science cannot resolve Banquo's dilemma, but research advances occasionally offer a shortcut.

My Norwegian student Arvid Ek submitted a thesis to Harvard University in 1952 describing the synthesis of 5-hydroxytryptophan. The availability of this novel amino acid enabled SIDNEY UDENFRIEND in 1953 to demonstrate its role as a substrate for "aromatic amino acid decarboxylase" and as the precursor for 5-hydroxytryptamine, or serotonin, an important neurotransmitter. The need to localize and assay serotonin was one of the reasons that ROBERT L. BOWMAN, now Chief of the Laboratory of Technical Development in the Heart Institute, developed a special instrument. The history of the Bowman-Aminco spectrophotofluorometer (SPF) reflects the importance and growing application of one of the most useful analytic tools in biological and clinical chemistry. Here Bowman explains some of its advantages (12):

In pharmacology, we often extract material from the liver of a mouse. We give the mouse a less than toxic dose of something relatively toxic (a few milligrams at the most). The amount that is in the liver might be 1% of that, and what you extracted might be again only 1%. Before fluorometry, the requirement was to use bigger animals. In pharmacology, you must use several animals. . . . So spectrofluorometry has led to simplified pharmacological experimentation and cost reduction. Where before dozens of larger animals were required, now only one or two small animals are needed. The savings in feed and housing alone are considerable.

Udenfriend states (13):

The instrument really revealed itself as a powerful research tool in the studies on 5-hydroxyindole metabolism which were being carried out in my laboratory at that time. With it, methods were developed for the assay of 5-hydroxytryptamine . . . in tissues at levels of 0.01-1.0 μg of tissue. Not only that, but identification of the amine could be made at the microgram level by comparing excitation and fluorescence spectra with those of the authentic compound.

The instrument surpassed all the design goals. Biological substances, including many not previously known to fluoresce, were readily identified and measured. One early application was in testing the hypothesis of serotonin-reserpine antagonism. As SEYMOUR KETY noted, the SPF greatly reduced the time and research necessary to demonstrate the fallacy of this concept, probably averting much unproductive investigation.

Several Nobel Prize winners have relied on the SPF as an important tool. For example, JULIUS AXELROD in collaborative studies identified labile metabolites of lysergic acid diethylamide (LSD), mescaline, and norepinephrine. In Axelrod's words (12):

> The SPF made it possible to measure noradrenaline and serotonin . . . practically. . . . This changed the direction of the whole field of neurobiology. . . Quantitative studies . . . established the relationship of the level of these substances to certain mental illnesses and aided in the development of mental tranquilizer and energizer drugs. Continued studies in this area will yield additional information on the chemical basis for mental illness.

Fluorinated Amino Acids and Neurotransmitters

Fluorination of a compound is the substitution of a fluorine atom for a hydrogen atom in the molecule. The first amino acid to be fluorinated in the Laboratory of Chemistry was proline, the precursor of hydroxyproline. These two amino acids are building-stones of collagen—the protein of connective tissue and the major protein constituent of vertebrates. Proline hydroxylase, the enzyme that converts bound proline to bound hydroxyproline, appears to be involved in wound healing, tissue regeneration, and clinical syndromes including rheumatoid arthritis, Paget's disease, acromegaly, and hepatoma. Investigators saw the heuristic and possible therapeutic value of controlling this enzyme. Accordingly, cis- and trans-4-fluoroprolines were incorporated into procollagen and hydroxylated to collagen in different degrees. Various effects (toxic) were displayed, especially in weanling, fast-growing rats. These promising early observations (1965) were extended to other fluoroamino acids, with surprising effects in various systems.

In 1968 the Section on Biochemical Mechanisms began a long-term project under LOUIS A. COHEN: the synthesis and biological evaluation of ring-substituted derivatives of histamine, histidine, and other biologically significant imidazoles. Few analogs or inhibitors of these metabolically critical compounds were then known, largely because of the inadequacy of synthetic methods.

Attention was first given to the fluorine substituent. Because of its small size, the fluorine atom, though highly electronegative, often substitutes for hydrogen. How hydrogen is replaced in the design of medicinals can be critical because a recognition site in an enzyme or receptor may not be able to bind a molecule much larger than the natural substrate. Physical and chemical properties are also important, for a drastic change in one or the other may have the effect of altering a normal metabolic process. After years of frustration in attempts to introduce fluorine by classical synthetic approaches, the problem was finally solved by the discovery of a photochemical method. A large number of fluoro analogs of biologically important imidazoles are now available.

The choice of fluorine for this effort proved fortunate. Many of the analogs have shown interesting and useful properties in metabolic systems. For example, 2-fluoro-L-histidine was found to compete with histidine in protein synthesis in both microorganisms and mammals. At the same time, this compound shows antibacterial, antiviral, and antileukemic properties at concentrations far below toxic levels in mice. It is noteworthy that the other ring-halogenated histidines, bearing much larger substituents, appear to have none of these properties.

Other new synthetic methods have led to imidazoles containing carboxy, cyano, nitro, azido, and trifluoromethyl substituents. The azidoimidazoles are useful in photochemical labeling of binding sites, while the nitro analogs show selective toxicity for cancer cells and are valuable sensitizers in radiation therapy. The trifluoromethylimidazoles have provided the key for a new direction in bioorganic research: the design of receptor affinity labels for use in vivo. At pH values above 9, these compounds lose hydrogen fluoride and become highly reactive intermediates that can form new covalent bonds at receptor and enzyme recognition sites. An analog of a histidine-containing peptide hormone may be capable of blocking a hormone receptor permanently.

Discovery of a multitude of biological uses for fluoroimidazoles stimulated research in the synthesis and pharmacology of other fluorinated medicinals. Ring-fluorinated analogs of the biogenic amines proved to be especially noteworthy. These amines play critical roles as hormones and chemical neurotransmitters. At least one phenolic group is necessary for them to exhibit their agonist properties, and fluorine could be expected to influence biological behavior through its electronegative effect on the phenolic group. Furthermore, a complex balance of biosynthesis, storage, release, interaction with postsynaptic receptors, and metabolism of the neurotransmitters is required for proper neuronal function. Fluorine could alter any or all aspects of this balance.

Beginning in 1975, ring-fluorinated analogs have been made of tyramine, dopamine, norepinephrine, serotonin, isoproterenol, and phenylephrine. As expected, the alteration in physicochemical parameters affects biological properties. Thus, the effect of fluorine substitution in the biogenic amines can be related to increased lipophilicity with respect to the action of monoamine oxidases A and B, while the activities of catechol-O-methyltransferase and phenol-sulfurtransferase reflect greater phenolic acidity.

To date the most striking effect of fluorine substitution involves the interaction of fluorinated norepinephrines (FNEs) with postsynaptic receptors. Norepinephrine (NE) is the neurotransmitter of the autonomic nervous system, and the α- and β-adrenergic receptors mediate its action. (Subsets of receptors are also known.) Development of agonists and antagonists for the specific types of adrenergic receptors continues to be an important area of research in neuropharmacology.

In 1978 Cohen, KENNETH L. KIRK, and CYRUS R. CREVELING discovered that fluorine substitution on the aromatic ring of NE results in a remarkable alteration in specificities for adrenergic receptors, depending on the site of substitution. Thus, 6-FNE is a specific α-adrenergic agonist, 2-FNE is a β-adrenergic agonist, and 5-FNE behaves similarly to NE itself. In studies of the central nervous system, these activities were found to be directly related to the binding of analog to receptor.

Additional analogs, fluoroisoproterenol and fluorophenylephrine, were synthesized and tested. It was found that fluorine in the 2-position of the aromatic ring invariably blocked α-adrenergic activity, while fluorine in the 6-position inhibited β-adrenergic activity.

Such clearcut specificities must result from fundamental differences in the mode of binding to the respective receptors. The mechanisms of action are under intensive investigation. It should also be noted that the structural similarities of the FNEs to NE itself have made these analogs extremely useful research tools. There is no limit in sight for the development of fluoro analogs of metabolites—analogs that may find important use in research and medicine.

Breakthrough for Protein Chemistry:
Cyanogen Bromide Degradation

The organic chemist, like Weber's Freischütz, is looking for magic bullets that may be directed to known targets,
or that nature directs to targets yet unknown. One of the
smallest and most effective of these bullets is cyanogen bromide, which I discovered with ERHARD GROSS (1928-1961) in the
Laboratory of Chemistry as a selective cleaving reagent.

The usefulness of cyanogen bromide consists in its ex-
clusive "search and cleave" action on methionyl peptide bonds.
The longest protein sequence worked out so far by this method
is the single chain of 1021 amino acids (MW 116,248) of β-galactosidase, an enzyme in *Escherichia coli*. The 24 peptides
formed by selective cleavage of the 23 methionyl bonds separate easily on a column of *O*-carboxymethylcellulose and are
then accessible to successive Edman degradations. Today these
are mostly done automatically on a "sequenator," with remarkable accuracy under optimal conditions.

Pehr Edman, shortly before his death in 1977, proudly
observed that the sequence of more than 80,000 amino acids
had been established. Even this is dwarfed, of course, by
the coding capacity of the mammalian germline, or genome—the
totality of operative genes comprising some 2 billion amino
acid units (14).

The cyanogen bromide method, introduced in 1961, has
proved its usefulness most recently and dramatically in the
genetic synthesis of important hormones (see Figure 1). The
final step in recovering the human hormone somatostatin in
such a process was a purely chemical reaction. A synthetic
gene for somatostatin, in order to be expressed in *E. coli*,
was linked to an indigenous gene. The gene for the enzyme
β-galactosidase was used, and the link was the codon ATG for
methionine, an amino acid not present in somatostatin. Hence,
the microorganism produced the peptide methionyl-somatostatin
linked to the enzyme. Cyanogen bromide broke the polypeptide
at methionine, liberating the hormone. Further, the approach
provided a safety factor in that the *E. coli* could not make
the hormone directly. This marks the first successful use
of recombinant DNA techniques to get a bacterium to produce
a polypeptide of a higher organism.

More recently the approach was extended to the chemical
synthesis of insulin. Synthetic genes for the A and B chains
of human insulin—peptides with 77 and 104 base pairs—were
linked by the methionine codon to a gene of *E. coli*. Again
cyanogen bromide split the genetic product at the foreign methionine link, liberating the two chains, or conceivably the
insulin precursor (pre)proinsulin. The method is now operative

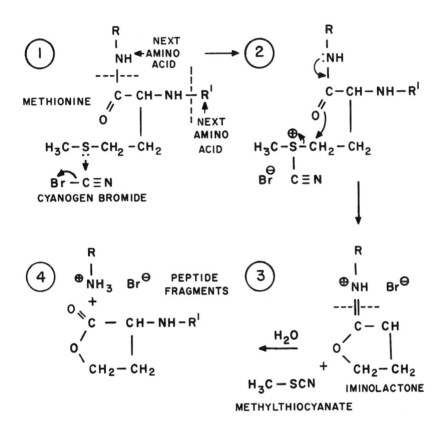

FIGURE 1.   Cyanogen bromide cleaves selectively the amino acid methionine, sketched here as linking R and R', unspecified remainders of a peptide sequence. (1) The cleavage reaction starts when the carbon atom of cyanogen bromide attracts electrons from the sulfur atom of methionine, freeing the bromine anion. (2) The sulfur now attracts electrons, which flow from a nitrogen atom through the methionine molecule. (3) The sulfur, separated, drops out as methylthiocyanate, an uncharged volatile compound. (4) The resulting iminolactone is unstable and, in aqueous solution, breaks down into two peptide fragments.

at a new Eli Lilly plant in Indianapolis for the production and testing of human insulin.

I reported on nonenzymatic methods for cleavage and modification of proteins in 1961 (15), concluding with these words:

There is a growing conviction among organic chemists that the scientific frontier of organic chemistry has moved from small molecules to the large entities that are involved in the process of the formation and preservation of the living cell. Consequently the skills of the organic chemist wisely should be applied to the design of special methods for the analysis, degradation, and synthesis of large molecules. A comparative macromolecular methodology will be written some day and will demonstrate the simplicity of the underlying concepts.

Certainly, all the reactions utilized for the selective cleavage of proteins are conceptually not new, and, in retrospect, surprisingly simple. This preview may serve a useful purpose in delineating, perhaps for the first time, the criteria and requirements that are essential to selective cleavage. In principle, all selective cleavages are, or must be, variations of a key theme, namely, intramolecular acceleration of displacement or elimination reactions to the point where they will occur under extremely mild conditions.

The formulation and recognition of this principle, so fruitful for protein chemistry, may stimulate and influence the search for better methods in neighboring fields.

Indeed, the revolutionary method for sequencing DNA reported in 1977 by A. M. Maxam and W. Gilbert (16) utilizes simple reagents, such as dimethyl sulfate or hydrazine, in cleavage reactions that are differentiated by dilute acid.* Dimethyl sulfate under properly controlled conditions selectively cleaves at guanine, adenine, cytosine, or thymine. Hydrazine, in the presence of sodium chloride, cleaves cytosine preferentially before thymine. Another small molecule, sodium borohydride, can be used under proper conditions to photoreduce bound uridine to dihydrouridine residues.

The sequencing of DNA has in many cases superseded the more laborious sequencing of the corresponding protein. DNA sequences such as those of bacteriophage $\phi\chi$ 174, with 5386 nucleotides, are rapidly being established. Eventually such methods will permit the sequencing of a complete DNA—e.g., that of adenovirus, with about 35,000 nucleotides. Protein sequences have been audited and corrected by means of the highly accurate DNA sequencing technique.

---

*Liberating N(3)-methylated adenine. Guanines methylate five times faster than adenines, at N(7), and can be released in turn.

Historically, cyanogen bromide cleavage was applied to audit the known sequence of such a "famous" protein as ribonuclease (ANFINSEN, Stein, and Moore, 1971 Nobel Prize). The method made possible the sequencing of immunoglobulin (Edelman), collagen (KARL PIEZ), and fibrinogen (Henschen).

Selective Toxins with New Targets

Novel toxins with unknown targets are supplied by nature. They are normally revealed by their high toxicity, and studies on their mechanisms of action have disclosed the targets.

The first such toxin we investigated (1940) was calabash curare, the arrow poison used by many South American Indians. That it was related to a degradation product from strychnine, the Wieland-Gumlich aldehyde, was established much later by Hans Schmid in the laboratory of Paul Karrer. Wieland, also interested in novel toxins, was the pioneer of toad venom. When I learned that amphibian venoms were used in western Colombia as arrow poisons, the two subjects coalesced and led to isolation of batrachotoxin, one of the strongest toxins known to man (17).

This steroidal ester, from the skin of the poison-arrow frog *Phyllobates aurotaenia,* opens the gates of sodium channels in nerve and muscle. It acts by lowering the transmembrane potential and preventing reclosure of the sodium channels more or less irreversibly. As a blocker of axonal transport of proteins and vital enzymes, it is about 1000 times as potent as vinblastine or colchicine.

Other toxins, such as saxitoxin (from a dinoflagellate comprising red tide), tetrodotoxin (from the Japanese pufferfish), and scorpion venom, help to identify and define special sites for regulation, recognition, and ion transport in the receptor complex. Credit for these discoveries belongs largely to WILLIAM A. CATTERALL.

Saxitoxin maintained by the Food and Drug Administration is distributed to scientists upon NIH approval of research applications. The small supply has a melodramatic background. Some time after extraction of the toxin from several tons of Alaskan butter clams (which concentrate the dinoflagellate in their siphons), batches from two laboratories found their way into CIA hands and were cached in Washington, D.C. In September 1975 the Senate Select Committee To Study Governmental Operations With Respect to Intelligence Activities was inquiring into the CIA's failure to destroy certain toxic materials under provisions of the Biological Weapons Convention. Urged by scientists to preserve the saxitoxin as a valuable research tool, the Committee explored the legality of such a move, with

Senator Charles Mathias, Jr., taking the lead. The Committee subsequently persuaded the CIA and the White House to turn the fated batches over to NIH. The Office of Intramural Affairs, Office of the Director, NIH, has responsibility for the saxitoxin distribution program.

The unique properties of histrionicotoxin and its congeners (from the skin of another Colombian frog) were established in collaborative studies with E. X. Albuquerque at the University of Maryland Medical School. These toxins block cholinergic postsynaptic effects, which depend on open channels—i.e., a critical minimum frequency of stimulation. The stimulation may be electrical or iontophoretic, but histrionicotoxin at micromolar concentrations that block the effects of iontophoretic acetylcholine does not alter the responses to spontaneously released acetylcholine from presynaptic vesicles. This observation is crucial in interpreting the effects of direct and indirect stimulation in neuro- and electrophysiology experiments.

Histrionicotoxin has been shown to inhibit the uptake of radioactive sodium by chick embryo muscle cells in tissue culture. This suggests that the toxin inhibits the nicotinic receptors by causing an increase in their affinity for agonists. Acting on the desensitized receptors, the toxin appears to stabilize the desensitized state.

The subject of such selective toxins is as fascinating as it is inexhaustible. For the opportunities to be realized, the time must often be right and the stage set by requisite advances in molecular biology.

Our latest "magic bullet" is an unusual tropane alkaloid, anatoxin-a, from blue fresh-water algae. This is an ideal agonist for nicotinic acetylcholine receptors. It is close to acetylcholine, the natural neurotransmitter, with regard to the opening time of the ion conductor channel (1.5 msec).

Control of ion transport by such novel agents has therapeutic implications for the future, inasmuch as neurotransmitters are suspected to be at the source of psychic disorders, sleep patterns, and memory.

From False Transmitters to
Chemical Sympathectomy

SIRO SENOH, my first collaborator from Japan, began a study in 1959 on nonenzymatic conversions of dopamine to norepinephrine (NE) and trihydroxyphenethylamines. What started out as a basic study in organic chemistry has led to one of the most interesting developments in the field of catecholamines.

The "Senoh-Witkop amine" (6-hydroxydopamine, or 2,4,5-trihydroxyphenethylamine) serves in low concentrations as a false transmitter—as an amine mimicking NE, replacing and releasing it from storage sites (e.g., in mouse heart). In higher concentrations the amine first impairs transmission functionally, then produces degeneration of the nerve terminal. We have shown that 6-hydroxydopamine has a very low oxidation potential and easily forms aminochromes. This instability confounds detection of the Senoh-Witkop amine as a labile metabolite of dopamine.

The Senoh-Witkop amine has been invoked in a hypothesis on the etiology of certain mental disorders. It is held that reduced activity of the enzyme dopamine β-hydroxylase results in release and autoxidation of dopamine, damaging adrenergic terminals and thus leading to schizophrenia, manic depression, or Parkinsonism. So far this hypothesis has not found much acceptance. An alternative process might be considered: enzymatic m-O-methylation of 6-hydroxydopamine by catechol-O-methyltransferase. The potential metabolite 2,4-dihydroxy-5-methoxyphenethylamine and the corresponding analog 6-hydroxynormetanephrine are much more stable than oxidation products of dopamine, and are isomeric with metabolites of mescaline (by demethylation) or of the false transmitter 3,4,5-trihydroxyphenethylamine (by remethylation).

Electron microscopy and tritiated substrates (compounds tagged with ^{3}H, or tritium, a radioisotope of hydrogen) enabled H. THOENEN and his collaborators to demonstrate that 6-hydroxydopamine can selectively destroy adrenergic neurons. This chemical sympathectomy provides a valuable new tool for investigation of the physiology and pharmacology of neurons, both peripheral and central. These findings led to the First International Symposium on 6-Hydroxydopamine in 1971.

Extending the above observations, H. G. Baumgarten and later JOHN W. DALY and Creveling created hydroxyserotonin derivatives capable of damaging serotonergic nerve centers.

[See Cohen's chapter, "Studies on the Etiology of Schizophrenia," and Kopin's on "Neurotransmitters and Neuropsychopharmacology."]

The Labile Metabolites

The challenge in studying labile metabolites is their instability and thus their brief, sometimes momentary life in vivo. My own interest in these evanescent metabolic products started with the synthesis of formylkynurenine by ozonization of tryptophan (1944) and the synthesis of 5- and 7-hydroxytryptophans (1953), the former of which is a substrate for aromatic decarboxylase (18). There was no reason to suspect in those days that hydroxylation of tryptophan to 5-hydroxy-tryptophan by soluble hydroxylases, or of tryptamine to 6-hydroxytryptamine by particle-bound microsomal hydroxyl-ases, involved a shift of hydrogen from positions 5 to 4 and 6 to 7, respectively. The rearrangement of a carbon skeleton by migration and degradation of the pyruvic acid side chain from p-hydroxyphenyl pyruvic to homogentisic acid is probably the first example of the rearrangement that Udenfriend later called the "NIH shift."

The NIH shift was an accidental discovery (see Figure 2). The search for a rapid, clinically useful assay of phenyl-alanine hydroxylase, the enzyme deficient in phenylketonurics, led Daly to the synthesis of p-[^{3}H]phenylalanine and the realization that the enzymatically formed tyrosine still re-tained more than 90 percent of its radioactivity. This obser-vation, at first interpreted as an experimental error, was confirmed after the advent of NMR (nuclear magnetic resonance) techniques and instrumentation. Repetition of the experiments with p-[^{2}H]phenylalanine gave m-[^{2}H]tyrosine with 60 percent retention of deuterium.

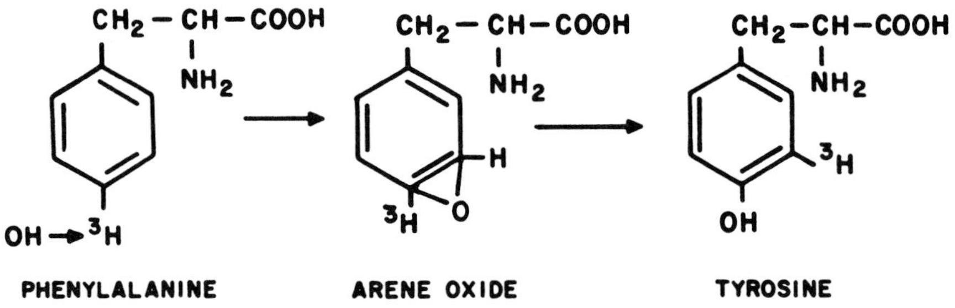

PHENYLALANINE   ARENE OXIDE   TYROSINE

FIGURE 2. The NIH shift was discovered in the search for a rapid assay for phenylalanine hydroxylase, a soluble enzyme system that converts the amino acid phenylalanine to tyrosine (parahydroxyphenylalanine). Genetic deficiency of the enzyme results in phenylketonuria, which can cause extreme mental re-tardation if not detected and treated. In metabolic hydroxyl-ation of phenylalanine, OH was thought to replace the H in the para position. But in an experimental hydroxylation of phenyl-alanine labeled with the radioisotope tritium (^{3}H), the re-sultant tyrosine was found to contain 90 percent of the ^{3}H, now shifted to the meta position. The "NIH shift" necessarily involved the formation of an extremely reactive (and poten-tially dangerous) intermediate, an arene oxide.

What started as serendipity was carried on by design. NIH scientists showed that arene oxides were substrates for the soluble hydrases of supernatant from liver microsomes. Up to that time, arene oxides were a chemical curiosity believed incapable of existence or too unstable to be isolated. The pioneer in their preparation was Emanuel Vogel in Cologne, who derided my request for a sample of the newly prepared 1,2-naphthalene oxide and my contention that this labile compound should be an intermediate in the enzymatic conversion of naphthalene to α-naphthol by liver microsomes. The discovery is now well known and affords one of the classical transformations proving the NIH shift (19).

Cancer-Inducing Polycyclic Hydrocarbons

Many groups have extended the concept of arene oxides as labile metabolites into drug metabolism, long-range toxicity studies, or the etiology of cancer caused by polycyclic aromatic hydrocarbons (PAHs). The metabolism of the carcinogen benzpyrene, found in smoke and smog, involves activation by mixed-function oxidases. Their role and regulation are being studied in several laboratories (20).

Almost 30 years ago ELIZABETH MILLER and CHARLES HEIDELBERGER showed a covalent binding of PAHs to proteins of mouse skin. There was some correlation between the binding and carcinogenicity, and Boyland speculated that an aromatic epoxide might be the reactive intermediate. After much investigation, however, the protein binding theory of carcinogenesis faded into the background for lack of evidence.

A major step forward was a 1964 report of correlation between the carcinogenic potency of benzpyrene and its level of covalent binding to mouse skin DNA (20). Until 1968 the metabolism of the carcinogen was generally believed to be merely a detoxification process unrelated to the carcinogenic action. This view was due largely to the fact that all the metabolites then known were noncarcinogenic.

Benzpyrene and similar PAHs are metabolized by liver microsomes in the presence of certain cofactors. The effective enzyme system was first called mixed-function oxidase or aryl hydrocarbon hydroxylase. This same kind of system was eventually solubilized, revealing the NIH shift in tagged (tritiated, deuterated, or halogenated) aromatic substrates. Intermediate, highly reactive arene oxides are involved.

At this time the new method of high-pressure liquid chromatography (HPLC) was introduced, first by HARRY V. GELBOIN, NCI, then by DONALD M. JERINA, formerly of the Laboratory of Chemistry. More than 40 metabolites of the PAHs were isolated. These included seven phenols, three not previously characterized; several diols; and a number of glucuronide, glutathione, and sulfate conjugates.

Research in this field was handicapped by the unavailability of PAH metabolites or derivatives. At NCI Gelboin developed a program, engaging J. F. Engel's and D. J. McCaustland's laboratory at Midwest Research and R. G. Harvey's at the University of Chicago, to produce these compounds for distribution to the general scientific community. More than 150 compounds synthesized by these laboratories and by Jerina and HARUHIKO YAGI were widely distributed. Since then, NCI has met requests for 3000 samples a year. The key intermediates of activation, the trans-diol and the diol epoxides, were first synthesized by McCaustland and Engel.

Six phenols, three diols, and the diol epoxides were tested for mutagenic activity. Gelboin published the first report showing that the diol epoxides were super mutagens— i.e., at least 1000 times more mutagenic than any of the other known metabolites. He investigated whether they were indeed formed by mammalian tissue. Using liver microsomes and HPLC, he isolated three optically active trans-diol intermediates, demonstrating the stereospecificity of the microsomal reactions.

What matters for the etiology of cancer is the effect of these highly specific arene oxide metabolites on DNA. Nucleophilic amino groups of guanine and, to a lesser degree, adenine residues open these epoxides to form covalent bonds. Such adducts have been studied and reported by Weinstein, TSUYOSHI KAKEFUDA (NCI), Calvin, Jerina, P. Brookes, ALAN M. JEFFREY, and others. PETER A. CERUTTI, a former member of the Laboratory of Chemistry, has classified the role of DNA repair enzymes.

The major current trend deals with the molecular biology of the process. How does the diol epoxide affect gene expression, the nature of the induced mutations, and gene transpositions? Monoclonal antibodies are used to identify specific enzymes determining metabolic pathways and may help to elucidate the genetic basis for carcinogen susceptibility.

A Chemist's Approach to
the Interferon Problem

Interferon is a natural substance produced by virus-infected mammalian cells in response to various natural or synthetic inducers. It is known to have antiviral and anti-tumor activity in animals and humans. Interferon occurs in minute amounts and shows species specificity. Until recently its scarcity severely hampered biomedical applications. Hence, the production of human interferon by recombinant DNA technology has generated much excitement, and fundamental studies on its mode of action are under way in many laboratories.

Interferon has been shown to induce two new proteins in cells. One of these is a kinase that phosphorylates eukaryotic initiation-factor 2 and thus blocks protein synthesis. The other, an enzyme called 2-5A synthetase, responds to stimulation with double-stranded RNA (an intermediate of RNA virus replication) to produce the trinucleotide 2-5A.* This substance, of a kind unique in nature, activates a latent cellular endoribonuclease, which degrades messenger RNA and thus inhibits protein synthesis.

PAUL TORRENCE and his associates in the Laboratory of Chemistry have synthesized 2-5A and derivatives. One of the latter, though not itself an inhibitor of protein synthesis, antagonizes 2-5A action. This derivative was used in extracts from interferon-treated cells to demonstrate that the 2-5A enzyme complex indeed inhibits protein synthesis generated by double-stranded RNA. Thus, it appears that interferon acts chiefly through the 2-5A system to block viral and tumor activity. The question arises, Could 2-5A be used directly, bypassing the interferon system? This could provide a new approach to virus chemotherapy and perhaps to the control of tumor cell growth and the immune mechanism, to the extent that 2-5A is involved in interferon's corrective functions.

Two fundamental problems arise. First, 2-5A has a short biological half-life and must be modified for greater durability. Second, it is not readily taken up by intact cells because of its negatively charged character and must be converted to a more lipophilic form. A newly synthesized analog of 2-5A is 10 times more active than the naturally occurring agonist, probably as a result of its increased lifespan. Continued application of chemical principles in this context may have therapeutic potential.

The theme of small molecules with large effects—i.e., agonists and regulators—is capable of many variations. Here is the "chink in the wall" that allows chemists to use their synthetic skills to advantage in the study of reactions proceeding through membranes.

Epilogue

Chemistry, especially in a biomedical environment, has become an ancillary science. Isolation, structure, and syn-

---

*5'-O-triphosphoryl-adenylyl(2',5'-adenylyl)2',5'-adenosine.

218   BERNHARD WITKOP

thesis of new natural products are prologue. The drama un-
folds when these children of nature—often venoms, toxins,
poisons—are used by man to probe the dynamics of life in
other systems. Many scientific disciplines are brought into
play. Yet the essentials of the marvelous phenomenon that
is life become more and more understandable in one language
only—that of organic chemistry.

References

1. Committee for the Survey of Chemistry, National Academy
   of Sciences. Basic Chemical Research in Government Laboratories, pp. 41-49. Washington: NAS-NRC, 1966 (56 pp.).
2. Witkop, B. Paul Ehrlich—His ideas and his legacy. In
   Proceedings, Nobel Foundation Symposium, Karlskoga, Sweden, 1981. Naturwissenschaftliche Rundschau 34:361-379,
   1981.
3. Horecker, B.L. Unraveling the pentose phosphate pathway. In Reflections on Biochemistry (pp. 65-72), A.
   Kornberg et al. (eds.). Oxford and New York: Pergamon,
   1976.
4. Witkop, B. Heinrich Wieland Centennial: His lifework
   and his legacy today. Angew Chem (international ed.)
   16:559-572, 1977.
5. Witkop, B. Erich Mosettig. Proc Chem Soc (London), Nov.
   1964, pp. 376-377.
6. May, E. Reminiscences and musings of a classical medicinal chemist. J Med Chem 23:225-232, 1980.
7. Mello, N.K., and J.H. Mendelson. Buprenorphine suppres-
   ses heroin use by heroin addicts. Science 207:657-659,
   1980.
8. Jasinski, D.R., J.S. Pevnick, and J.D. Griffith. Human
   pharmacology and abuse potential of the analgesic buprenorphine: A potential agent for treating narcotic addiction. Arch Gen Psychiatry 35:501-516, 1978.
9. Merz, H., and K. Stockhaus. N-[(Tetrahydrofuryl)alkyl]
   and N-(alkoxyalkyl) derivatives of (-)-normetazocine,
   compounds with differentiated action profiles. J Med
   Chem 22:1475-1483, 1979.
10. Atwell, L., and A.E. Jacobson. The search for less harm-
    ful analgesics, pp. 43-47. Lab Anim, Sept.-Oct. 1978.
11. Rice, K.C. Synthetic opium alkaloids and derivatives.
    A short total synthesis of (±)-dihydrothebainone, (±)-
    dihydrocodeinone, and (±)-nordihydrocodeinone as an ap-
    proach to a practical synthesis of morphine, codeine,
    and congeners. J Org Chem 45:3135-3137, 1980.

12. Axelrod, J. Fluorescence News (Silver Spring, Md.: American Instrument Company) 8:1, 1974.
13. Udenfriend, S. Fluorescence assay in biology and medicine, Vols. I and II. New York: Academic Press, 1962, 1969.
14. Witkop, B. The chemist's magic bullets. In Science and Scientists, pp. 351-360; M. Kageyama et al. (eds). Tokyo: Japan Scientific Press, 1981.
15. Witkop, B. Nonenzymatic methods for the preferential and selective cleavage and modifications of proteins. Adv Protein Chem 16:221-321, New York: Academic Press, 1961.
16. Maxam, A.M., and W. Gilbert. A new method for sequencing DNA. Proc Natl Acad Sci USA 74:560-564, 1977. [A fuller and highly instructive presentation is given in Gilbert's Nobel Lecture, December 8, 1980: Les Prix Nobel, pp. 120-138. Stockholm: Almquist & Wiksell, International, 1981.]
17. Witkop, B. New directions in the chemistry of natural products: The organic chemist as a pathfinder for biochemistry and medicine. Experientia 10:1121, 1971.
18. Witkop, B. Forty years of trypto-fun. Heterocycles 20: 2059-2075, 1983. Summarizes the attempts to catch and characterize labile tryptophan metabolites.
19. Guroff, G., et al. Hydroxylation-induced intramolecular migrations: The NIH shift. Science 158:1524-1530, Sept. 1967.
20. Gelboin, H.V., and P.O.P. Ts'o. Polycyclic Hydrocarbons and Cancer, Vol. 3. New York: Academic Press, Inc., 1981.

DEVELOPMENT OF ENZYMOLOGY

The origins of the National Institutes of Health are rooted in the study of infectious diseases, and for this reason there was greater emphasis on microbiology than on biochemistry in the early days. Prominent biochemists, however, were members of the Hygienic Laboratory. These included WILLIAM MANSFIELD CLARK, a major contributor to the study of the hydrogen ion concentration and the oxidation-reduction potential, and CLAUDE HUDSON, a sugar chemist of high distinction.

Despite the important contributions of some eighteenth century scientists such as Lavoisier and Priestley, the development of biochemistry depended upon the concurrent growth of organic chemistry, and this occurred mostly in Germany. It is therefore not surprising that the preeminent school of biochemists were largely Germanic, including Embden, Meyerhof, Von Euler, Lohmann, Schuster, and a host of others. In the United States biochemistry grew slowly at first, but received a strong impetus as a result of the immigration of scientists from Germany just before and during World War II.

Once started, the science grew rapidly in many countries. In the NIH Clinical Center, one can see biochemical equipment in use and biochemical procedures under way in almost every laboratory module. Biochemistry has become a tool fundamental to most other approaches in biomedical science, and biochemists abound in all of the Institutes.

The chief peculiarity that distinguishes biochemistry from the rest of chemistry is the fact that chemical reactions occurring in living tissues are almost always catalyzed. The catalysts of biochemistry are called enzymes. So far all enzymes have been found to be proteins, and a vast number of them have been discovered, studied, named, and cataloged over the past half-century. Many have been isolated in a high state of purity, and the detailed structures of a few have been determined. Much of biochemical research today involves such enzymology.

Typical questions confronting the enzymologist include, Is the enzyme constitutive or is it induced? Is it highly *specific or does it act on a variety of substrates? What cofactors, if any, are required to elicit maximum catalytic activity? What factors regulate the amount and activity of enzymes and how do they perform their function?*

It has often developed that the product of one enzymatic reaction serves as the substrate for another, and if such relations recur we have what is termed a metabolic pathway. Such was the classical glycolytic pathway delineated by Embden and Meyerhof and the tricarboxylic acid cycle discovered by Krebs. The following pages recount the investigation of the pentose phosphate pathway, which was largely worked out by BERNARD HORECKER at NIH.

The reader will also find accounts of other early investigations in three NIH laboratories largely dedicated to the pursuit of enzymology. Later work is described in many other chapters. It is hoped that these early examples of NIH biochemical research will give the lay reader a sense of what biochemistry is and what the biochemist does. The scientist may find them interesting as history.

D. S.

12

DEVELOPMENT OF ENZYMOLOGY

I. Early Enzymological Research

Herbert Tabor

Enzymological research at the National Institutes of Health started with the work of SANFORD ROSENTHAL and CARL VOEGTLIN in the early 1930s in the Hygienic Laboratory at 25th and E Streets, N.W., Washington, D.C. They were concerned with the importance of heavy metals in the oxidation of sulfhydryl groups, particularly those of glutathione. Little work in the discipline, however, was carried out at NIH until the early 1940s, when an enzymological research program began in the National Cancer Institute. ALTON MEISTER describes that program in an accompanying section.

A little later, enzymological research was instituted in another NIH laboratory by BERNARD HORECKER. He had published, with Haas and Hogness, an important paper on a new "yellow enzyme," cytochrome *c* reductase. Horecker was extremely well-trained in modern enzymology, and his background and experience with enzyme purification surpassed that available in most departments of biochemistry in the United States. When he first came to NIH, he worked in the Division of Industrial Hygiene, part of which was later incorporated into the Experimental Biology and Medicine Institute (EBMI). He was assigned certain war-related problems, such as detection of CO-hemoglobin in blood and the metabolism of DDT. For the CO-hemoglobin project, he employed an automatic recording spectrophotometer constructed by FREDERICK BRACKETT. This instrument, then the only one of its kind in the world, enabled him to discover the infrared bands of hemoglobin.

Immediately after the war Horecker returned to enzymatic research. He recognized the advantage of the spectrophotometer and the opportunity it afforded enzymologists to perform

HERBERT TABOR, M.D., Chief, Laboratory of Biochemical Pharmacology, National Institute of Arthritis, Diabetes, and Digestive and Kidney Diseases.

rapid, multiple assays and kinetic analyses, where formerly
they had depended on single colorimetric determinations or
cumbersome manometric measurements. The Beckman spectrophotometer was still hard to obtain, since it had just been
introduced, and the only one at NIH was available to Horecker
in Building 2.

Meanwhile, in Building 4, the Division of Physiology
(later incorporated into EBMI) was engaged in various nutritional studies. ARTHUR KORNBERG, working with FLOYD DAFT and
W. HENRY SEBRELL, was involved in establishing the importance
of folic acid in blood regeneration. On assignment as a Commissioned Officer of the Public Health Service, he had arrived
at NIH in 1942 after serving as a medical officer in the Coast
Guard. Earlier he had studied the occurrence of jaundice
(later recognized as Gilbert's disease) in normal medical students at the University of Rochester School of Medicine, but
had had no formal research training.

Kornberg's nutritional studies were very productive, and
he was most enthusiastic about his work and the techniques
used. However, at a Gibson Island Conference (later called
Gordon Conference) on vitamins, he heard of the exciting work
of E. E. Snell, D. W. Woolley, and I. C. Gunsalus in defining
the role of pyridoxal phosphate as a coenzyme. He immediately
realized the potential of enzymatic approaches to the study
of metabolism. Deciding to gain expertise in enzymology, he
asked NIH to send him to an enzyme laboratory for additional
training—a most unusual request, for NIH usually trained its
investigators within the institution. Credit should be given
to Sebrell, Daft, and ROLLA DYER (Director of NIH at the time)
for realizing the merit of Kornberg's request, even though
they were not personally experienced in enzymology. They
agreed to support him for a few months' stay with Severo Ochoa
at New York University, and the visit was stretched to a year.
He then spent some eight months with Carl and Gerty Cori at
Washington University in St. Louis.

Typically, Kornberg had felt that it was important for him
to become familiar with the enzymatic literature and techniques *before* he went to Ochoa and the Coris, so as not to
waste precious time in those laboratories. He arranged to work
first with Horecker for six months, and this was the beginning
of a long and fruitful association.

NIH was a small institution in the early 1940s, and appointments were infrequent. In particular, only a few new
Commissioned Officers came each year (probably fewer than
three). All were M.D.'s and usually had little research experience; they were assigned to NIH shortly after their internship. One exception was LEON A. HEPPEL.

Heppel had done an outstanding study on the substitution

of Na$^+$ for K$^+$ in the tissues of animals on a K$^+$-free diet, as part of his Ph.D. studies with C.L.A. Schmidt at the University of California at Berkeley. After receiving his Ph.D., he entered medical school at the University of Rochester (where he and Kornberg were classmates and close friends). There he held a part-time fellowship with Wallace Fenn and carried out pioneer studies on the electrolytes of muscle. He was among the first to establish, contrary to prevailing views, that both Na$^+$ and K$^+$ could cross a biological membrane. After his graduation from medical school and his internship, Heppel came to NIH in 1942 and was assigned to work under PAUL NEAL in the Division of Industrial Hygiene. He was an indefatigable worker and quickly completed a variety of studies on the toxicity of chlorinated hydrocarbons. After the end of the war, he directed these studies toward enzymatic work on the dehalogenation process, performing experiments that are still classic in the field.

Since Horecker, Kornberg, and Heppel were good friends and the only established biochemical investigators in EBMI, it was natural that they should have lunch together frequently and discuss their experiments. I was pleased to join them and participate in their enthusiastic discussions. We soon converted these spontaneous meetings into a more formal journal club. Each day, at lunch, one of us would report in depth on a paper or a series of papers. A luncheon seminar was most unusual at that time, and our colleagues predicted that we would all develop ulcers. Fortunately, they were wrong.

The formal presentations were constantly interrupted by a multitude of questions. We were intent on learning as much as possible about the new and exciting work being done in enzymology. I remember, in particular, one series of daily meetings in which we covered each paper in Warburg's *Die Schwermetallen*. More important than the formal presentations was the opportunity to discuss our own work and the papers in the literature.

After several months in Horecker's laboratory, Kornberg went to New York, where he studied the enzymatic decarboxylation of β-keto acids and participated in the discovery of the "malic" enzyme responsible for converting malic to lactic acid. In St. Louis, in the course of studies of aerobic phosphorylation, he became interested in coenzyme metabolism and the biological role of inorganic pyrophosphate.

Just before Kornberg returned to Bethesda, a rather unusual event occurred at NIH. The scientists in Building 2, including Horecker and Heppel, were told that their jobs were abolished, since the positions were needed for a new PHS laboratory of industrial toxicology in Cincinnati. It should be emphasized that such administrative catastrophes have been surprisingly rare at NIH; and this one, fortunately, was swiftly resolved, with an important outcome for enzymology at NIH. It permitted Kornberg to persuade Sebrell, Director of EBMI (and later of NIH), to organize a unit in the Institute with Kornberg as Chief and Horecker and Heppel as independent investigators. The group moved into new quarters on the first floor of Building 3 and started what proved to be an extremely productive phase of research in enzymology.

A few of us still remember the three scientists, Horecker, Heppel, and Kornberg, carting equipment and chemicals from Building 2 to Building 3 on New Year's Eve 1948 while a Commissioned Officers' dance was in full swing in Wilson Hall. It was hard to be selective on a cold winter's night, with the result that the new quarters were stocked not only with useful reagents but also with an exotic collection of chromium, molybdenum, uranium, and other metal salts used for toxicological studies. Many years later Heppel discovered a young man, recently arrived from Iran, in the enzyme section stockroom carefully copying down the names of all these odd salts, which still remained on the shelves. He had been sent there by MARSHALL NIRENBERG, who thought that a fine way to start his new enzyme chemistry laboratory would be to inventory this particular stockroom and duplicate it.

The daily seminar discussions continued with even greater intensity, especially since Kornberg could now contribute from the background he had received during his work with Ochoa and the Coris. The intensity of the group's interest was in evidence the day we all lined up on F Street, at 7:30 a.m., to buy tickets to the Budapest Quartet concert at the Library of Congress. Heppel presented an entire seminar as we stood in line, thus enabling us to work through the lunch hour and compensate for the time spent in obtaining tickets. (The topic was Jacob Stekol's work on methyl group transfer.) The luncheon seminar also served as a convenient forum for talks by the many visitors who came to Bethesda to consult with Kornberg, Horecker, and Heppel.

Kornberg recently told me of a visit he had about 1949 from Gerty Cori, who was in Washington for a committee meeting. She expressed concern for his having a promising scientific career blunted by being relegated to a government laboratory. He tried to explain, perhaps unsuccessfully, that her concerns were unwarranted—that his place and group at NIH provided an excellent academic environment. Time has certainly proved his evaluation to be correct.

During the next few years, the work of this group was extensive, and we were all excited by the interesting results obtained in a variety of fields with the newly developing enzymatic techniques. Although each person worked on his own problem, there was a continual interchange of ideas, techniques, and materials. An important aspect of this cooperation was our preparation in NIH laboratories of large amounts of coenzymes and enzymes for use as reagents, since they were unavailable commercially.

The collaborative studies of these three investigators illustrate the value of their association. In one of these studies, Horecker and Heppel purified xanthine oxidase and discovered that it catalyzed the reduction of cytochrome c, but only in the presence of oxygen. The observation later led Fridovich and Handler at Duke University to discover the role of superoxide anion in biological systems. Horecker and Heppel also succeeded in isolating the NAD* and NADP** cytochrome c reductases from mammalian liver. A short time later Horecker and Kornberg collaborated in the publication of a classic paper on the extinction coefficients of NAD and NADP—information requisite to quantitative enzymological work with these coenzymes.

It was during this period that Horecker developed the concept of the pentose pathway and the hexose monophosphate shunt. He has summarized these experiments and discoveries in the following section.

Meanwhile Kornberg carried out his important work on the enzymatic synthesis of the coenzymes NAD, NADP, and FAD.*** WILLIAM PRICER served as a research assistant and ANTHONY SCHRECKER as a postdoctoral fellow. From these studies emerged the structural assignment of the third phosphate of NADP, the concept of pyrophosphorolysis, and above all, the impetus to explore the biosynthesis of nucleic acids and their nucleotide precursors.

There were other notable developments in Kornberg's work during this lively interval (1948-1952). He studied NAD-dependent isocitric dehydrogenase, enzymatic synthesis of phospholipids, and adenosine kinase. With the assistance of postdoctoral fellows, he studied pyrimidine metabolism by means of enzymes obtained from enrichment culture (OSAMU HAYAISHI), the biosynthesis of orotic acid (IRVING LIEBERMAN), and choline kinase (JONATHAN WITTENBERG). In 1959, only seven years after leaving NIH, Kornberg was awarded the Nobel Prize in medicine.

Heppel's main work in the early period included discoveries of the enzymatic metabolism, in vitro, of such toxic and pharmacological agents as halogenated hydrocarbons, inorganic nitrite, and nitroglycerine. Studies on the purifica-

_____

*NAD: nicotinamide adenine dinucleotide.
**NADP: nicotinamide adenine dinucleotide phosphate.
***FAD: flavin adenine dinucleotide.

tion and properties of yeast inorganic pyrophosphatase, 5'-nucleotidase, and pork liver nucleases led rather naturally to an interest in ribonucleic acid (RNA) biochemistry. Stimulated by reports of exciting new discoveries in Todd's and Markham and Smith's laboratories, Heppel spent a sabbatical year in England in 1953. There he carried out pioneer studies that helped to establish the nature of the internucleotide linkage in RNA. He also demonstrated polynucleotide synthesis via a transnucleotidation catalyzed by ribonucleases.

After his return to NIH Heppel spent the next 11 years on RNA biochemistry. The enzymatic techniques and tools he developed during this period were invaluable aids in subsequent studies at NIH and elsewhere on RNA biosynthesis and the nature of the genetic code. His associates were RUSSELL HILMOE, VIRGINIA PORTERFIELD, WILLIAM BYRNE, and HENRY KAPLAN (of Stanford University).

I was in another laboratory in Building 4 with Sanford Rosenthal, working on the electrolyte changes in traumatic shock and burns* and, subsequently, on the metabolism of histamine. Stimulated by the activities of the Heppel-Horecker-Kornberg group, I purified diamine oxidase (histaminase) and demonstrated the in vitro and in vivo conversion of histamine to imidazoleacetic acid and its riboside. These studies were later extended (with Hayaishi and ALAN MEHLER) to the enzymes involved in histidine metabolism. We showed that urocanic acid and formiminoglutamate were intermediates in the metabolism of histidine, and (with JESSE RABINOWITZ) that folic acid was involved in the further metabolism of formiminoglutamate.

Although Rosenthal's background was in pharmacology, he

---

*I was particularly fortunate to be able to work with Rosenthal on these studies, which provided the experimental basis for the present treatment of traumatic and burn shock. Rosenthal's work showed the importance of fluid and electrolytes and led to the recommendation that therapy should emphasize the administration of large amounts of saline (particularly the Na^+) rather than plasma during the acute shock period. My experiments were largely concerned with studying the mechanism of these therapeutic findings—namely, the demonstration that large changes occur in the Na^+, K^+, and water content of traumatized tissues. Subsequently, Rosenthal continued these studies with R. CARL MILLICAN and KEHL MARKLEY. The work was very controversial at the time, since accepted therapy was based on the concept that replacement of plasma protein was the important aim. Subsequent studies have proved Rosenthal correct, and current treatment within 24 hours after a serious burn involves the administration of large amounts of saline without plasma.

was always interested in new ideas and new techniques. He believed that the best postdoctoral training was obtained by doing independent work. As an example, when JACK STROMINGER joined our group with no prior laboratory experience, Rosenthal encouraged him to work on his own problem. This was the beginning of Strominger's well-known studies on uridine nucleotides and the mechanism of penicillin action. Subsequently, LEONARD WARREN joined our laboratory and carried out his studies on sialic acid, ROBERT SCHIMKE initiated his work on the factors regulating the levels of enzymes in mammalian tissues, and BRUCE AMES continued his investigation of histidine biosynthesis.

In 1948 the National Heart Institute was founded, and a large number of promising young investigators arrived from various universities. CHRISTIAN B. ANFINSEN, EARL and THRESSA STADTMAN, and DANIEL STEINBERG were housed temporarily, all in one room, in Kornberg's space in Building 3. The proximity of this group led to an exciting and valuable expansion of our intellectual environment. Earl Stadtman had published his classic work with H. A. BARKER on acetyl phosphate and acetyl coenzyme A and had just spent a postdoctoral year with Fritz Lipmann. The Stadtmans introduced us to the field of anaerobic organisms and their significance for biochemical research. Most important, we all became close friends and exchanged ideas, information, and materials.

Kornberg left NIH in 1953 to become Chairman of the Department of Microbiology at Washington University in St. Louis. Horecker stayed at NIH until 1959, and Heppel until 1967. After Heppel left, GILBERT ASHWELL took his place as Chief of the Laboratory of Biochemistry and Metabolism. I continued to work in the Laboratory of Pharmacology in Building 4.

During the entire period, we were fortunate to be associated with many visitors and postdoctoral fellows, most of whom are now well-known investigators in biochemistry. The seminar group, which continued to have representatives from both the Building 3 laboratory (later in Building 10) and the Building 4 laboratory, included over the years Ames, Ashwell, SIMON BLACK, Byrne, ROBERTA COLMAN, GAVIN CROWLEY, ANTHONY FURANO, VICTOR GINSBURG, Hayaishi, EDWARD HEATH, HOWARD HIATT, JERARD HURWITZ, WILLIAM JAKOBY, GRAHAM JAMIESON, HERMAN KALCKAR, Kaplan, CLAUDE KLEE, LEONARD KOHN, DAVID KORN, KIYOSHI KURAHASHI, LORETTA L. LEIVE, MARIE LIPSETT, PAUL MARKS, ROBERT MARTIN, Mehler, EDITH MILES, HAROLD NEU, NANCY NOSSAL, Rabinowitz, Schimke, JAY SEEGMILLER, MAXINE SINGER, Strominger, CELIA TABOR, Warren, REED WICKNER, and others.

Subsequently many groups have been involved in enzymological research at NIH in addition to those mentioned in this section. The techniques of enzymology became widespread, and enzymological studies form the basis of many of the investigations reported in other chapters of this book.

In considering the evolution of enzymology and biochemistry at NIH, it is pertinent to consider aspects of the milieu that led to their explosive expansion. What factors contributed to NIH's position as one of the most outstanding institutions in these areas? The most important, of course, was the recruitment of a number of gifted, dynamic investigators. For a variety of reasons, most of which are beyond the scope of this article, they were interested in biomedical research —especially biochemistry and enzymology—and wanted to come to NIH. University departments were still small and poorly funded, and NIH was particularly attractive to graduates of medical schools who wanted to carry out investigative studies but had little if any formal background in this area. Some had read *Arrowsmith* or *Microbe Hunters* in high school—books that had an impact on many young people during the 1920s and 1930s. Others were influenced by traditions of scientific inquiry absorbed during their undergraduate and graduate training. A most important factor was the military draft, since NIH afforded medical graduates an opportunity to do research rather than routine clinical or administrative work. In addition, NIH was expanding at that time and, unlike most universities, was not encumbered by existing departmental structures: new sections could easily be organized and old ones reorganized. NIH was also free of some of the prejudices that were still present in many university departments.

The NIH administration deserves much credit for selecting so many outstanding people. An essential element in the success of NIH during this period was the willingness of its administration under Dyer, Sebrell, and JAMES A. SHANNON to support these new investigators and permit them to work without constraints or concern for immediate practical implications. Their productivity proved the wisdom of this policy.

Finally, of course, we cannot separate the developments at NIH from the dramatic expansion of biochemistry and enzymology elsewhere, largely as a result of the NIH extramural program and congressional funding of basic research. Not only were NIH investigators influenced by publications from other laboratories, but they encouraged visits and communication from investigators throughout the world. One source of contacts was the extramural study section system: members of the study sections would visit colleagues at NIH while meeting in Bethesda. As a result of all these factors, NIH scientists lost their isolation and engaged in a vital, continuing interchange of ideas and personnel with the rest of the academic community.

DEVELOPMENT OF ENZYMOLOGY

II. Elucidation of the
Pentose Phosphate Pathway

Bernard L. Horecker

When these studies were initiated, the glycolytic pathway for the metabolism of carbohydrates had been defined; but another pathway, possibly more important in respiration, appeared to begin with the direct oxidation of glucose 6-phosphate to 6-phosphogluconate, a reaction discovered by OTTO WARBURG many years earlier. Warburg had also shown that 6-phosphogluconate was further oxidized to yield CO_2 and a substance that appeared to be a 5-carbon sugar phosphate. Both of these oxidations required TPN (NADP), which was then thought to be the coenzyme of respiration. [TPN = triphosphopyridine nucleotide, now called NADP = nicotinamide adenine dinucleotide phosphate.]

Neither TPN nor 6-phosphogluconate was then commercially available. ARTHUR KORNBERG needed the coenzyme for studies on isocitrate metabolism, and in 1948 we collaborated in a crash program, working around the clock, to prepare a stock of it. We owned the world's supply of TPN and were flattered to fill a request for 25 mg from Warburg himself. Phosphogluconate was also prepared, and I was ready to begin the study of its oxidation by an enzyme as yet unknown, to be called 6-phosphogluconate dehydrogenase. After months of frustration, a preparation was finally available that yielded quantities of CO_2 and pentose phosphate stoichiometric to the quantities of 6-phosphogluconate consumed. The studies were made possible by the knowledge of the precise extinction coefficient of TPN, established earlier in collaboration with Kornberg. My collaborator during all of this work was PAULINE SMYRNIOTIS, who is still at NIH. We were joined by HANS

BERNARD L. HORECKER, Ph.D., Head, Laboratory of Molecular Enzymology, Roche Institute of Molecular Biology. Formerly Chief, Laboratory of Biochemistry and Metabolism, National Institute of Arthritis and Metabolic Diseases.

KLENOW, my first postdoctoral fellow, who participated in the early work on the pentose phosphate pathway.

Identification of the pentose phosphate required its separation from other components of the reaction mixture. During a visit to Oak Ridge, Kornberg observed Waldo Cohn's beautiful nucleotide separations achieved by the new technique of ion-exchange chromatography. Kornberg suggested that I use this to isolate the pentose phosphate formed from 6-phosphogluconate. His valuable suggestion led to the separation of two pentose esters, one formed very early in the reaction and later identified as a new pentose phosphate, D-ribulose 5-phosphate, and the other as the sugar previously identified in nucleotides, D-ribose 5-phosphate. The time course established ribulose 5-phosphate as the first product of 6-phosphogluconate oxidation and led to the discovery of another new enzyme, pentose phosphate isomerase.

Dische had shown that ribose phosphate from nucleotides was converted to triose and hexose phosphates. The next goal was the isolation of the enzyme(s) that catalyzed this conversion and the elucidation of the mechanisms involved. Almost simultaneously, our laboratory and Racker's at the Public Health Research Institute in New York isolated a new enzyme, later named transketolase, and showed that it contained thiamin pyrophosphate.

One product of the reaction was glyceraldehyde 3-phosphate, but the fate of the 2-carbon fragment remained unknown. A clue to its identity was provided by Calvin's discovery of the 7-carbon sugar sedoheptulose phosphate as a product of CO_2-fixation in plants. On Christmas Eve 1951, a time when even Kornberg and LEON HEPPEL were absent from the laboratory, I succeeded in demonstrating that the product formed from pentose phosphate in the transketolase-catalyzed reaction was identical to an authentic sample of sedoheptulose provided by NELSON RICHTMYER of the NIH Laboratory of Chemistry. The chromatograms with the blue sedoheptulose spot hung on our Christmas tree that evening.

An important intermediate in the conversion of pentose phosphate to sedoheptulose 7-phosphate was xylulose 5-phosphate, which was first isolated and identified in NCI by GILBERT ASHWELL and shown by Racker and by JERARD HURWITZ in our laboratory to be the C_2-donor in the reaction catalyzed by transketolase.

JAY SEEGMILLER in our laboratory had confirmed the formation of hexose phosphate from 6-phosphogluconate, and we assumed that it was derived from sedoheptulose 7-phosphate by removal of the last carbon atom. This, however, proved to be incorrect. Sedoheptulose 7-phosphate, when generated from pentose phosphate, was rapidly converted to hexose-monophosphate, but this did not happen when sedoheptulose 7-phosphate was isolated and added to the same reaction mixture in the absence of pentose phosphate. The requirement for pentose phosphate was traced to the formation of triose phosphate. Then, following a suggestion from H. A. BARKER, working across the hall in Kornberg's laboratory, we were able to demonstrate that hexose phosphate was formed by a three-carbon transfer from sedoheptulose 7-phosphate to glyceraldehyde. With PAUL MARKS and HOWARD HIATT, we identified the other product of the reaction as a new 4-carbon sugar, D-erythrose 4-phosphate. The enzyme was named transaldolase, since it catalyzed the breakage and synthesis of aldol linkages.

To prove that these reactions were really involved in the conversion of pentose phosphate to glucose 6-phosphate, I spent the summer of 1951 at the Brookhaven National Laboratory with Martin Gibbs, who had developed a method for microbiological degradation of glucose to yield each carbon atom in a different product. With this technique we degraded glucose 6-phosphate formed from radioactive precursors—$[1-^{14}C]$—and $[3,4-^{14}C]$-ribose 5-phosphates—and showed that the distribution of carbon in the hexose followed the predictions of the transketolase-transaldolase pathway. To account precisely for the labeling pattern, it was necessary to add one more reaction to this pathway, in which a second molecule of xylulose 5-phosphate donated a C_2 fragment to the erythrose 4-phosphate. Thus three equivalents of pentose phosphate would yield two of hexose phosphate and one of triose phosphate. The prediction of this reaction from the isotope data was later confirmed in Racker's laboratory. The cycle had now been completed and the reactions of the pentose phosphate pathway established.

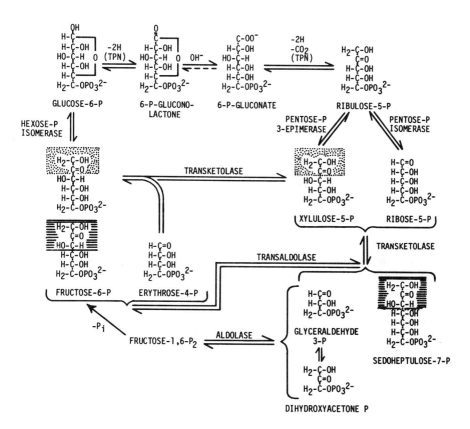

THE PENTOSE PHOSPHATE PATHWAY serves as an important source of sugars and other essential compounds. It is here repre- sented as beginning with (1) oxidation of glucose 6-phosphate by TPN (triphosphopyridine nucleotide) and proceeding through several steps to the formation of (2) a pentose ester, ribu- lose 5-phosphate. This is converted to (3) ribose 5-phosphate and (4) another ester, xylulose 5-phosphate. Ribose 5- phosphate (with the aid of transketolase, an enzyme containing vitamin B_1) yields (5) a seven-carbon sugar, sedoheptulose 7-phosphate, which contributes three carbon atoms to form (6) glyceraldehyde 3-phosphate and (via transaldolase) four carbon atoms to form (7) a sugar, erythrose 4-phosphate. Xylulose 5-phosphate and erythrose 4-phosphate yield (via transketolase) fructose 6-phosphate. Isomerization of the latter (9) yields glucose 6-phosphate, which may now reenter the sequence. The stippled and striped areas represent frag- ments transferred in the transketolase and transaldolase re- actions.

DEVELOPMENT OF ENZYMOLOGY

III. Recollections About Enzymology and Amino Acid Biochemistry at NCI

Alton Meister

I joined the Laboratory of Biochemistry at the National Cancer Institute in 1947. JESSE P. GREENSTEIN, Chief of the Laboratory and the most noted biochemist at NIH at that time (1), had been working on the enzymology of tumors and was beginning to turn his attention to the chemistry and biochemistry of the amino acids and peptides. Amino acid biochemistry expanded rapidly after 1950 (2), and many of the significant new developments came from the NCI intramural program.

The early history of enzymology and amino acid biochemistry at NIH revolves almost entirely about Jesse Greenstein and his group. Before coming to NCI, Greenstein had done research on the chemistry and biochemistry of amino acids, peptides, and proteins in Edwin J. Cohn's laboratory at Harvard and in Max Bergmann's laboratory in Dresden. Bergmann at that time was developing his carbobenzoxy method of peptide synthesis, and Greenstein used this procedure for the preparation of lysylglutamic acid and lysylhistidine. He made fundamental contributions to the physical chemistry of amino acids and peptides. In his work on protein structure and denaturation, he used porphyrindin for determination of the sulfhydryl groups of native and denatured proteins. He discovered the powerful action of guanidinium salts as denaturing agents for proteins and examined the titratable sulfhydryl groups of a number of proteins, such as myosin and egg albumin.

In 1939 CARL VOEGTLIN, the first Director of the National Cancer Institute, offered Greenstein a position with an exceptionally able group, which Greenstein later described as

ALTON MEISTER, M.D., Professor of Biochemistry, Cornell University Medical College. Formerly Section Head, Laboratory of Biochemistry, National Cancer Institute.

"something of a unique experiment in the organization of cancer research. Several independent groups of professional investigators trained in various disciplines, such as pathology,
genetics, physics, and chemistry, were brought together under
one roof and encouraged to undertake voluntarily, on a mutually independent basis, cooperative research on problems
which interested them, and which could only be solved by effort from several directions."

Tumor Enzymology

Greenstein systematically studied many enzyme activities
of a variety of tumors and normal tissues. These investigations led him to conclude, as summarized in his monograph
Biochemistry of Cancer (3), that (a) each normal tissue is
characterized by an individual pattern of enzymatic activities
that serves to distinguish it from other tissues, (b) tumors
possess qualitatively the same enzymes as normal tissues,
(c) a tumor's pattern of enzyme activity is largely independent of its age, growth rate, and the strain of the host, and
(d) the functional activities of normal tissues decrease or
disappear when they become neoplastic. The range of enzymatic
values for tumors usually lies between the extremes for the
corresponding normal tissues, and is much narrower among tumors. Greenstein concluded that tumors tend to converge, enzymatically, to a common type of tissue.

His findings and the conclusions he drew from them, which
are supported by later work, constitute a classic landmark in
the field of cancer research. These generalizations apply also
to the well-known earlier work of OTTO WARBURG, who discovered
the characteristic high aerobic glycolysis of tumors. As Sidney Weinhouse has pointed out (4), tumors consume oxygen at
rates that fall within the wide ranges displayed by the normal
tissues of origin and apparently possess the same electron
transport systems that occur in those tissues. They can carry
out oxidation of glucose and fatty acids at rates that are
well within the normal ranges.

Greenstein also observed that tumors produce essentially
similar systemic effects in the host. He studied in some
detail the marked decrease in liver catalase activity that
occurs in animals bearing rapidly growing tumors. In these
studies a direct effect of tumors on liver catalase was shown.
It was demonstrated in mice that the catalase activity returned rapidly to normal when the tumor was removed. The tumor was implanted in the tail and was removed by cutting the
tail off.

Greenstein spent many years doing cancer research and

achieved an outstanding reputation in this field. Indeed, his cancer studies, judged in the context of that period, were of the highest quality. It should be noted that few laboratories were engaged in work on enzymes. Although research at NIH was excellent in certain areas, such as infectious diseases, the Institutes were little interested in biochemistry. Greenstein assembled an active group of biochemists at the Cancer Institute and encouraged other Institutes to do likewise (1), thus contributing significantly to the developments that soon placed NIH at the forefront of biochemical investigation.

At the completion of his work on the enzyme activities of tumors and normal tissues, Greenstein chose not to continue biochemical studies on cancer. He commented that "cancer research has been the graveyard of many scientific reputations." Although not pessimistic, he felt that the combined efforts of several disciplines would ultimately be needed for full comprehension of the neoplastic transformation. He believed that many basic discoveries, in biochemistry as well as other fields, would be required before the cancer problem could be directly attacked. In about 1947 Greenstein decided to return to his earlier interests in amino acids, peptide chemistry, and enzymology. During the period 1947 to 1955, he and his group published more than 100 important papers on these subjects.

Glutaminases, Peptides, and Pure Amino Acid Isomers

Greenstein, with CHARLES CARTER, MAURICE ERRERA, VINCENT PRICE, FLORENCE LEUTHARDT, and others, characterized the mammalian glutaminases. Two types of glutaminase activity were found. One was activated by inorganic phosphate (glutaminase I)(Figure 1), the other by adding α-keto acids (glutaminase II).

Greenstein's group carried out an extensive series of investigations on the synthesis and properties of dehydropeptides and other peptides. Initially the dehydropeptides were assumed to be split by separate peptidases, but the group later found that the usual peptidases catalyzed the reactions.

They studied the oxidation of the dipeptide L-cysteinyl-L-cysteine, which Greenstein had synthesized in 1937. He was interested in this substance because of its relationship to naturally occurring peptides, such as insulin and oxytocin. He isolated a number of products of its oxidation, including the cyclic disulfide derivative of L-cysteinyl-L-cysteine. The crystalline dimeric product of such oxidation was found to

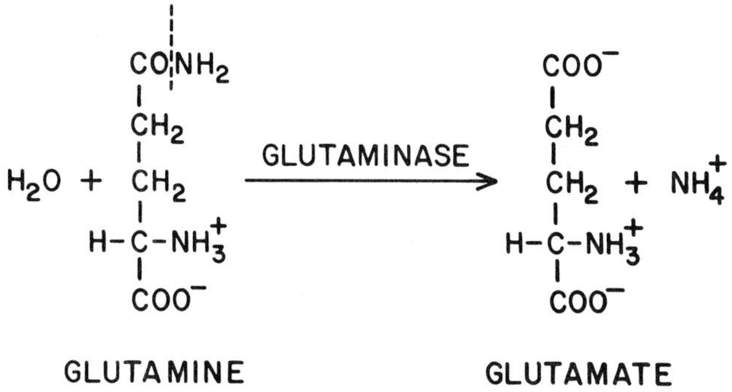

$$H_2O + \begin{array}{c} CO\!\cdot\!NH_2 \\ | \\ CH_2 \\ | \\ CH_2 \\ | \\ H-\overset{+}{C}-NH_3 \\ | \\ COO^- \end{array} \xrightarrow{\text{GLUTAMINASE}} \begin{array}{c} COO^- \\ | \\ CH_2 \\ | \\ CH_2 \\ | \\ H-\overset{+}{C}-NH_3 \\ | \\ COO^- \end{array} + NH_4^+$$

GLUTAMINE   GLUTAMATE

FIGURE 1. Glutaminase I, which is activated by inorganic phosphate, catalyzes the hydrolysis of glutamine to form glutamate and ammonium ion. The deamidation of glutamine that is stimulated by α-keto acids ("glutaminase II") is explained by two reactions; see below.

consist mainly of parallel cystinylcystine, with the two free amino groups adjoining one disulfide group and the two free carboxyl groups adjoining the other (5). Greenstein examined the problems involved in preparing unsymmetrical open–chain derivatives of cystine and the complications introduced by disulfide interchange reactions. He synthesized monoglycyl-L-cystine for the first time.

Greenstein made a major contribution to the chemistry of amino acids and to the study of metabolism and nutrition by developing methods for the preparation of optically pure L- and D-amino acids (6). This work was conducted in collaboration with PAUL FODOR, Price, JAMES GILBERT, LEON LEVINTOW, DOUGLAS HAMER, DANIEL RUDMAN, ROBIN MARSHALL, SANFORD BIRNBAUM, S.-C.J. FU, K. R. RAO, M. CLYDE OTEY, and others. It should be remembered that at that time (early 1950s) the commercially available preparations of L-amino acids were generally of poor quality, often expensive, and difficult to obtain. Resolution of racemic amino acids (DL mixtures) by the diastereoisomer separation procedure was far from ideal in terms of operation and yield. Greenstein therefore sought good general methods of resolution. He finally adopted procedures in which enzymes isolated from kidney—renal acylase I and renal amidase—were used. These hydrolyzed only the L isomers of N-acetylated DL-amino acids and DL-amino acid amides, respectively. This permitted separation and preparation of both the L and D isomers from a racemic amino acid in high yield, with optical purities greater than 99.9 percent (Figure 2).

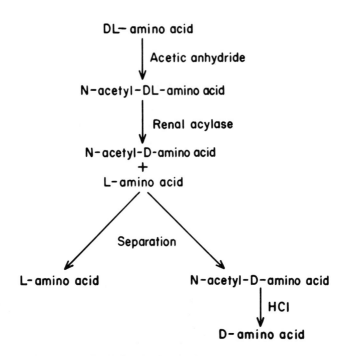

*FIGURE 2. Outline of J. P. Greenstein's procedure for re-
solving DL-amino acids using renal acylase (1949).*

Realizing that the polarimetric method was not a sufficiently sensitive test of optical purity, Greenstein used
enzymes—for example, the D- and L-amino acid oxidases and
the L-specific amino acid decarboxylases—as reagents to detect minute amounts of optical isomers present as impurities.
By 1954 these procedures had been applied to the preparation
of the L and D isomers of more than 60 racemic amino acids.
This led to an immediate increase in the quality of amino
acids available for scientific research and had a tremendous
impact on biochemical studies. The work on resolution of
amino acids also facilitated important studies on the stereo-
chemical configurations of the diasymmetric amino acids, including isoleucine, threonine, and hydroxyproline, and on the
chemistry of peptides such as arginylarginine.

A significant aspect of these investigations dealt with
nutritional and metabolic studies of amino acids in experimental animals. Research was conducted on the toxicity of
amino acids, on the function of arginine in combating the
toxic effects of ammonia, and on the development of a water-
soluble chemically defined diet. These studies led ultimately
to the amino acid preparations now used in hospitals through-

out the world. It can truly be said that the work of Greenstein and his colleagues, including PIERO GULLINO, MILTON
WINITZ, Birnbaum, JEROME CORNFIELD, Otey, J. P. duRUISSEAU,
and TAKASHI SUGIMURA, made intravenous alimentation a practical procedure.

One of Greenstein's last accomplishments was a comprehensive treatise on amino acid chemistry (7). Its three volumes,
written in collaboration with Winitz, stand as a major contribution to the field and continue to be inestimably valuable in
many investigations.

Greenstein in the Laboratory

Greenstein was a prodigious worker; he spent long hours
in the laboratory and could be found there on most evenings
and weekends. He enjoyed being in the laboratory and, even
when his group became rather large, never gave up working at
the bench. I recall one Saturday morning when we both arrived
at Building 6 at about the same time and found the electricity
turned off so that repairs could be made. I picked up a book
and went home. When I returned later that day, Greenstein was
doing an evaporation, using a water pump and a gas burner,
with barely enough light to see by. He commonly carried out
scientific discussions while doing a procedure in his laboratory, and rarely sat down except to write a paper. He hardly
ever stayed away from the laboratory because of illness. A
few days after his cholecystectomy in about 1953, he was hard
at work as usual, stopping occasionally to empty the biliary
drainage bottle he had strapped to his body.

Greenstein was exceedingly careful about the purity of
compounds he used, whether they were made in his laboratory
or obtained elsewhere. I recall an occasion on which he requested a sample of the barium salt of adenosine triphosphate
from a very distinguished scientist. In those days ATP was
not available commercially, but had to be isolated, usually
from muscle, by a rather tedious procedure. Before using the
sample he had been given, Greenstein checked it and found that
it did not contain "labile phosphate" or nitrogen. Indeed, it
turned out to be barium phosphate. We then spent about a week
isolating ATP from rabbit muscle.

Greenstein carried out many catalytic hydrogenations and
took extensive precautions to avoid explosions and fires.
These included the dousing of his inevitable cigar. Nevertheless, one day the dreaded event did occur. Returning from an
errand, I saw that everyone was running out of the building,
and someone said that Greenstein's laboratory was on fire. I
rushed in to see him vainly spraying CO_2 from an extinguisher

on a violently burning tank of hydrogen. We exhausted several extinguishers, but the fire was spreading and the tank seemed hot enough to explode at any moment. I nervously suggested that we leave, if necessary by the second-story window. Greenstein, however, managed somehow to close the red-hot valve with his bare hand. We then extinguished several secondary fires that had started on the lab benches. Greenstein sustained a severe burn, but continued to work regularly with a messy loose bandage on his right hand. After several months the burn healed with some scarring. I truly believe that without his heroic action, the laboratory might well have been destroyed, together with its two terrified occupants. (Ever since, I have kept an asbestos glove handy during hydrogenations.)

Greenstein himself wrote almost all of the papers that bear his name, in a style distinguished by elegance, conciseness, and superb use of language. He would sit down at his desk with a pad of lined paper and write the article, from title page to references, together with figures and tables, often finishing the same day. The words flowed freely and he seldom had to make corrections. The paper was usually typed and ready for the journal within a few days.

During that period Greenstein's laboratory was indeed a busy place. About 50 investigators worked there from about 1947 to Greenstein's untimely death in 1959. These included young Ph.D.'s and M.D.'s as well as visiting scientists from all over the world. Morale and motivation were high. Greenstein and his group supplied advice and compounds to other groups at NIH and to many other laboratories.

The laboratory attracted many distinguished visitors. Some that I recall were Hans Krebs, K. U. Linderstrøm-Lang, Leslie Hellerman, Esmond Snell, Carl Neuberg, John Edsall, Otto Warburg, David Rittenberg, Erwin Brand, James Sumner, Albert Lehninger, Wendell Stanley, Vincent duVigneaud, DAVID SHEMIN, Jakob Stekol, David Green, Van Potter, Sidney Weinhouse, and Edward Doisy. Linderstrøm-Lang spent about a month with us, giving a number of informal seminars that stimulated some memorable discussions. Otto Warburg came to the Cancer Institute to work with DEAN BURK on photosynthesis (1948-1949), but spent a good deal of time with Greenstein's group. My own contacts with him, often initiated by his need for a compound, were rewarding and instructive.

Hans Krebs made his first visit to NIH in 1951. He arrived without prior notice and modestly asked someone in Building 1 if he could visit the biochemistry laboratories. Greenstein was out of town giving a lecture, and I was told that an English biochemist had shown up and wanted to visit. I had the pleasure of meeting Krebs for the first time, and invited him

to give an informal seminar. He spoke about his work on glutamate transport. Krebs received the Nobel Prize for physiology and medicine in 1953 and returned to NIH the following
year to give a major lecture.

When Greenstein died in 1959 at the age of 57, his accomplishments were equivalent to those of several average scientific lifetimes. His research did much to develop the prestige
of the National Cancer Institute and of the later-organized
NIH, which incorporated NCI. He stimulated and trained many
younger scientists. His contributions were acknowledged by a
number of major awards both in this country and abroad. He
was proud to be a scientist in the service of the Government.
As Chief of the Laboratory, he commanded the respect and ad-
miration of the distinguished senior scientists on his staff
as well as of his own research group.

The Laboratory of Biochemistry

Our laboratory in 1947 was relatively well equipped for
the times. We did not have air-conditioning, and I recall
using a refrigerated bath to obtain a temperature of 37°C
during the summer of 1948. We had one Beckman spectrophotometer and one subscription to the *Journal of Biological Chemistry*; we took turns in using these essentials. We had cold
rooms, warm rooms, a mass spectrometer, radioactive counting
facilities, an analytical ultracentrifuge, and a Tiselius apparatus. The fume hoods worked, but were not entirely satisfactory. The odors of chemicals and animals that permeated
Building 6 may well have led to the decision to move the NCI
administrative offices to another building.

CLAUDE HUDSON, in the Experimental Biology and Medicine
Institute, had the only polarimeter at NIH, so we took our
samples to him. Hudson was a distinguished sugar chemist, an
impressive scientist, and a fine person. He was very cooperative, but rarely let anyone touch his precious apparatus. He
insisted on making the measurements himself and allowed us
only to look through the eyepiece and to read the dial settings. After several years our laboratory got its own polarimeter, and also newer types of equipment, such as a recording
spectrophotometer, flash evaporator, and fraction collectors.
Our microanalyst was ROBERT KOEGEL, whose efforts were super-
lative. One could often get analyses for carbon, hydrogen,
and nitrogen within a few hours.

"Acylpyruvase"

Greenstein's discovery that addition of pyruvate markedly accelerates the deamidation of glutamine by liver extracts led to some interesting developments. One was made possible by the gift of a sample of acetylpyruvate (2,4-diketovalerate), from Albert Lehninger, who had studied the metabolism of this compound in his doctoral research. We found that acetylpyruvate, like pyruvate, stimulates the deamidation of glutamine. We then discovered that it is quantitatively converted by liver extracts to pyruvate and acetate. These findings had not been anticipated from earlier separate studies on acetylpyruvate by Breusch, Krebs, and Lehninger. We found that this conversion is also catalyzed by extracts of other tissues. I then prepared a series of 2,4-diketo acids and found that these were also split enzymatically. We purified the enzyme from liver and called it acylpyruvase (8a).

The work was extended to 3,5-diketohexanoic acid (triacetic acid), and it was found (8b,c) that acylpyruvase splits 3,5-diketo acids as well. I prepared triacetic acid as the δ-lactone from dehydroacetic acid, which was obtained by heating gaseous ethyl acetoacetate at about 450° in an iron pipe according to the directions published by Collie in 1891. Later we hung the pipe on the wall, where it attracted amused attention for a number of years. Acylpyruvase activity proved to be identical to that which normally cleaves fumaryl acetoacetate to fumarate and acetoacetate (8d). This activity is markedly diminished in hereditary tyrosinemia (8e).

Transamination, Alpha Keto Acids, and Vitamin B_6 Phosphates

Greenstein found that most of the added pyruvate could be recovered at the end of the pyruvate-stimulated glutamine deamidation reaction, as determined by the formation of the α-keto acid 4-dinitrophenylhydrazone. I later found that pyruvate does disappear, as determined with lactate dehydrogenase, and that α-ketoglutarate is formed. Thus, the total α-keto acid concentration remains constant. This suggested that the pyruvate-stimulated glutaminase phenomenon involves transamination. We confirmed this, with Sarah Tice (Eastman) (9a), in experiments showing that glutamine transaminates with a variety of α-keto acids to form the corresponding amino acids. These were initially identified by paper chromatography (a procedure introduced into our laboratory by HERBERT SOBER) and later quantitated by microbiological assay.

With most α-keto acids, the reaction occurred more rapidly

with glutamine than with glutamate, indicating that appreciable hydrolysis of glutamine to glutamate did not occur. When glutamine labeled with ^{15}N in the amide group (prepared by MAX BERENBOM and JULIUS WHITE) was used, all of the isotope was recovered in the ammonia formed. Transamination of glutamine would be expected to yield α-ketoglutaramate, the α-keto acid analog of glutamine; and hydrolysis of this compound would give α-ketoglutarate and ammonia. To test this, α-ketoglutaramate was prepared. However, it was only deaminated slowly by liver extracts. It was then found that α-ketoglutaramate existed in two interconvertible forms, only one of which is hydrolyzed by the amidase.

We were not able at that time to separate the amidase from the transaminase. We examined more than 20 compounds structurally related to glutamine in the hope of finding one that would participate in transamination but whose α-keto analog would not be split by the amidase (9b). Two such compounds were found. In the reaction between γ-methylglutamine and α-keto acids, the formation of α-keto-γ-methylglutaramate was demonstrated. These and related studies showed that glutamine deamidation stimulated by α-keto acids occurs in two steps: transamination, followed by deamidation of α-ketoglutaramate catalyzed by α-keto acid-ω-amidase (Figure 3).

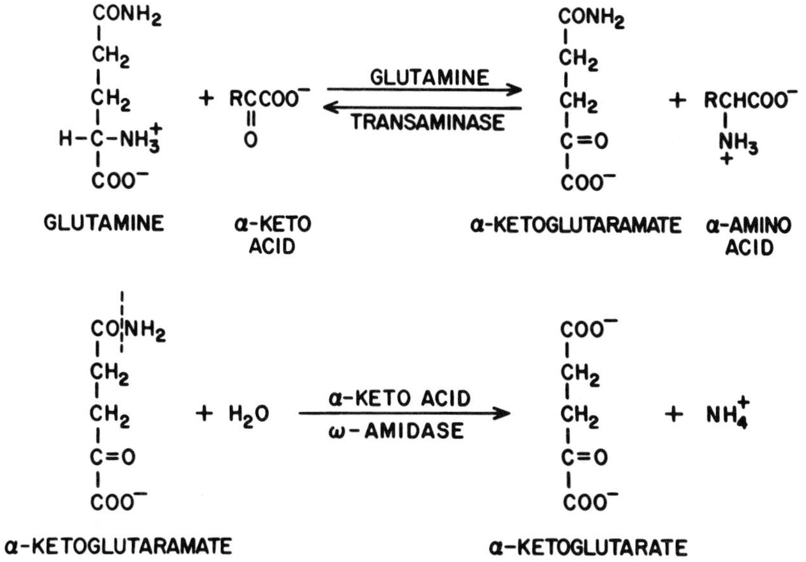

FIGURE 3. The two enzyme-catalyzed reactions involved in the α-keto acid-mediated deamidation of glutamine (1950).

The finding that glutamine participates in transamination was most interesting because at that time it was generally believed that only three amino acids participated: glutamate, aspartate, and alanine (10). Braunstein and Kritsmann (11), the first to demonstrate enzymatic transamination, originally reported that such reactions take place with many amino acids; but it was soon apparent from the work of P. P. Cohen that this conclusion was based on inadequate analytical procedures. Later work by Cohen (12) and by Braunstein (13) led to the revised view that only the three amino acids mentioned above participate significantly in transamination, and that the reactions are catalyzed by two enzymes: glutamate-aspartate transaminase and glutamine-alanine transaminase.

Rudolf Schoenheimer and his colleagues had found that when ^{15}N-amino acids (or ^{15}NH$_4^+$) are given to rats, the isotope appears subsequently in almost all of the amino acids. In commenting on these and related studies, Schoenheimer stated (14): "Only glutamic acid, aspartic acid, and alanine, but none of the other amino acids, have been shown to take part in . . . [transamination]. The occurrence of the isotope in the other amino acids of our rat proteins can thus be attributed to neither the enzyme of Von Euler (glutamate dehydrogenase) nor that of Braunstein. Other mechanisms must be investigated."

The findings on glutamine transamination (9), together with studies on transamination of glutamate (15), stimulated other developments in amino acid metabolism, and it soon became apparent that virtually all of the naturally occurring amino acids participate in transamination reactions. Moreover, there are a number of separate transaminases (2). Additional stimulation came from the important suggestion by Esmond Snell (16) that vitamin B$_6$ might be an enzyme-bound cofactor for transaminases.

Although the new developments emphasized the importance of α-keto acids, only a few were known and could be prepared by methods described in the literature. We devised a general procedure in which purified amino acid isomers (abundantly available in our laboratory) were oxidized by optically specific oxidases to yield the corresponding α-keto acids (17). These were purified by distillation or ion exchange chromatography and crystallized as free acids or salts. More than 40 α-keto acids were prepared in this manner, including the α-keto analogs of L-isoleucine, L-alloisoleucine, arginine, ornithine, lysine, and citrulline as well as glutamine and asparagine. It was recognized that the α-keto analog of glutamine could exist in both open-chain and cyclic forms and that the α-keto analog of asparagine could exist in a dimeric form. Transamination between ornithine and α-keto acids was

shown to involve the δ-amino group; and the ornithine-glyoxy-
late reaction, in which an aldehyde is both a reactant and a
product, was studied.

It was found that most α-keto acids interact with lactate
dehydrogenase. Five of these—pyruvate, glyoxylate, β-mercap-
topyruvate, β-hydroxypyruvate, and α-ketobutyrate—were found
to be highly reactive with this enzyme (2,18). Studies on β-
mercaptopyruvate led to the discovery of an enzyme that converts this α-keto acid to pyruvate and elemental sulfur (19).
In the presence of a reducing agent, the rate of conversion is
increased and hydrogen sulfide is formed rather than sulfur.
Later this enzyme was found to catalyze the transfer of sulfur
to a number of different substrates, such as sulfite and cya-
nide (20).

The work on transamination and α-keto acids led to a number of almost simultaneous developments in which several members of our laboratory participated. Tests of Snell's hypothesis had shown that animals and microorganisms deficient in
vitamin B_6 exhibited decreased transamination, and it was also
found that apotransaminases could be activated by impure preparations of pyridoxal phosphate. A finding by Umbreit, O'Kane,
and Gunsalus (21), however, cast doubt on Snell's theory: although pyridoxal phosphate activated glutamate-aspartate apotransaminase from pig heart, pyridoxamine phosphate under the
same conditions did not. Because of our interest in this problem and in a newly discovered enzyme, aspartate β-decarboxyl-
ase (see below), and because only impure preparations of pyridoxal and pyridoxamine phosphates were available at the time,
ELBERT PETERSON, Sober, and I undertook to prepare pure pyridoxamine 5'-phosphate (22).

This effort, thanks particularly to Peterson's excellent
work, led rather quickly to crystalline pyridoxamine 5'-phos-
phate. Oxidation of these beautiful rhombic plates with man-
ganese dioxide gave ammonia in stoichiometric amounts and
pyridoxal 5'-phosphate, which was crystallized. I recall that
shortly after this work was published, Karl Folkers (then at
Merck) made a visit to our laboratory to see the crystals with
his own eyes. Apparently Merck was much interested in these
compounds but had not as yet obtained them in pure form.

We found that both pyridoxamine 5'-phosphate and pyridoxal
5'-phosphate activated glutamate-aspartate apotransaminase
purified from pig heart (23). Activation required preincuba-
tion of enzyme with coenzyme prior to the addition of substrate. In these studies ^{32}P-labeled coenzymes were also prepared for the first time, and their binding to the enzyme was
determined. It was also demonstrated that 4'-deoxypyridoxine
5'-phosphate and pyridoxine 5'-phosphate (prepared later by

Peterson and Sober)(24) did not activate the apotransaminase but prevented its interaction with the natural cofactors.

An opportunity to examine the multiplicity of transaminases arose as a result of the isolation of an interesting mutant of *Escherichia coli* by Bernard Davis, then a Public Health Officer stationed at the Kips Bay Building near the Cornell Medical Center in New York City. I went there to learn the penicillin method for isolation of mutants, which he (and independently Joshua Lederberg) had invented, and brought the mutant back to Bethesda. It required L-isoleucine for growth, but in contrast to other isoleucine-requiring mutants, growth was not supported by the α-keto analog of L-isoleucine—i.e., d-α-keto-β-methylvalerate. L-Valine, in addition to L-isoleucine, was required for maximal growth, but valine could not be replaced by its α-keto analog α-ketoisovalerate.

Daniel Rudman (now Professor of Medicine at Emory University), an exceedingly capable man, had just joined our group after receiving his medical degree. He found that preparations of the mutant, in contrast to those of the wild strain, did not catalyze transamination between glutamate and α-keto-β-methylvalerate (25). But neither did the mutant catalyze transamination between valine and α-ketoglutarate; though valine augmented growth, considerable growth occurred in its absence. We therefore concluded that either valine was synthesized by a route not involving transamination, or the mutant had another enzyme capable of catalyzing transamination with valine. Rudman examined a large number of possible amino donors and found that only L-alanine and L-α-aminobutyrate could transaminate with α-ketoisovalerate in the presence of extracts of the mutant strain (Figure 4).

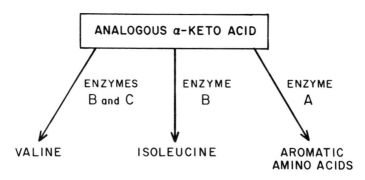

FIGURE 4. *Transamination reactions in* Escherichia coli. *In contrast to isoleucine, which is formed by a single transaminase (B), valine can be formed by two enzymes (B and C). Enzyme A acts predominantly to form aromatic amino acids.*

These experiments showed that at least three transaminases are present in the wild strain: an enzyme (B) that catalyzes transaminations involving glutamate, isoleucine, valine, and several other aliphatic amino acids; an enzyme (A) that catalyzes reactions involving glutamate, aspartate, tryptophan, tyrosine, and phenylalanine; and a valine-alanine (or α-aminobutyrate) transaminase (C). Failure of the mutant to exhibit an absolute requirement for valine was ascribed to the presence of the valine-alanine transaminase. Confirmation of these results was obtained by separation of the three enzymes from extracts of the wild strain, and by the finding that the valine requirement of the mutant could be met with equivalent amounts of either L-alanine or L-α-aminobutyrate. *E. coli* thus has two transaminases that can catalyze valine formation from α-ketoisovalerate, but only one that can utilize *d*-α-keto-β-methylvalerate for isoleucine formation. These enzymes, designated simply A, B, and C, have been studied extensively over the years, providing the basis for further work on their genetic origins.

I recall that Rudman did much of his work at night. Our laboratory was very crowded, and he enjoyed the peace and quiet—and the space available—between the hours of 11 p.m. and 8 a.m. I would arrive in the morning to find him bleary-eyed, and often every piece of clean glassware in the laboratory had been used.

Aspartate Beta Decarboxylase

We tried to determine the activity of glutamate-aspartate transaminase by measuring the glutamate formed in a reaction mixture containing enzyme, α-ketoglutarate, and aspartate. The procedure was that of Ernest Gale, who had proposed a method for determining glutamate based on its quantitative decarboxylation by *Clostridium welchii* cells. Both Gale and Krebs had reported that this organism was inactive toward L-aspartate. It was unlikely, however, that they had tested the cells on aspartate in the presence of α-keto acids.

We found formation of carbon dioxide in control vessels containing α-ketoglutarate, aspartate, and *C. welchii* cells (26). The cells produced equivalent amounts of carbon dioxide from aspartate at a slow rate, but when pyridoxal 5'-phosphate or small quantities of various α-keto acids were added, the rate was greatly enhanced. Using paper chromatography, we set out to determine the product formed from aspartate. For several days we erroneously believed it to be β-alanine. Indeed, studies with four different solvents supported this conclusion. But Sober insisted on running a fifth solvent (77 per-

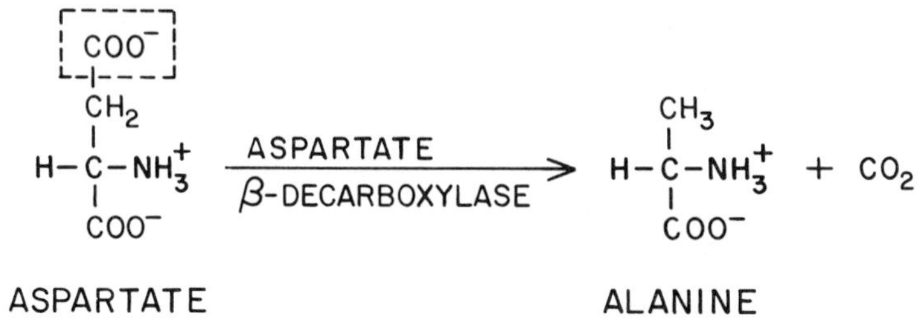

FIGURE 5.   β-Decarboxylation of aspartate to yield alanine.

cent ethanol), which showed that the product was not identical with β-alanine (Figure 5).   In those days (before the amino acid analyzer), paper chromatography was a valuable tool, but we became aware of its limitations.

A cell-free preparation of the organism irradiated with ultraviolet light showed little activity when either pyruvate or pyridoxamine 5'-phosphate was added separately, but a significant increase in activity was observed when these were added together or when pyridoxal 5'-phosphate was added alone. With paper chromatographic procedures and [2-^{14}C]pyruvate, evidence was obtained for transamination between pyridoxamine 5'-phosphate and pyruvate to yield alanine and pyridoxal 5'-phosphate.   The possibility that the added α-keto acid might transaminate with aspartate to yield the corresponding amino acid and oxaloacetate, which would decompose under these conditions to yield carbon dioxide, was excluded by studies with [2-^{14}C]pyruvate.   Although we did not fully understand the mechanism at the time, the work demonstrated the activity of an enzyme that directly decarboxylates aspartate at the β-carboxyl group (Figure 5) and provided evidence for the conversion of pyridoxamine 5'-phosphate to pyridoxal 5'-phosphate by enzymatic transamination (27)(Figure 6).

Biosynthesis of Glutamine

Our continuing interest in glutamine metabolism and the availability of the optical isomers of amino acids led to studies on the enzymatic synthesis of glutamine. Leon Levintow and I found that glutamine synthetase catalyzes the amidation of D-glutamate to form D-glutamine, but the rate of this reaction was about 30 percent of that found with L-glutamate (28). Such an experiment had not been done before, undoubtedly because D-glutamate was then a rare compound.   Of particular interest was the fact that when ammonia was replaced with hy-

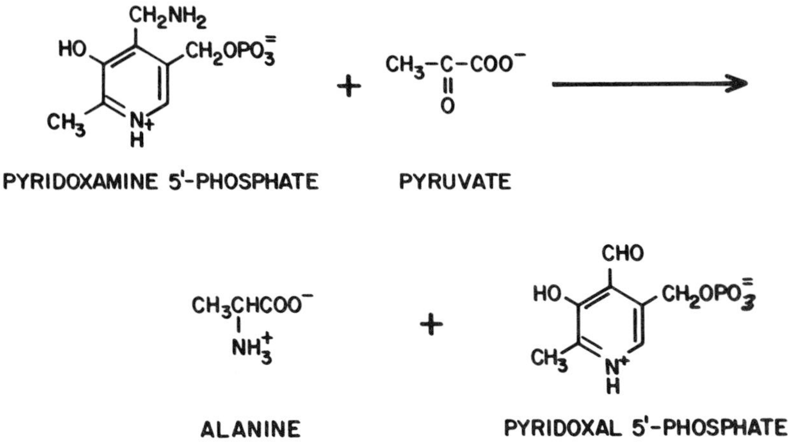

FIGURE 6. *Conversion of pyridoxamine 5'-phosphate to pyridoxal 5'-phosphate by transamination with pyruvate.*

droxylamine, the corresponding hydroxamic acids formed at about the same rate with L- and D-glutamate. This led us to suggest that the glutamine synthetase reaction involves two steps: (a) an initial activation of glutamate, which is of low optical specificity, and (b) a more specific reaction with ammonia, which becomes rate-limiting in the case of D-glutamate. Such a limitation is not noted with hydroxylamine, which reacts nonenzymatically with such compounds as acylphosphates and thiol esters.

In attempting to isolate enzymatically formed D-glutamine, we incidentally discovered that the glutamine synthetase reaction is freely reversible. This finding was of some interest because it made possible a good estimation of the value for the free energy of hydrolysis of ATP. Glutamine synthetase couples two reactions (Figure 7). From the equilibrium constant of the overall reaction that we determined, we deduced (with Manuel Morales, then at the Naval Medical Research Institute in Bethesda) that the standard free energy for the hydrolysis of ATP to ADP and inorganic phosphate is about -8000 calories per mole, on the assumption that the free energy of hydrolysis of glutamine is -3500 calories per mole (28,29).

These and other investigations on glutamine synthetase in 1953 and 1954 provided the basis for later work on the mapping of the active site of this enzyme, and demonstrated that enzyme-bound γ-glutamyl phosphate is an intermediate (30). The work on glutamine synthetase led to later studies on glutathione synthesis and function (31).

(1) Glutamate + Ammonia ——→ Glutamine

(2) ATP ——→ ADP + Inorganic Phosphate

FIGURE 7. The two half-reactions that are coupled by glutamine synthetase.

Other Studies

In early 1955 I participated in an interesting collaboration between SIDNEY UDENFRIEND, then at the Heart Institute, and Samuel Bessman, then at the Department of Pediatrics at the University of Maryland Medical School (32). We were interested in examining the role of transamination in phenylpyruvic oligophrenia, now commonly called phenylketonuria. Bessman had access to a number of patients with this disease, and Udenfriend had pioneered in the methodology needed. Relatively large amounts of glutamine were available at this time from Merck, which had prepared the compound synthetically with a view to its possible use in epilepsy. In the newly built Clinical Center, we gave two phenylketonuric patients oral doses of glutamine, glutamate, asparagine, glycine, succinate, or glucose and followed their urinary excretion of phenylpyruvate. (We had previously ingested the various compounds ourselves. Only glutamine affected me adversely, producing slight nausea.) We found that the administration of glutamine reduced the patients' excretion of phenylpyruvate and phenyllactate to about one-third of the control levels. Glutamate and asparagine had similar but less marked effects. We concluded that the decrease in phenylpyruvate excretion under these conditions is due to transamination, and that the reverse of this reaction is responsible for phenylpyruvate formation from the patients' accumulated phenylalanine.

Another collaborative project involved ROBERT GREENFIELD, who was examining the effects of tumor extracts on liver catalase. His object was to isolate from tumors a substance that would lower liver catalase as observed earlier by Greenstein. Greenfield also studied a few serum enzymes in patients at the George Washington Hospital. He made the interesting observation that a number of patients with heart and liver diseases had elevated values of serum lactate dehydrogenase. Unfortunately, we were so busy with other things that this work was allowed to slide. Later, of course, the determination of various serum enzymes proved to be of significant clinical value.

I recall that we became interested in a tricarboxylic amino acid, α-aminotricarballylic acid, and that CARL BAKER and I converted it to isocitrate by treatment with nitrous acid. I wanted a fair quantity of the natural d-isocitric acid, which had been isolated from plants by H. B. Vickery. GEORGE HOGEBOOM and I were both interested in the compound, which at that time was exceedingly rare. Since NIH had plenty of open land in those days, we easily acquired about one-fourth of an acre (now most likely covered by a building or a parking lot) and grew large numbers of bryophyllum plants. At the end of the summer, we harvested the leaves and isolated about 20 grams of pure d-isocitric acid. The collaboration with Hogeboom was enjoyable, and I incidentally learned a great deal about subcellular fractionation, an area in which Hogeboom and his co-worker WALTER SCHNEIDER were very active.

Ambience and Associations

I have attempted to set down here some of my recollections about the exciting and rewarding period I spent at NIH, tending, however, to select work in which I was personally involved. Our research was carried out in a highly favorable environment, the most significant features of which were Greenstein himself and the senior scientific staff. Collaborations were easy to arrange—for example, nutritional studies with Julius White and experiments with HAROLD MORRIS on vitamin B_6 deficiency in animals. Ideas were exchanged freely and the projects and results widely discussed. The constructive criticisms and suggestions that flowed back and forth were efficient catalysts, and the atmosphere was charged with enthusiasm and interest. Today I miss a time when funds, while not abundant, were certainly not the limiting factor, nor dependent upon long hours of writing grant applications.

During the period between 1947 and 1955, the Laboratory had a number of investigators who were authorities in their fields. Herbert Sober and Elbert Peterson were primarily involved in the application of chromatographic methods to the separation and analysis of proteins and other macromolecules. In collaboration with GERSON KEGELES, an authority on physicochemistry of macromolecules, they conducted fundamental studies on the use of cation exchange resins for the frontal analysis of proteins.

Sober and Peterson carried out pioneering work on the development and use of modified celluloses, such as DEAE- and

CM-cellulose. Their initial studies, reported in 1954 (33), had a significant effect on the work of scientists throughout the world; and the modified celluloses, now commercially produced, are used in virtually all biochemical laboratories. After Greenstein's death, Sober became chief of the Laboratory of Biochemistry, NCI.

Morris and his colleagues, especially ELIZABETH and JOHN WEISBURGER, were involved in studies on the role of vitamins, amino acids, fats, and other dietary constitutents in the origin and development of tumors. Their studies on carcinogenesis, especially on the mechanism of action of 2-acetylaminofluorene, were of the highest caliber.

MARY MAVER studied cathepsins and other proteinases of tumors and normal tissues. JOSEPH SHACK investigated the isolation and characterization of proteins, using a variety of biophysical and physicochemical approaches. Julius White and his colleagues conducted metabolic studies on the fate of amino acids and carcinogenic agents in normal and tumor-bearing animals—investigations involving the synthesis of carcinogens containing isotopes, both radioactive and stable. C. DONALD LARSEN discovered that urethan (ethyl carbamate) induces lung tumors in certain strains of mice.

Dean Burk and his colleagues, employing elegant manometric, polarographic, and spectroscopic techniques, conducted a number of studies relating to the metabolism and diagnosis of neoplasms. Otto Warburg spent a year with Burk investigating the quantum yield in photosynthesis.

The environment was further enriched by an influx of young scientists who worked in the various sections and units. Greenstein arranged for some members, especially the younger ones, to have 6-12 month sabbaticals in other laboratories, including, for example, those of HERMAN KALCKAR (Copenhagen), Fritz Lipmann (Boston), Melvin Calvin (Berkeley), Jacques Monod (Paris), and K. U. Linderstrøm-Lang (Copenhagen). This added much to the intellectual atmosphere; new ideas and approaches were constantly discussed. Although we did not have teaching responsibilities, the opportunity to teach younger colleagues informally and to learn from the more senior ones was invaluable.

As biochemistry developed in other areas of NIH, important new interactions became possible and intramural seminars became more frequent. I remember with much pleasure my significant contacts with CHRISTIAN ANFINSEN, EARL STADTMAN, THRESSA STADTMAN, DANIEL STEINBERG, ALAN MEHLER, BRUCE AMES, SIMON BLACK, OSAMU HAYAISHI, JACK STROMINGER, JESSE RABINOWITZ, WILLIAM JAKOBY, GILBERT ASHWELL, Hogeboom, Schneider, Udenfriend, Kalckar, and other "newcomers," as well as with ARTHUR

KORNBERG, BERNARD HORECKER, CELIA TABOR, HERBERT TABOR, LEON HEPPEL, and others whose research had begun to flourish.

The NIH of 1955, in striking contrast to that of 1947, had become one of the world's most active and productive research centers. I recall a visit to New York in 1949, when few of my colleagues there had heard of the National Institutes of Health. One of my former professors, a very distinguished man, strongly advised me to leave the Government, which "did not attract the best minds." The remarkable rise in NIH's reputation after about 1950 is a great tribute to its leaders and to others in the Government who supported them. I was fortunate in being at NIH during that exciting period.

Notes and References

1. Other biochemists then at NIH included Herbert Tabor, who worked with Sanford Rosenthal in the Division of Physiology; Leon Heppel and Bernard Horecker, members of the Division of Industrial Hygiene; and Arthur Kornberg, who worked with Floyd Daft and Henry Sebrell in the Division of Nutrition. These young men were in their formative years; they became well known for later contributions. Greenstein was active in building his own laboratory and urged that independent biochemical activities be supported in all of the Institutes. A list of Greenstein's publications is given in the Journal of the National Cancer Institute (January 1960), vol. 24, no. 1, pp. xv-xxx, and in Amino Acids, Proteins, and Cancer Biochemistry, J.T. Edsall (ed.), pp. 213-227, New York: Academic Press, 1960.
2. Meister, A. Biochemistry of the Amino Acids, second edition, volume 1 (711 pages), volume 2. New York: Academic Press, 1965 (first ed., 1957).
3. Greenstein, J.P. Biochemistry of Cancer, second edition. New York: Academic Press, 1954.
4. Weinhouse, S. Enzyme activities and tumor progression. In Amino Acids, Proteins, and Cancer Biochemistry, J.T. Edsall (ed.), p. 109, New York: Academic Press, 1960.
5. Greenstein, J.P., R. Wade, and M. Winitz. Studies on polycysteine peptides and proteins. Configurations of the peptides of L-cystine obtained by oxidation of L-cysteinyl-L-cysteine. J Am Chem Soc 78:373, 1956. Greenstein, J.P., et al. Preparation and disulfide interchange reactions of unsymmetrical open-chain derivatives of cystine. J Am Chem Soc 81:1729, 1959.

6. Greenstein, J.P. The resolution of racemic α-amino acids. Adv Protein Chem 9:121, 1954.

7. Greenstein, J.P., and M. Winitz. The Chemistry of the Amino Acids (three volumes). New York: Wiley, 1960.

8. (a) Meister, A., and J.P. Greenstein. Enzymatic hydrolysis of 2,4-diketo acids. J Biol Chem 175:573-588, 1948. (b) Meister, A. Metabolism of 3,5-diketohexanoic acid and its δ-lactone by tissue homogenates. J Biol Chem 178:577-589, 1949. (c) Witter, R.F., and E. Stotz. The metabolism in vitro of triacetic acid and related diketones. J Biol Chem 176:501, 1948. (d) Ravdin, R.G., and D. Crandall. The enzymatic conversion of homogentisic acid to 4-fumarylacetoacetic acid. J Biol Chem 189:127, 1950. (e) Kvittingen, E.A., E. Jellum, and O. Stokke. Assay of fumaryl-acetoacetate hydrolase in human liver; deficient activity in a case of hereditary tyrosinemia. Clin Chim Acta 115:311-319, 1981.

9. (a) Meister, A., and S.V. Tice. Transamination from glutamine to α-keto acids. J Biol Chem 187:173-187, 1950. (b) Meister, A. Studies on the specificity and mechanism of the glutamine α-keto acid transamination-deamidation reaction. J Biol Chem 210:17-35, 1954.

10. Meister, A. The enzymatic transfer of α-amino groups. Science 120:43-50, 1954. (Paul Lewis Award in Enzyme Chemistry Address).

11. Braunstein, A.E., and M.G. Kritsmann. Uber den- und Aufbau von Aminosauren durch Umaminierung. Enzymologia 2:129, 1937.

12. Cohen, P.P. Transamination. In The Enzymes 1:1040, 1950.

13. Braunstein, A.E. Transamination and the integrative functions of the dicarboxylic acids in nitrogen metabolism. Adv Protein Chem 3:2,1947.

14. Schoenheimer, R. The dynamic state of body constituents. Cambridge: Harvard University Press, 1949.

15. Cammarata, P.S., and P.P. Cohen. The scope of the transamination reaction in animal tissues. J Biol Chem 187:439, 1950. Feldman, L.I., and I.C. Gunsalus. The occurrence of a wide variety of transaminases in bacteria. J Biol Chem 187:821, 1950.

16. Snell, E.E. The vitamin activities of "pyridoxal" and "pyridoxamine." J Biol Chem 154:313-314, 1944.

17. Meister, A. Enzymatic preparation of α-keto acids. J Biol Chem 197:309-317, 1952; Methods Enzymol 3:404-414, 1957. See also Cooper, A.J.L., J.Z. Ginos, and Meister. The α-keto acids. Chem Rev 83:321-358, 1983.

18. Meister, A. Reduction of α, γ-diketo and α-keto acids catalyzed by muscle preparations and crystalline lactic dehydrogenase. J Biol Chem 184:117-129, 1950.

19. Meister, A., P.E. Fraser, and S.V. Tice. Enzymatic de-
     sulfuration of β-mercaptopyruvate to pyruvate. J Biol
     Chem 206:561-575, 1954.
20. Hylin, J.W., and J.L. Wood. Enzymatic formation of poly-
     sulfides from mercaptopyruvate. J Biol Chem 234:2141-
     2144, 1959. Fasth, A., and B. Sorbo. Protective ef-
     fect of thiosulfate and metabolic thiosulfate precursors
     against toxicity of nitrogen mustard (HN$_2$). Biochem Phar-
     macol 22:1337-1351, 1973.
21. Umbreit, W.W., D.J. O'Kane, and I.C. Gunsalus. Function
     of the vitamin B$_6$ group: Mechanism of transamination. J
     Biol Chem 176:629, 1948.
22. Peterson, E.A., H.A. Sober, and A. Meister. Crystalline
     pyridoxamine phosphate. J Am Chem Soc 74:570, 1952.
23. Meister, A., H.A. Sober, and E.A. Peterson. Studies on
     the coenzyme activation of glutamic-aspartic apotransam-
     inase. J Biol Chem 206:89-100, 1954.
24. Peterson, E.A., and H.A. Sober. Preparation of crystal-
     line phosphorylated derivatives of vitamin B$_6$. J Am Chem
     Soc 76:169, 1954.
25. Rudman, D., and A. Meister. Transamination in *Escherichia
     coli*. J Biol Chem 200:591-604, 1953.
26. Meister, A., H.A. Sober, and S.V. Tice. Enzymatic de-
     carboxylation of aspartic acid to α-alanine. J Biol Chem
     189:577-590, 1951.
27. Later the enzyme was highly purified from several sour-
     ces. The mechanism is now known to involve formation
     of an aspartate aldimine, which tautomerizes to the
     ketimine. After β-decarboxylation of the ketimine, the
     resulting alanine ketimine may tautomerize to the cor-
     responding aldimine, which hydrolyzes (the normal cata-
     lytic pathway), or the alanine ketimine may hydrolyze to
     give the pyridoxamine form of the enzyme and pyruvate.
     Aspartate β-decarboxylase was the first of the vitamin
     B$_6$ enzymes shown to have multiple catalytic capacities.
     See Tate, S.S., and A. Meister, L-Aspartate β-decarboxy-
     lase: Structure, catalytic activities, and allosteric
     regulation, Adv in Enzymol 35:503-543, 1971.
28. Levintow, L., and A. Meister. Enzymatic synthesis of D-
     glutamine and related hydroxamic acids. J Am Chem Soc
     75:3039, 1953; Reversibility of the enzymatic synthesis
     of glutamine. J Biol Chem 209:265-280, 1953.
29. Edsall, J.T., and J. Wyman. Biophysical Chemistry, vol.
     1, p. 210. New York: Academic Press, 1958.
30. Meister, A. Glutamine synthetase of mammals. In The
     Enzymes (third edition) 10:699-754, 1974.

31. Meister, A. On the cycles of glutathione metabolism and transport. In Symposium on Biological Cycles (honoring Sir Hans A. Krebs). Curr Top Cell Reg 18:21-57, 1981.

32. Meister, A., S. Udenfriend, and S.P. Bessman. Diminished phenylketonuria in phenylpyruvic oligophrenia after administration of L-glutamine, L-glutamate, or L-asparagine. J Clin Invest 35:619-626, 1956.

33. Peterson, E.A., and H.A. Sober. Chromatography of proteins on cellulose ion-exchangers. J Am Chem Soc 76: 1711-1712, 1954.

Introduction

STUDIES ON PROTEINS

The primary structure of all proteins was ascertained many years ago to be a linear array of amino acids, of which about 20 occur in nature, linked to each other by what is known as a peptide bond. Imposed upon this simple linear structure are a number of possible linkages that connect one chain to another or bridge various portions of the same chain. The best known of these linkages is the disulfide bond (-SS-) connecting two half-cystines, as in the ribonuclease and insulin molecules. Disulfide bonds form spontaneously whenever a pair of sulfhydryls (-SH) close to each other are oxidized. This phenomenon occurs spontaneously but can be greatly accelerated by an appropriate enzyme. The presence of disulfide bridges stabilizes the conformation, or shape, of protein molecules, and it is important to understand how they arise.

We know that the sequence of amino acids in the polypeptide chain during protein formation is carefully regulated by messenger RNA, which in turn derives its information from DNA of the gene. But the subsequent establishment of disulfide bonds within the chain is not directed by any outside agent; it is determined by the primary amino acid sequence. If this sequence contains multiple half-cystines, then the mathematical permutations would suggest various possible bridges. In actual fact, however, the amino acid sequence dictates specifically which disulfide bridges arise. These turn out to be the ones that provide a conformation with the lowest free energy. The conformation that is most comfortable is the one achieved, and all other possibilities are rejected. This discovery led to C. B. ANFINSEN's receiving the Nobel Prize for chemistry. Some of his studies on the synthesis and folding of proteins are explained in the accompanying chapter.

Over the past two decades, there has been enormous improvement in our ability to determine the sequence of amino acids in polypeptides and proteins of high molecular weight and to synthesize polypeptides of predetermined structure. Development of these skills was essential to our understanding of what proteins truly are and how they are formed in the body.

This chapter includes descriptions of studies relating to collagen, a family of proteins that hold together the various structures of the body by virtue of their remarkable tensile strength. Also described are studies of the contractile proteins, which are prominent in muscle but occur in many other cells as well. Clearly, it is among their functions to provide motility to the organism and its parts. Elsewhere this book describes research on other proteins, of which the enzymes are perhaps the most widely studied.

D. S.

13

STUDIES ON PROTEINS

I. The Synthesis and Folding of Protein Chains

C. B. Anfinsen

Many of the basic studies on chain-folding and on disulfide bond formation in proteins were carried out during
the late 1950s and early 1960s in the Laboratory of Cellular
Physiology and Metabolism, National Heart Institute. The
vigor and productivity of this work attests strongly to the
merits of the Clinical and Research Associate Programs. Much
of the research in protein chemistry and related fields involved the collaboration of the particularly well-qualified
M.D.'s who came to NIH as an alternative to military service.

Prior to the studies described here, a fairly primitive
body of knowledge existed on the biosynthesis of proteins in
tissue slices and minces. Little was known about how amino
acids were assembled into polypeptide chains. In the case of
hemoglobin synthesis, Bishop and Schweet had provided preliminary evidence that the NH_2-terminal valine residues, following short pulses of reticulocytes with labeled valine, were
less highly labeled than the average valine in the rest of
the molecule. Dintzis and colleagues then showed that the
specific radioactivity of residues increased uniformly along
the chains from the NH_2-terminus to the COOH-terminus. At
NIH, CANFIELD and ANFINSEN, who had determined the amino acid
sequence of egg white lysozyme, studied the specific activity
of leucine residues along its chain after brief incubation of
hen's oviduct minces with $[^{14}C]$leucine. Here again, in a well-
characterized protein, specific activity increased in an N–C

*C. B. ANFINSEN, Ph.D., D.Sc., Professor of Biology, The Johns
Hopkins University. Scientist Emeritus and former Chief, Lab-
oratory of Chemical Biology, National Institute of Arthritis,
Metabolism and Digestive Diseases.*

fashion, supporting the conclusion that protein chains were assembled on polysomes* from the NH_2-terminal amino acid residue to the COOH-.

How the extended, newly synthesized chain becomes a specific three-dimensional structure emerged as a major problem. In the case of bovine pancreatic ribonuclease, random formation of the 4 disulfide bonds from 8 SH groups would yield 105 possible isomers. In 1957 SELA, WHITE, and Anfinsen reported in *Science* on the reductive cleavage of the SS bridges and on the reformation of enzymatically active ribonuclease by air oxidation of the reduced protein.

This early work was followed by a long series of studies on the precision and kinetics of SS bond formation in a number of protein structures. HABER and Anfinsen worked out conditions for quantitative conversion of fully reduced ribonuclease to the active, native protein. Then Anfinsen, Sela, and COOKE showed that all but 3 of the 11 ε-amino groups of the protein could be "polyalaninated"—i.e., embellished with approximately 60 alanine residues on the "outside" of the molecule—and that such a protein could be fully reduced and reoxidized, with complete regeneration of enzyme activity. Only the side chains "inside" the RNase molecule were required for proper folding and SH-pairing.

A particularly interesting discovery was an enzyme in the endoplasmic reticulum of cells that could catalyze the formation of SS bonds and rearrange incorrect bonds to yield the native protein. Whereas the most rapid conversion of reduced RNase to native RNase in the absence of this catalyst took approximately 20 minutes, enzyme-catalyzed SS bond formation occurred in about 2 minutes, the time required for polypeptide chain synthesis in the polysomal system of the cell.

These studies, by GOLDBERGER, EPSTEIN, and Anfinsen, were extended by a number of other colleagues, including FUCHS, De LORENZO, GIVOL, and STEERS. The enzyme was isolated and studies were carried out on its mechanism of action. The single SH group in the interchange enzyme was essential to rearrangment of incorrect SS bonds and for catalysis of SS bond formation. Givol and others showed that this enzyme would inactivate insulin, yielding a precipitate composed of a network of randomly cross-linked chains.

The work meshed beautifully with the discovery of proinsulin by Steiner and colleagues, and indicated that the required information for SS bond formation in insulin was no longer available when the "spacer" peptide was cleaved out

---

*Clusters of ribosomes assembled within the cell by messenger RNA filaments bearing the genetic information for biosynthesis of peptides.

of the cross-linked proinsulin molecule to yield the two-chained insulin structure. Similar observations were made on chymotrypsin, whose three-chained structure is derived from the single-chained chymotrypsinogen precursor by two proteolytic cleavages.

STUDIES ON PROTEINS

II. Protein Conformation and Dynamics

Alan N. Schechter

The discovery from C. B. ANFINSEN's laboratory in the National Heart Institute in the late 1950s that the reduction of disulfide bonds in proteins was reversible under certain conditions led to the postulate that the pairing of half-cystine amino acid residues was guided primarily by the amino acid sequence and not external template mechanisms. Anfinsen and his colleagues soon extended this hypothesis to the more general conclusion that the conformation of a protein—its three-dimensional structure—was specified by the information in the amino acid sequence and the solvent. The experimental verification for these conclusions came from Anfinsen's studies of a variety of proteins, in collaboration with MICHAEL SELA, FRED WHITE, ED HABER, CHARLES EPSTEIN, BOB GOLDBERGER, and others.

The significance of this work was vast. The "central dogma" of molecular biology is that the genetic information in the nucleotide chain of DNA is transferred to the nucleotide chain of RNA, which then determines the amino acid sequence of each protein. However, it was also clear by the 1950s that the biologically significant forms of proteins were highly folded, complex structures. The mechanism of this folding that occurs after protein biosynthesis was not understood until Anfinsen and his colleagues demonstrated the simplest answer: that the native structure of a protein represents the form that is the most thermodynamically stable under physiological conditions.

During 1962–1963 Anfinsen spent a year as a professor of biological chemistry at Harvard, but returned to NIH in 1963 to establish the Laboratory of Chemical Biology in the Na-

A. N. SCHECHTER, M.D., Chief, Laboratory of Chemical Biology, National Institute of Arthritis, Diabetes, and Digestive and Kidney Diseases.

tional Institute of Arthritis and Metabolic Diseases. The scope of the laboratory was broadly defined, and a vast range of problems were approached over the next 20 or so years. It was clear, however, that Anfinsen was committed to exploring the implications in protein chemistry of the "thermodynamic hypothesis." To this end he recruited—relying heavily on the Research Associate Program he had helped devise—a group of very dynamic and productive medical scientists. These included HIROSHI TANIUCHI, PEDRO CUATRECASAS, SARA FUCHS, DAVID ONTJES, ALAN SCHECHTER, GILBERT OMENN, HENRY EPSTEIN, IRWIN CHAIKEN, DAVID SACHS, and BRUCE FURIE.

One of the main thrusts of this group in the early years was the study, reviewed in the previous section, of the enzyme that catalyzes disulfide interchange and allows the spontaneous folding of proteins in vivo at biologically relevant rates. The primary objective of the new laboratory was to synthesize functional proteins chemically, having predicted their three-dimensional conformation. Functional proteins should be makable, since they would fold spontaneously, and their conformation predictable from knowledge of the amino acid sequence. To this end a comprehensive study of the extracellular nuclease of *Staphylococcus aureus* was initiated. This phase lasted over a decade and led to more than 100 papers.

The sequence of the 149 amino acids in this protein was determined by Anfinsen, Taniuchi, and their colleagues. In collaboration with Cuatrecasas, Fuchs, Omenn, and others, they determined its fundamental enzymological, physical, and immunological properties. Studies by Taniuchi and Schechter showed that substrates and cofactors affected both the conformation of the active site and the general mobility, or dynamics, of the protein. Physical techniques, including stopped-flow and nuclear magnetic resonance spectroscopy, were developed by Schechter and Epstein, in collaboration with the Heart Institute's Laboratory of Technical Development and the Division of Computer Research and Technology, to show that the refolding of the protein could be accomplished in milliseconds and to study the molecular mechanism of refolding.

These studies pushed available technology to the limit in analyzing conformational transitions. With the assistance of laboratory alumni—Michael Sela, Sara Fuchs, and their colleagues, now at the Weizmann Institute of Science in Rehovot, Israel—Anfinsen and his group developed between 1970 and 1975 a new, immunologic approach to study the folding and unfolding of proteins and peptides. Sachs and Schechter, with the aid of ANN DEAN, showed that one could use monospecific antibodies to the native staphylococcal nuclease to measure the folding of peptide fragments from it. The antibodies' decrease in

affinity for the fragments as compared with the affinity for
the immunogen (the native protein) was a good index of the
degree of folding.

In collaboration with Furie, these workers showed, further, that monospecific antibodies made to the fragments
themselves could be used to measure the unfolding or dynamics
of the native protein. Other laboratories have now applied
these methods to a great many proteins. And these applications have been markedly extended in recent years by the advent of monoclonal antibody technology, which facilitates
the preparation of the monospecific antibodies needed for
meaningful association constants in soluble systems. These
immunologic techniques allow the detection and quantitation
of conformational states and transitions not otherwise demonstrable.

To determine experimentally the detailed rules that govern
the thermodynamically guided folding of proteins, Anfinsen
and colleagues, during the late 1960s and early 1970s, also
undertook the chemical synthesis of nuclease, using the Merrifield solid-phase technique. Although it was never possible to
synthesize the entire protein in a biologically active form,
large fragments were produced and deletions or substitutions
of individual amino acids made in order to examine the roles
of different residues in folding. This work has led, at NIH
and elsewhere, to hundreds of studies on the use of synthetic
peptides in biomedical research, including practical pharmacological applications. The work in the Laboratory of Chemical Biology is summarized by Chaiken in an accompanying section.

By the mid 1970s the several investigators who constituted the Laboratory of Chemical Biology made use of these
experimental and conceptual analyses of protein conformation
and dynamics to move into new fields of biomedical research.
Anfinsen, before his retirement in 1981, developed methods
to purify the human interferons and obtained the earliest
structure-function analyses of these proteins, including partial amino acid sequences.

Taniuchi and colleagues initiated elegant, detailed studies of the conformational dynamics of nuclease, ribonuclease,
lysozyme, and cytochrome *c*. They developed fragment systems
in which folding could be studied independently of denaturing
perturbants and showed the importance of "global, cooperative
interactions" in the three-dimensional structure of proteins.
Schechter and his colleagues applied immunological techniques
to develop radioimmunoassays specific for different human
hemoglobins. In addition, the realization from the nuclease studies that even short peptides could have significant
amounts of folded structure led Schechter and his colleagues

to a new approach to a therapy for sickle cell disease based on use of stereospecific peptides to inhibit the polymerization of deoxyhemoglobin S. Although this effort has not yet yielded a compound suitable for human trials, it has been the foundation of much current work in sickle cell therapy and has enabled the Laboratory of Chemical Biology to clarify the molecular and cellular pathophysiology of this genetic disorder. [These studies are detailed in the Schechter-Eaton section of the chapter "Genetic Diseases."]

Many of the studies that originated in the Laboratory of Cellular Physiology and Metabolism of the National Heart Institute and the Laboratory of Chemical Biology of the Arthritis Institute, including the career paths of many of the alumni of these laboratories, are summarized in *The Impact of Protein Chemistry on the Biochemical Sciences: A Symposium in Honor of Christian B. Anfinsen,* edited by A. N. Schechter, A. Dean, and R. F. Goldberger, to be published in 1984 by Academic Press. Among the many honors that came to Anfinsen for his work on proteins, covered in this and adjacent sections, was the Nobel Prize in chemistry for 1972.

STUDIES ON PROTEINS

III. Synthesis, Semisynthesis, and Protein Function

Irwin M. Chaiken

The National Institutes of Health has provided a singularly hospitable environment for the multidisciplinary study of proteins by chemical synthesis and semisynthesis. Modifying proteins through the synthesis of sequence-variant analogs continues to be a powerful approach to understanding how these macromolecules form and maintain their active, correctly folded structures. These efforts use a wide variety of technologies, including peptide and protein chemistry, enzymology, endocrinology, spectroscopy, X-ray crystallography and, increasingly, molecular genetics. Thus, carrying out such research is not an activity one easily performs in isolation; access to the talents of scientific neighbors can mean the difference between the ordinary and the pace-setting. NIH, with its highly diverse scientific community, offers a natural haven for peptide and protein engineering.

An early appreciation of the value and limitations of synthesizing proteins developed from pioneer efforts in Bethesda on the synthesis of peptides. Starting in the 1940s and 1950s, the research groups of J. P. GREENSTEIN and B. WITKOP synthesized a variety of peptides and described many of their physicochemical and functional properties. In the laboratories of Greenstein and J. FOLK, this work led to the use of synthetic peptides as substrates for studies of the active sites of proteases and transglutaminases. A *Washington Post* reporter, in 1976, saddled Folk with "doing basically the same type of experiment over and over . . . for 24 years . . . in a laboratory cluttered with test tubes and paraphernalia." Happily, the reporter overcame this first perception of Folk's work and duly recognized its noble purpose: "attempting to un-

IRWIN M. CHAIKEN, Ph.D., Senior Investigator, Laboratory of Chemical Biology, National Institute of Arthritis, Diabetes, and Digestive and Kidney Diseases.

ravel the mysteries of enzymes, the molecules that are vital
to all life processes." Peptide synthesis has continued to
occupy NIH scientists in mapping antibody- and protease-active
sites and other biological recognition surfaces and in developing new synthetic procedures and clinically useful reagents.
These activities have attracted numerous international visitors, including N. IZUMIYA, A. PATCHORNIK, M. WILCHEK, A. FON-
TANA, M. FRIDKIN, M. OHNO, and H. YAJIMA. Interest in chemical synthesis and semisynthesis has led to the establishment
of an NIH Peptide Discussion Group and to several symposia on
the chemical synthesis of peptides and proteins.

Chemical synthesis of large polypeptides, including parts
of proteins themselves, became a goal and a reality in research programs begun at NIH in the mid 1950s. By the early
1960s, seminal experiments by C. B. ANFINSEN and colleagues
on bovine pancreatic ribonuclease had shown that the information required for protein folding and resultant biological
function resides largely in the covalent structure, the amino
acid sequence. Thus, changes made in individual residues in
the structure would be expected to perturb local and perhaps
overall properties, giving clues to how sequence directs folding and function; and therein lay the promise of understanding
proteins through site-specific mutagenesis.

Yet there were limitations on how large a polypeptide
could be chemically synthesized routinely enough to make an
adequate collection of analogs. These limitations included
low solubility and coupling efficiency of large polypeptide
intermediates and the difficulty of purifying intermediate
and final polypeptides from closely related side products.
Thus, despite limited though important achievements in total
chemical synthesis (as for pancreatic ribonuclease in the laboratories of R. F. Hirschmann, R. B. Merrifield, and Yajima),
increased attention was given to semisynthesis. By the late
1960s a few key fragment complexes, enzyme-derived, were
available, including those made by H. TANIUCHI and Anfinsen
from staphylococcal nuclease. Here, one of the native polypeptide fragments could be removed, then replaced by a synthetic counterpart. These complexes formed the basis for
semisynthesis studies aimed at describing the roles that particular amino acids play in folding and catalysis. From the
late 1960s into the 1970s, such efforts resulted in a broad
series of studies of semisynthetic staphylococcal nucleases
by Anfinsen, D. A. ONTJES, A. R. ZEIGER, I. PARIKH, G. R.
SANCHEZ, G. A. HOMANDBERG, A. KOMORIYA, and Chaiken.

A sine qua non of both synthesis and semisynthesis is
that the amino acid sequence of the native protein be known.
Judging from the number of automated sequencing instruments
at NIH, there has been a strong commitment to acquire this

type of information. Importantly, defining the correct sequence is not a matter of approximation for someone putting polypeptides together residue by residue. Semisynthesis of a noncovalent fragment complex of staphylococcal nuclease started precariously in the late 1960s with the preparation of a sequence in which glutamic acid residue 43 was mistaken to be glutamine. Only when the correct identification was ultimately made was the first semisynthetic nuclease realized. The inadvertent and inactive Gln 43 peptide became the first nuclease analog. By 1972 the reasons for lack of catalytic activity of this sequence became clear. Chaiken, Sanchez, Ontjes, and Anfinsen put in sufficient labor at the solid-phase synthesis shaker to show that Glu 43 in native nuclease is an integral component in the catalytically active site, probably as a ligand for the essential calcium ion.

It was thus appreciated early that synthesis could allow directed study of catalytically important residues through minimal synthetic modification. This led B. M. DUNN, C. Di-BELLO, K. L. KIRK, L. A. COHEN, H. C. TAYLOR, Komoriya, Homandberg, and Chaiken in the 1970s to develop 4-fluoro-L-histidine analogs of semisynthetic ribonuclease, which helped define the functional roles of amino acid residues His 12 and 119 in bovine pancreatic ribonuclease. The functions of critical, nonactive-site residues also have been investigated, including those in semisynthetic studies of cytochrome c by Taniuchi, M. JUILLERAT, and D. VELOSO.

Development of the semisynthesis approach was aided in part by bad penmanship. Glu had been mistakenly written to resemble Gly on a schedule sheet for synthesizing ribonuclease S-peptide. Consequently, Gly 9 semisynthetic ribonuclease-S was made in 1973 and found to be somewhat of a dud in forming a stable protein conformation. Undaunted belief in the validity of one's own results led to further syntheses. And Dunn and Chaiken eventually concluded that ribonuclease prefers naturally occurring Glu over Gly at position 9 because it needs the residue to help stabilize an α-helical framework normally provided by S-peptide residues 3-13.

These results ultimately led Komoriya, T. KANMERA, and Chaiken to consider the information content of proteins to consist, as a first approximation, of sequences producing a conformational framework containing a limited number of residues that provide either noncovalent contacts to stabilize structure or active (or recognition) site elements. To test this, a set of greatly simplified model S-peptides was designed and synthesized. The peptides contained poly-alanine helical frames in which were embedded a small subset of native residues predicted to be essential, most notably Phe 8, His 12, and Met 13. The catalytic activities observed for this

series of modeled peptides when added to S-protein have provided a graphic expression of how different parts of the protein sequence contribute mechanistically to biological function.

Methodological developments that improved semisynthetic
and synthetic studies of proteins have been a bright and continuous theme at NIH. In the 1960s and 1970s classical advances in methodology were made in the laboratories of E.
GROSS, Witkop, and J. K. INMAN for the synthesis of small
peptides. And L. CORLEY, D. H. SACHS, and Anfinsen introduced a rapid solid-phase synthesis method for larger fragments.

Development of nonsynthetic methods has also been important. In 1961 Gross and Witkop reported the selective cleavage
of proteins at methionyl bonds by cyanogen bromide [see Witkop
chapter]. While the value of this method for protein sequencing was quickly recognized, the impact on semisynthesis became
apparent more gradually as the demand increased for limited
cleavage products. Other selective chemical cleavage methods
followed, including that of Fontana, G. OMENN, and Anfinsen,
in which the bromine adduct of 2-(2-nitrophenylsulfenyl)-3-
methylindole is used for cleavage at tryptophanyl residues.

Methodological advances from Chaiken's group in the 1970s
helped to bring the study of semisynthetic proteins fully into
the realm of protein chemistry by providing analogs that could
be studied rigorously by the full array of techniques available for native proteins. In the early 1970s, methods were
developed for fractionating solid-phase-derived semisynthetic
proteins to essentially full functional purity. Given such
products, M. PANDIN, E. A. PADLAN, and Taylor crystallized
semisynthetic ribonuclease-S and showed it to be of the same
structure as the native enzyme. Taylor, H. AMMON, and Komoriya
followed by crystallizing several analogs of semisynthetic
ribonuclease-S. Some of these, including the 4-F-His 12 and
model S-peptide analogs of ribonuclease-S, have become subjects of high-resolution structural analysis, using X-ray
diffraction, by Taylor, J. S. RICHARDSON, and D. C. RICHARD-
SON. Therein the structural evaluation of semisynthetic ribonuclease mutants has reached the level of atomic resolution.

Starting in 1978, Homandberg, Komoriya, and Chaiken utilized procedures for enzymatically restitching synthetic and
native fragments to yield covalently intact semisynthetic
proteins. It thus became possible to define effects of sequence engineering not just in noncovalent fragment complexes
but also in reconstructed covalent forms, thereby allowing
assertions with greater precision about the roles of particular amino acids in folding and function of mutant proteins.
The potential to reconstruct proteins from fragments, both

enzymatically and chemically, has been used by Kanmera and Chaiken to begin building semisynthetic analogs of biosynthetic precursors of hormones by putting together synthetic pieces with those that are formed proteolytically during the in-vivo generation of biologically active peptides. The promise seems reasonable to use such precursor analogs to evaluate molecular mechanisms involving the precursors, many of which cannot be normally obtained in large amounts as native macromolecules.

Progress in recombinant DNA methods in the early 1980s has enabled this technology to be used for producing native proteins and site-specific analogs. Indeed, genetic engineering for making structural variants of proteins offers an attractive complement to direct chemical synthesis and semisynthesis, especially for large polypeptides and proteins. NIH has become an important center for development and use of recombinant DNA methods. One can envision with optimism NIH research activity using the expanding technologies of both genetic engineering and chemical synthesis for inquiry into the structural basis of protein function.

Selected References

Anfinsen, C.B. Principles that govern the folding of protein chains. Science 181:223-230, 1973.

Chaiken, I.M. Semisynthetic peptides and proteins. CRC Crit Rev Biochem 11:255-301, 1981.

Greenstein, J.P., and M. Winitz. Chemical procedures for the synthesis of peptides. Chapter 10 in Chemistry of the Amino Acids, vol. 2. New York: Wiley, 1961.

Rich, D.H., and E. Gross (eds.). Peptides—Structure, Synthesis, Function. Rockford, Ill.: Pierce Chemical Co., 1981.

Shortle, D., D. DiMaio, and D. Nathans. Directed mutagenesis. Annu Rev Genet 15:265-294, 1981.

STUDIES ON PROTEINS

IV. Sequence Analysis

Bryan Brewer

The 1960s ushered in a new era at NIH in the determination of the primary sequence of proteins. The stage was set to bring together a group of investigators with diverse personalities and research expertise that would dramatically change the analysis of protein structure. The world of the protein chemist had been electrified by Pehr Edman's report of the first automated instrument for sequence analysis—the "sequenator." Few people in the scientific community had actually seen the machine, but tales of long, uninterrupted degradations were circulating everywhere. Edman, a brilliant chemist, was a quiet, soft-spoken Scandinavian with a penchant for secrecy in his research, and the development of the sequenator had been shrouded in mystery. Only a few associates were permitted the complete details of the phenylisothiocynate procedure, and even fewer were privy to Edman's future plans.

HUGH NIALL, a member of Edman's group, came to NIH in late 1967 to join the rapidly growing laboratory of JOHN POTTS in the National Heart Institute. Potts' interests were in the area of polypeptide hormones. He had been trained in CHRIS ANFINSEN's laboratory, which was regarded as the center of protein research at NIH and was staffed with many future stars in academia. Potts and Niall presented an interesting contrast in personalities. Potts, dynamic, outgoing, political, had recruited Niall, a soft-spoken Australian with many of Edman's characteristics, including his secrecy and aloofness. Soon after arriving at NIH, Niall set up the Edman procedure and began to discuss the merits of the new automated device.

BRYAN BREWER, M.D., Chief, Molecular Disease Branch, Division of Intramural Research, National Heart, Lung, and Blood Institute.

NIH: AN ACCOUNT OF RESEARCH
IN ITS LABORATORIES AND CLINICS

271

ISBN 0-12-667980-0

An advance of major importance to the field of protein sequencing was developing just around the corner from Potts, Niall, and colleagues. For years JOHN PISANO had been interested in analytical techniques for identification of the phenylthiohydantoin (PTH) amino acids obtained from the Edman degradation. He had developed an excellent new gas chromatographic method for their quantitative determination. Niall immediately recognized the tremendous potential of this new method and rapidly incorporated it for identification of the PTH derivatives.

Initial research in Potts' laboratory, which included Niall and two younger colleagues, BRYAN BREWER and HENRY KEUTMANN, focused on calcitonin, a recently discovered thyroid hormone involved in calcium homeostasis. After Brewer had isolated the hormone from pigs, Niall rapidly sequenced it by the manual Edman method and quantitated the PTH amino acids by Pisano's gas chromatographic technique. The effectiveness of this combined approach was readily apparent. Potts, quickly perceiving the full potential, contacted the Beckman Instrument Company in California for possible development of a commercial instrument incorporating gas chromatography.

Over the next 18-20 months, a group of dedicated, talented chemists and machinists at Beckman developed a prototype sequencer. This instrument differed in many respects from the original Edman sequenator, particularly in the ability to degrade peptides. The prototype instrument worked very well, and a few custom-built models were placed in the field for trial. Neurath's laboratory in Seattle, for one, provided a great deal of practical information on performance. With the development of a commercial sequencer, gas chromatography as introduced by Pisano became the method of choice for PTH identification.

Potts, Niall, and several co-workers left NIH, as Potts had accepted a position at the Massachusetts General Hospital in Boston. The availability of a commercial instrument for the automated degradation of proteins and peptides had an explosive effect on the number of proteins sequenced. Several Beckman sequencers rapidly appeared in laboratories throughout NIH. The area of immunology quickly became a veritable caldron of research activity. BILL TERRY and LEROY HOOD in NCI were among the first to look at the variable region of the immunoglobulin light chains by amino-terminal sequence analysis [see Paul-Waldmann chapter], and ETTORE APPELLA also began a detailed analysis of immunoglobulins.

The advent of a new technology often produces instant competition. This was the case with Appella and STUART RUDIKOFF. These investigators shared adjacent laboratories at NIH. They were careful to avoid direct confrontations, but were exquisitely aware of each other's progress and new acquisitions in intrumentation. A new modification in sequence methodology by Beckman might be quickly installed at both ends of the hall to maintain the competitive edge.

Bryan Brewer stayed on after Potts' laboratory shifted to Boston. Continuing the study of polypeptide hormone in the Heart Institute, Brewer and his co-worker ROSEMARY RONAN determined the structure of the parathyroid hormone by automated sequence analysis. Shortly thereafter, Potts and JERRY AURBACH announced *their* sequence determination of the structure. The attempts to establish priority took on the intrigue of a James Bond movie. Brewer's announcement of the structure at an international meeting in Wisconsin was followed rapidly by Aurbach's in New York City. The fierce competition between the groups illustrates the explosive nature of this field in the wake of new methodology.

Progress in the sequence analysis of proteins continued over the next few years at NIH. HENRY FALES and colleagues adapted mass spectroscopy for analysis of PTH derivatives, and the method was used extensively by Brewer, Ronan, and FAIRWELL THOMAS for elucidation of the amino acid sequence of several plasma apolipoproteins, the protein constituents of plasma lipoproteins. Pisano, continuing to pursue the identification of PTH derivatives, replaced the gas chromatographic technique by high-speed liquid chromatography. This became the method of choice in most sequence laboratories.

STUDIES ON PROTEINS

V. Collagen Research

Karl A. Piez

The study of collagen chemistry began at NIH in 1952 when KARL A. PIEZ, a newcomer to the National Institute of Dental Research (NIDR), set up a recently developed procedure for ion exchange chromatography of amino acids and modified it to separate hydroxyproline and hydroxylysine. These amino acids are virtually unique to collagen. Piez and ROBERT L. LIKINS first applied the procedure to collagen in a study of the biosynthesis of hydroxylysine, following in concept an earlier study of the biosynthesis of hydroxyproline by MARJORIE R. STETTEN. Piez's supervisors, unable to judge his work, sent his manuscript to Stetten, who gave it her approval. She and her husband, DeWITT STETTEN, Jr., had recently come to NIH from Columbia University.

In the mid 1950s, determination of the amino acid composition of a protein was a major event. Jerome Gross at Harvard, having studied collagen for some time, had many samples. He and Piez were brought together by BERNHARD WITKOP, who worked in the laboratory next to Piez's in Building 4. Piez and Gross published amino acid analyses of a variety of vertebrate and invertebrate collagens, beginning a collaboration that has had a continuing influence.

The next step in the project was to determine the chain structure of the collagen molecule. This was made possible by the development of cellulose ion exchangers at NIH in 1956. Aware of this major advance by HERBERT SOBER and ELBERT PETERSON and aided by their advice, Piez and his colleagues MARC S. LEWIS and GEORGE R. MARTIN prepared carboxymethyl-cellulose and used it to separate the polypeptide chains of collagen.

KARL A. PIEZ, Ph.D., Director, Connective Tissue Research Laboratories, Collagen Corporation, Palo Alto, California. Formerly Chief, Laboratory of Biochemistry, National Institute of Dental Research.

They found that the major collagen of higher animals, now called type I collagen, contained two kinds of chains designated α1 and α2, with the molecular formula $α1_2α2$. Covalently crosslinked dimers and trimers were present in varying amounts.

This discovery and the ion exchange procedure enabled the research group to make a series of rapid advances in the 1960s. They determined the chain structures and other properties of various collagens and studied collagen biosynthesis. With Gross and his colleagues, they showed that the toxic condition known as lathyrism resulted from an inhibition of aldehyde formation and thus crosslinking by the active agent, β-aminopropionitrile.

Since the α1 and α2 chains of collagen contain over 1000 amino acids each, further advances depended on having a specific cleavage procedure to prepare smaller peptides suitable for amino acid sequencing and other chemical and physicochemical studies. This procedure also came from NIH researchers. In 1961 ERHARD GROSS and Bernhard Witkop developed a method for specific cleavage of polypeptide chains using cyanogen bromide [see Witkop chapter]. In 1965 PAUL BORNSTEIN and Piez applied the method successfully to collagen. They were able to prepare and separate cyanogen bromide peptides from α1 and α2 chains and from crosslinked α1 and α2 dimers.

A very productive period ensued in which ANDREW H. KANG, YUTAKA NAGAI, EDWARD J. MILLER, JOSEPH M. LANE, WILLIAM T. BUTLER, PETER P. FIETZEK, JENS VUUST, MERRY R. SHERMAN, ROBERT C. SIEGEL, JOHN R. DANIELS, and ERVIN H. EPSTEIN as well as Martin, Bornstein, and Piez participated. Between about 1965 and 1970, they isolated the first covalent crosslink from collagen, identified it as an aldol arising from lysine-derived aldehydes in the α1 and α2 chains, and showed that these aldehydes were located in nonhelical end regions. They characterized a variety of collagens from different species and began amino acid sequencing. They also studied various aspects of collagen biosynthesis.

The ability to characterize a collagen by its peptide pattern through cyanogen bromide cleavage led Miller, VICTOR J. MATUKAS, Epstein, and Piez, in 1969-1971, to show that collagen was not a single protein but a family of different gene products. In addition to type I collagen, which they had been studying up to that time, they identified type II as unique to hyaline cartilage and type III as a constituent of skin and other tissues. Types IV, V, and others were later identified elsewhere.

Many of the investigators involved in these projects developed their own research programs on collagen and other aspects of connective tissue biochemistry when they left NIH.

These include major laboratories established by Bornstein at the University of Washington, Miller and Butler at the University of Alabama, Kang at the University of Tennessee, Fietzek in Munich and later at Rutgers University, and Nagai in Tokyo. Martin established his own laboratory in NIDR, with an active program in developmental biology of connective tissue. He and Bornstein, working independently, showed in 1970 that collagen is synthesized as a larger molecule, procollagen, which is converted to collagen outside the cell. Through these people, their collaborators, and now a third generation of investigators, research beginning at NIH in 1952 has had a major impact on connective tissue biochemistry throughout the world.

Since 1972 Piez has studied the structure of the collagen fibril and its mechanism of assembly. X-ray diffraction provides limited information about fibril structure, so other methods have had to be developed. These include molecular modeling, beginning with known primary and secondary structures, and electron microscopy of reconstituted fibrils and intermediate aggregates. Nuclear magnetic resonance techniques are also being applied to collagen fibril structure by DENNIS A. TORCHIA and his colleagues. Fibril assembly is being studied by various physicochemical methods as well as by electron microscopy. The earlier work on collagen chemistry has made these studies on higher-level structures possible.

STUDIES ON PROTEINS

VI. Muscle Research

Robert S. Adelstein

This is a personal account of muscle research at NIH since 1961. As such, it makes no claims to objectivity, completeness, or importance—particularly since a single paper resulted from the first five years (published in *Biochemical and Biophysical Research Communications* in 1963) and 50 percent of that was wrong. The right part was the molecular weight of actin, which was 57,000 at the end of the 1950s and which WAYNE KIELLEY and I later pushed down to 43,000. There it will probably stay, since we now know the amino acid sequence. But I am getting ahead of myself.

I arrived at NIH in July 1961. At that time Wayne Kielley and BILL HARRINGTON had just published their paper showing that myosin was made up of three polypeptide chains, each of approximately 200,000 daltons. It is quite possible that this paper taught me more about science than any I would read in the next 20 years. First of all it showed that you could do excellent science and still come out wrong. Second, it set before me two important examples of how to handle an honest error. There was that of Bill, who never faltered, as I see it, but continued, indeed continues, to produce outstanding work. On the other hand, Wayne never got over the triple-stranded model of myosin, and though I learned a great deal about science from Wayne, who certainly had tremendous impact on my work from 1961 to 1967, I did not learn when to quit and go on to something else.

There were a number of us besides Wayne and Bill working on contractile proteins at that time. There was MIKE YOUNG, DAVE KOMINZ, RICHARD PODOLSKY, BILL CARROLL, and later ED KORN

ROBERT S. ADELSTEIN, M.D., Chief, Laboratory of Molecular Cardiology, Division of Intramural Research, National Heart, Lung, and Blood Institute.

and EVAN EISENBERG. Previously, ELEMER MIHALYI and KOLOMAN
LAKI had also worked in this area.

The 50 percent of my 1963 paper that was wrong reported
that actin was made up of two subunits, which could be dissociated by 5M guanidine hydrochloride or 8M urea. To this day
I keep the results of the Model E runs and have been known to
pore over them every now and then (when no one is around).

Having been dealt a low blow by actin, I was ready to seek
my revenge. In 1967 MIKE KUEHL and I decided to isolate the
cyanogen bromide peptides of actin as the first step in determining the primary structure. When we discovered that
Marshall Elzinga of the Boston Biomedical Research Institute
had similar ideas, we decided to divide the work: we would
isolate and arrange the cyanogen bromide fragments, and he
would sequence them. This joint effort yielded the complete
primary structure of rabbit skeletal actin—but not before we
had experienced a number of exciting events. There was the
bottle of ninhydrin, for instance, that blew up all over us
in Building 3. Then, of course, there was the problem of the
missing peptide. . . .

We had convinced ourselves and Marshall (not to mention
the referees of a paper we published in *Biochemistry*) that
there was a 16-residue peptide, "CB-14." It took the better
part of a year for Marshall to convince us that we had created
this peptide with our own little ion-exchange column—that CB-
14 simply doesn't exist. It was a glorious day when we finally
put the sequence together. And it convinced us of one thing—
that we never wanted to work on primary structure again.

The year was 1970 and there were three of us—MARY ANNE
CONTI (a technical assistant), Mike, and I. At a meeting
of our journal club, which included Wayne Kielley and Evan
Eisenberg among others, Mike summarized a paper from the Weizmann Institute on the presence of myosin in platelets. We had
two successive impressions. The first was that the protein
they had purified (or thought they had, from the amino acid
analysis) was probably fibrinogen. The second was that they
were probably right and platelets do contain myosin.

For a number of years I had felt rather isolated in working exclusively with the proteins of biceps and heart muscle.
(No one understood smooth muscle at that time.) The Weizmann
paper indicated that myosin, and by inference the reciprocal
protein actin, if really present in nonmuscle cells, must be
doing something very important at a cellular level. The idea
was not original. Years before, Ariel Lowey had suggested
that nonmuscle cells contain an actomyosinlike* substance;

*Actomyosin: a protein complex composed of actin and myo-
sin; the essential contractile substance of muscle.

and E. F. Luscher had shown that platelets contain an actin-like and myosinlike protein. But no one had yet isolated and characterized purified myosin from nonmuscle cells so that it could be directly compared to the well-characterized myosin molecule of rabbit skeletal muscle. Myosin was appealing because it was the "motor" molecule of contraction and had a unique ATPase activity that could easily be quantitated.

We spent the next few years isolating and characterizing myosins from all sorts of vertebrate nonmuscle cells: human platelets (with Mike Kuehl and TOM POLLARD), mouse fibroblasts (with DICK OSTLUND, GEORGE JOHNSON, and IRA PASTAN), glial cells (with STAN SCORDILIS and JEFFREY ANDERSON), and prefusion myoblasts (with Stan Scordilis) among others.

In 1971 I attended the American Society of Biological Chemists meeting in San Francisco to present our observation that human platelet myosin bore a marked resemblance to skeletal muscle myosin in structure and function. Just prior to our presentation, a paper was given on the phosphorylation of troponin—the initial report on phosphorylation of a muscle protein. Such was the interest in this topic that the room was packed to overflowing. Needless to say, it emptied out before and during our platelet report, and by the time we had reached the conclusion, equilibrium had been restored. We managed, however, to maintain our objectivity, and in our first experiment upon returning to NIH, we dropped some $(\gamma-^{32}P)$-ATP into our platelet myosin preparation. In a sense, we never looked back—until now.

Simply stated, our work over the past 10 years has concerned the following: All vertebrate eukaryotic cells contain actin and myosin, and phosphorylation of the light chain of myosin regulates the interaction of these two proteins. The phosphorylation is in turn regulated by a specific Ca^{2+}-dependent kinase, which requires for activity the calcium-binding protein calmodulin. (This dependence was first shown in smooth muscle cells by DAVE HARTSHORNE.) CLAUDE KLEE and I have characterized myosin kinase from smooth muscle cells, which are an excellent model for nonmuscle cells, since the interaction of actin and myosin is dependent on phosphorylation of myosin in both. Others involved in this research have been MARY PATO, JIM SELLERS, PRIMAL deLANEROLLE, DAVE HATHAWAY, JOHN TROTTER, and Stan Scordilis.

In June 1979 Jacques Demaille was talking to Claude and me about the Gordon Conference he had recently attended. Phil Cohen had reported the observation that calmodulin was a subunit of the enzyme phosphorylase kinase. The significance for us was as follows: Phosphorylase kinase is a well-known substrate for cyclic AMP-dependent protein kinase; and perhaps myosin kinase, which resembles phosphorylase kinase in some but not all its properties, would also be a substrate. We tried the experiment. Unlike most that I was ever involved in, it worked the first time. Of course, the stoichiometry took a while to get right—2 mols of phosphate, not 1, are incorporated.

The significance of this recent work is in the suggestion of how cAMP might affect muscle and nonmuscle cells. Since it decreases the activity of myosin kinase, a rise in cAMP would be expected to result in *relaxation* of smooth muscle and a decrease in contractile activity (motility, cytokinesis, possibly transformation) in nonmuscle cells such as fibroblasts and macrophages. Whether this idea is right or wrong remains to be seen.

Of course, NIH investigators have made many advances in the field of contractile proteins during the past 20 years. Ed Korn and his associates analyzed the contractile proteins of *Acanthamoeba* and characterized in this ameba the various isoenzymes of myosin. One of these myosins appears to be unique in being a trimer and not a hexamer. Ed and his associates also characterized the regulatory systems that control the assembly of actin and myosin filaments in *Acanthamoeba* and, in the case of one particular ameba myosin, showed that phosphorylation *decreases* the actin-activated MgATPase activity by dissociating the myosin filaments.

Dick Podolsky and his colleagues have advanced muscle mechanics through X-ray analysis of muscle fibers. And Evan Eisenberg has made major contributions to our understanding of the kinetics of the myosin ATPase activity in the presence and absence of actin. Recent work by LOIS GREENE and JOE CHALOVICH in Evan's laboratory has changed our thinking about how troponin-tropomyosin regulates actin-myosin interaction. It now appears that tropomyosin, instead of blocking the formation of a noncovalent bond between actin and myosin, prevents an alteration in the angle of attachment, inhibiting the actin and myosin filaments from sliding past each other.

In closing at this point, I should stress my omission of other important work on contractile proteins by NIH scientists. This brief and highly personal summary is meant only to convey a flavor of what life was like in one laboratory.

A REVISIONIST VIEW OF
THE BREAKING OF THE GENETIC CODE

The science of genetics became molecular with Watson and Crick's publication in 1953 of the structure of DNA (deoxyribonucleic acid). It was entirely plausible that the sequence of nucleotides comprising the very long DNA molecules dictated the sequences of amino acids in the various proteins of the body. For this purpose the nucleotides afforded a four-letter alphabet—A, G, T, C (adenine, guanine, thymine, cytosine)—which could be postulated to spell up to 64 three-letter words. A major question, however, remained: Which of these words coded for which of the 20 amino acids that are incorporated into protein chains? This problem in biological cryptanalysis was solved almost entirely in the laboratories of the National Institutes of Health.

The momentous event is engagingly related in the following chapter. ROBERT MARTIN was an active participant in the "cracking of the code." He not only describes first-hand the major scientific steps, but also gives us insight into the turbulence and interactions, some productive, some not, that marked the process of discovery. Noteworthy are his thumbnail sketches of the major actors in the drama, including MARSHALL NIRENBERG, LEON HEPPEL, and GORDON TOMKINS.

In The True History of the Conquest of New Spain, *Bernal Díaz managed to capture the aura of excitement that accompanied Cortés's troops because he was reminiscing about an extraordinary personal adventure (1519–1521). In much the same way, Dr. Martin recaptures the excitement on the NIH campus as several scientists, variously situated in the Bethesda laboratories, tabled their own work to help Nirenberg press forward in the face of potent outside competition. In many ways, this was their finest hour.*

D. S.

14

A REVISIONIST VIEW OF
THE BREAKING OF THE GENETIC CODE

Robert G. Martin

There is an apocryphal story of an elderly Harvard professor of history who was asked by one of his students about
the Schleswig-Holstein affair. The professor's eyes sparkled.
"Only three people in the world ever fully understood the
machinations of that intrigue. Professor X from Tübingen, but
he died before he could finish his treatise. Professor Y in
Paris, but he's senile. And myself." The professor smiled.
"And I've forgotten."

A definitive history of the breaking of the genetic code
may never be told. Partly because the participants disagree
or simply forgot. Partly because scientists don't generally
think in historical perspective. And even the most well-
intentioned and hard-working historians of science may miss
the backstage gossip or fail to appreciate the undercurrents
of their subject matter.

The Breaking of the Code as History

Only one serious attempt has been made to put the discovery into the broader context of the midcentury revolution in
molecular biology. Horace Judson's book *The Eighth Day of
Creation* is an amazing study. For 600 pages Judson weaves a
myth of Olympian proportions. Then, in an epilogue of merely
12 pages, he comes close to destroying the myth and almost
reaches the truth. But the impression of the previous text
has been too strong, and one could hardly escape the conclusion that after the Eighth Day, Francis Crick rested.

Judson's accuracy is not in question. His exposition and
documentation are impressive. And he clearly and forcefully
describes the thrill of scientific discovery. André Lwoff's

*ROBERT G. MARTIN, M.D., Chief, Microbial Genetics Section,
Laboratory of Molecular Biology, National Institute of Arthritis, Diabetes, and Digestive and Kidney Diseases.*

account of his technician, so involved in an experiment as to identify with the bacteria, saying "Sir, I am entirely lysed" when disintegration of cells indicated that phage (bacterial virus) had been induced by ultraviolet light; Max Perutz's realization, on examining the X-ray scatter of mercury-tagged hemoglobin, that the basis for completely defining the structure of a protein was at last in hand; even Crick's unusually subdued "We're the only two [who] know it's a triplet code" as he and Leslie Barnett scanned their Petri plates—these are what keep a scientist at the bench. The discoveries are not always of such moment, of course. But the flash of recognition after long and tedious labor as a gel stain shows the predicted pattern, a scintillation counter detects the anticipated radioactivity, or the dim light of a darkroom reveals the telling image is indeed our principal reward.

At one point Judson laments that he, as a historian, will be vilified "like the damned eighteenth-century Dutchman who made Rembrandt's *Night Watch* smaller to fit a smaller room." A better analogy might be that of the eighteenth-century muralist who redid the ceiling of the Sistine Chapel, obscuring the original Michelangelos for 200 years. Not that the truth is so much more fascinating than the portrait Judson paints; it's just that his world is filled with giants and pygmies, while most molecular biologists, by my perception, have stood between four-foot-ten and six-foot-one. I don't deny that molecular biology has had its leaders, some far brighter than others. But they have rarely achieved their status through science alone. Equally important have been their facility with the written word, their eloquence of speech, their political savvy, their caustic wit—and plain luck. Too often the "leaders" have slowed scientific progress.

*The Eighth Day of Creation,** a paean to Crick and Jacques Monod, is a classic of the Great Man theory of history. Yet much of the evidence disproving that theory is clearly presented. To take the art analogy one step further, the history of molecular biology from the late 1950s on is like a Brueghel canvas, crowded with active groups following their own pursuits, yet drawn together by a central theme, a common interest.

Science vs. the Scientist

It is misleading to write science history without some mention also of political history, as the two are inextri-

---

*Judson, H. F. *The Eighth Day of Creation: The Makers of the Revolution in Biology.* New York: Simon and Schuster, 1979.

cable. In the fourth decade of this century, one of the most rational and creative societies of modern times—the society that gave us Einstein, Warburg, Freud, Mann, Heisenberg, Gropius, and Mahler—also gave us Hitler. From the devastation he wreaked was born a new, if short-lived, era of optimism and rationalism. In addition, the end of the second world war, with the bombing of Hiroshima and Nagasaki, raised the public's awareness of scientific progress to new heights.

The National Science Foundation was created (1950), and the National Institutes of Health was rapidly expanded. Young men and women returning from the war and youths emerging from high school found professions in the sciences not only respectable but even promising of financial security. Quite clearly, the seeds for the harvest that was to be molecular biology had been planted before the war, both here and abroad. Science tended to be an esoteric profession whose members were of a different breed than those who came afterward.* Research was still done in "schools" or groups, with scholars huddled about one or two masters to keep out the chill of general disinterest. War and the bomb changed all that.

Financial support not only led to a great expansion in the population of biochemists, physical chemists, microbiologists, and geneticists; it also fostered America's entry into the international community of science. While it may be argued that the influx of European scientists just before the war had already guaranteed that entry, there can be little question that fellowship support had a profound influence. The dollar was strong in Europe. What bright young American would spend his or her postdoctoral years in Bloomington or Pasadena when Paris was not only accessible but cheap? And with all due respect to the French scientific ambience, it is hard to imagine failure with the talents of Ames, Beckwith, Cohen, Hogness, Pardee, Miller, Stent, Tomkins, Yarmolinsky, and many others.

My thesis is that by the mid to late 1950s, American molecular biology had attained a critical mass. The fuse was set on October 4, 1957, when Russia launched Sputnik I. Now money burst into basic research as well as space technology. The chain reaction was in motion and there was no stopping it. No longer was one scientist or a small handful needed to keep the reaction going. Ideas were repeatedly and independently formulated (and as often forgotten); discoveries were sometimes made simultaneously in several laboratories.

---

*See, for example, *Phage and the Origins of Molecular Biology*, edited by J. Cairns, G. Stent, and J. D. Watson. New York: Cold Spring Harbor Laboratory of Quantitative Biology, 1966.

Although tempers flared over priorities, the priorities did not exist, because the logic of one set of experiments led inexorably to the next.

Fueling this growth from the intellectual side was, of course, the most important discovery of molecular biology—the elucidation of the structure of DNA. But even this achievement, largely responsible for the expansion of the field, would probably not have been delayed by more than two or three years if James Watson and Francis Crick had never been born.

Science set the course.

In the mid 1950s Millislav Demerec and his students began mapping *Salmonella typhimurium* mutants that required amino acids in the culture medium. They quickly noticed that genes of related functions were often adjacent on the chromosome. BRUCE AMES and PHILIP HARTMAN extended this work, developing quantitative assays for the enzymes of histidine biosynthesis. Ames soon perceived that the genes for these enzymes were activated coordinately—that they were derepressed as a unit. At an NIH Christmas party at the Horeckers' in 1958, he explained his ideas to Monod, who happened to be visiting. Ames's paper appeared in the *Proceedings of the National Academy of Sciences* the following summer. Soon afterward, François Jacob and Monod, using the cleverest of genetic tricks, isolated a class of mutants that regulated the expression of adjacent genes. The theory of the operon—a group of coordinate genes and an operator gene—was launched.

When the course was set by the scientists rather than by science itself, the direction was often wrong. In the summer of 1961, at the Cold Spring Harbor Symposium on Regulation, Monod presented his conclusions that the lactose operon was negatively controlled—that the genes for lactose degradation were controlled by a repressor rather than an activator. (MARSHALL NIRENBERG, not a member of the inner circle, was denied admission to this meeting, though, unknown to that group, he had already cracked the code.) Monod had a proclivity for generalization and concluded that all control was of the "negative type." Ellis Englesberg, not a member of the club, not an accomplished speaker like Monod, presented data to the effect that control of the arabinose degradative genes was positive. His data were considerably less extensive than Monod's, but sound nonetheless. Before the session ended, Englesberg retreated nearly in tears, crushed by Monod's onslaught.

It was the near destruction of Englesberg's concept of positive control that made the repressor, predicted by the notion of negative control, so terribly important. If all biological control worked via repressors, their isolation was imperative. But of course, as we now know, negative control is but one of many kinds; there is no universality of control mechanisms. That this should be the case seems now so obvious that it is hard to understand Monod's vehemence in arguing against positive control, except that the concept made his work appear less universal, less important.

Nirenberg and Company

When Marshall Nirenberg arrived at NIH in the summer of 1957, it was ostensibly to work with HANS STETTEN as a postdoctoral fellow. Stetten, as director of intramural research of the rapidly growing Arthritis Institute, was more and more absorbed by administrative obligations. To have some time at the bench, he would spend his summers at Woods Hole. So Nirenberg, lanky, shy, and quiet, even somewhat hesitant in his speech, but with fairly definite ideas about what he wished to do, set himself to work until Stetten returned. Their relationship was friendly, but Marshall worked largely alone.

Around the corner from Nirenberg's lab was LEON HEPPEL's. Intense, excitable, birdlike, Heppel is a person whose delight in scientific research is only exceeded by his enthusiasm for life. I can recall his summoning scientists from their laboratories and leading them down a long corridor, like the Pied Piper, to view the setting sun emblazoning the autumn leaves. "Just look at that view! Isn't it fantastic?" And for five minutes he would chant the beauties of nature. Then (jokingly): "O.K., everyone, back to work."

Heppel reveled in his own compulsive idiosyncrasies. The following routine was a daily occurrence when I came to Heppel's lab in February 1960. BARBARA GARRY, Ames's technician, would arrive at 8:05 a.m.; Heppel, 15 minutes later. Glass micropipettes were in wide use at the time, and Heppel would wash his own each morning, but he had to be first lest someone accidentally contaminate the cleaning solutions. The pipettes were carefully rinsed, then placed in a suction device 16 at a time. Now the tips were dipped twice in a soap solution, five times in tap water, five times in two successive beakers of distilled water, and finally in acetone. Garry would stalk her prey each morning. Pipettes in hand, she would emerge from her lab the moment Heppel arrived.

"No, no, no!" Heppel would cry, "Just a minute, just a minute!"

"I can't wait all day, Leon." And Barbara would walk slowly toward the prep room.

Heppel would break into a run and disappear into his lab, slamming the door behind him. He had to change into khaki work pants before he could do anything else. Seconds later, he would emerge in a white coat, grasping the pipettes in one hand and holding up his pants with the other. Barbara would time it so that they arrived at the pipette washer in a dead heat. Neither ever tired of the game.

The candy dispenser was the site of another incident recalling Heppel's microphobia. "Gee, you know, Martin," he said (calling me, as usual, by my last name), "there's a Charleston Chew. I haven't seen one of those in twenty years. Gee, it'd be nice to have some. Twenty years! Wow!" It was an ingenuous remark devoid of calculation. I went to the dispenser and brought back the candy bar, unopened. Leon hesitantly agreed to accept a small piece—his way. He went to the sink, pulled down a paper towel and discarded it: it might have been contaminated by the air. He washed his hands and wiped them with the next towel. I started to open the candy bar, but he asked me to wait a moment. He went over to his bench where there was a box of tissues. The first tissue followed the towels—bad air again; the second he held in his hand while I unwrapped the bar, using my best sterile technique to make sure I didn't touch it. Only then did he break off a piece of the candy with the tissue and happily munch away.

Leon set the tone for the lab: careful, meticulous, childish, and screwy, but always calculatedly so. A member of the NIH staff since 1942, Leon had done much to clarify the structure and metabolism of nucleic acids—work that was fundamental to ARTHUR KORNBERG's discovery of an enzyme that synthesizes DNA. It was characteristic of him to keep a freezer full of polynucleotides he had synthesized over the years—a freezer he never failed to inspect daily.

Nirenberg, trained mainly in biochemistry, started a collaboration with WILLIAM JAKOBY, in Heppel's lab, because he wanted to learn from Bill about enzymatic induction and bacterial adaptation. Although Leon was the titular head of the lab, most of the investigators were entirely independent. Marshall and Bill collaborated for about a year. Then Marshall started looking for a permanent job.

During one of those first years, he took a course from ROBERT DeMARS on phage genetics. He still thinks it was the most influential course he ever had. The night school at NIH, where DeMars taught, was particularly active. Several of the physical chemists—DAVID DAVIES, for one—took a course that Ames gave in biochemical genetics. Perhaps it was the night school, perhaps for some scientists the common background of Cal Tech or Harvard, or perhaps it was just that NIH was smaller then, but geneticists and biochemists, crystallographers and physical chemists, endocrinologists and microbiologists were not only talking to one another, they were tennis partners and friends.

Nonetheless, the classical biochemists had an ingrained distrust of the data that the geneticists insisted were compelling. It was hard for them to accept proofs that involved the abstractions of microbial genetics.

And the more conservative approach was not without justification. Consider the remarkable fact that molecular biologists initially came up with the wrong answer to nearly 50 percent of the problems admitting of only two solutions—left to right or right to left. For example, the sequence of genetic elements in the operon was first proposed to be the operator, followed by the promoter, and then the first structural gene. Indeed, the "proof" of the promoter's existence was based on this arrangement, but it was incorrect. Again, it was first believed that protein synthesis started from the 3' end of messenger RNA (ribonucleic acid); that the repressor was RNA, not a protein; that phage RNA polymerase worked in both directions (this was even confirmed by a second lab); and that frameshift mutants were absolutely polar. All of these concepts were later found to be invalid.

Not that there is anything inherently wrong with the techniques of molecular biology. Rather, the impetuous and creative new breed of scientist often went off half-cocked on inadequate data. But the molecular biologists were sufficiently numerous and competitive that their conclusions, if not credits, were usually straightened out in short order. Whether this expense of spirit wouldn't have been better directed toward obtaining sounder initial data remains a moot point.

Studying the Flow of Intracellular Information

Somewhere along the way, Nirenberg met GORDON TOMKINS. Gordy had just been appointed a laboratory chief in the Arthritis Institute. Before that, he was a section chief in Heppel's lab (succeeding HERMAN KALCKAR), though on a different floor and at the other end of the Clinical Center, the large structure otherwise known as Building 10.

Tomkins was something special. After college he had struggled with himself over whether to study medicine or become a jazz musician. He never did decide. Flute. Medical school. Saxophone. Ph.D. Clarinet. His interests were catholic and his knowledge astonishingly diverse. He was perfectly comfortable discussing X-ray crystallography—Fourier transforms and differential Pattersons—18th-century chansons, physical chemistry—light scattering and optical rotatory dispersion—fauvism, endocrinology, tennis, molecular biology, cool jazz, mammalian control mechanisms, cell biology. . . .

But what Gordy said seemed to matter less than how he said it, for his wit and charm were ebullient and contagious. A whole generation of scientists has adopted his speech mannerisms. It is a tribute to his memory that associates continue to regale acquaintances with stories of Gordy's humor and how unfortunate they are not to have met him.

Tomkins loved to travel. He was frequently invited to give seminars and was often away from the lab, to the consternation of some of his NIH colleagues. When he left NIH for the University of California some years later, he invited his friends to his other job—playing jazz at the Hawk and Dove, a bar on Capitol Hill. "Don't worry about my leaving," he said. "Just remember, now when I'm traveling, I'll be here."

And his enthusiasm was infectious. He would meet an investigator doing something mundane and, in an instant, through his flights of fancy, would embellish and embroider the work until both were certain they were onto some fundamental discovery. Then Gordy would offer the person a job.

Gordy hired Marshall Nirenberg and gave him a small lab. Marshall went to work on protein synthesis. Planning to study the process in a cell-free system, he knew he would need a sensitive assay to detect protein. To measure net synthesis in bacterial extracts that would be full of protein was unrealistic. And radioactive amino acids, not yet commercially available, would have been impractical to produce in a one-man lab.

So Marshall decided to start by inducing cell-free synthesis of the enzyme penicillinase. It was known that certain bacteria produce this enzyme when penicillin is added to the culture medium. The idea, then, was to make bacterial extracts, add penicillin and whatever else might be needed for protein synthesis, and assay for the new protein (the enzyme) on the basis of its ability to degrade penicillin. Since minute quantities of penicillin could be easily measured biologically, the assay should be very sensitive.

The central dogma that DNA is copied into "messenger RNA" by a process called transcription and that mRNA then directs protein synthesis by the process of translation had not yet been formulated. Or if it had, Marshall had never heard of it. He certainly believed that DNA coded for protein synthesis, but the intermediate steps were murky at best.

He had a bible, the newly published symposium collection *The Chemical Basis of Heredity.* If, as Stent has claimed,

Schrödinger's *What Is Life?* inspired the first generation of molecular biologists, then *The Chemical Basis of Heredity* was the second generation's New Testament.

From the work of George Palade, Paul Zamecnik, and others, it was clear that protein synthesis went on in subcellular particles known as microsomes. These had been shown to contain large amounts of high-molecular-weight RNA. Also, Mahlon Hoagland and Zamecnik had discovered that a small RNA molecule, "transfer RNA" (tRNA), was involved in protein synthesis. This discovery was made in complete ignorance of Crick's deduction that protein synthesis would require an "adapter" molecule to utilize the genetic information. Thus, the adapter hypothesis, though clearly a brilliant insight, played no role whatever in the discovery of the adapter, tRNA. To whom should the historian award the kudos?

Almost every morning, Gordy Tomkins and David Davies would drive to work together. Gordy was always bubbling. He had hired this fantastic young guy who was really doing great stuff. One morning it would be an experiment that just needed a final control to be complete. The next morning it would be something else, the control having ruined the whole hypothesis. There were so many ups and downs that David is not quite sure he believed it when Gordy told him a year later that HEINRICH MATTHAEI and Nirenberg had broken the code.

The penicillinase experiments really never worked. But a paper by Alfred Tissières and his colleagues in the *Proceedings of the National Academy of Sciences* demonstrated that protein synthesis in a cell-free extract from the bacterium *Escherichia coli* was dependent on DNA. The experiments were simple in nature. The bacteria were ground with alumina in a little buffer and the extracts clarified by centrifugation. Radioactive amino acids were added and the mixtures incubated at body temperature for several minutes. The demonstration of protein synthesis made use of the fact that amino acids are soluble in certain warm acids but most proteins are not. By stopping the process with acid, collecting any insoluble material on filters, and measuring its radioactivity, the investigators could determine the amount of protein synthesis that had occurred.

Marshall soon switched to the *E. coli* system. In mid 1959 Matthaei presented himself on the threshold of Nirenberg's lab and was adopted as a postdoctoral fellow. The two worked closely, both literally and figuratively: there was almost no bench space.

A Glimpse of the Missing Link

Marshall and Heinrich first worked on improving the system developed by Tissières and Zamecnik. They found that the system was active when freshly made and that, upon dialysis, activity was lost. But more important, they found that protein synthesis was renewed when RNA from microsomal particles was added to the dialyzed extracts. So RNA could stimulate protein synthesis! But the effect was relatively small. They needed a better RNA preparation—one not so heavily contaminated with ribosomal RNA.

Nirenberg would discuss his experiments with Gordy, who would turn them into wondrous stories for David Davies the next morning. Always flowing with ideas, Gordy also gave Marshall suggestions and advice. It was probably in one of those sessions early in 1960, when Marshall was getting low stimulation of protein synthesis with exogenous RNA, that Gordy recommended (if he really did) that some synthetic polynucleotides be used as negative controls. Other polyanions had been found to stimulate, and Gordy was only suggesting that Nirenberg's stimulation by RNA might be nonspecific.

David Davies remembers the story a little differently. According to one theory of the code prevalent at the time— the "comma-less code"—polynucleotides of a single base should not have stimulated protein synthesis. Thus Gordy suggested the experiment, expecting a negative result. Whatever.

In subsequent years Gordy embellished the story to the effect that he had proposed using polynucleotides to break the code—an idea that Marshall and Heinrich strongly deny.

There was blissful ignorance of the messenger RNA hypothesis at NIH in the summer and fall of 1960. But a postdoctoral fellow of Leon Heppel's, AUDREY STEVENS, had apparently isolated an enzyme that made RNA from the activated precursors ATP, UTP, GTP, and CTP. Moreover, this enzyme worked only when provided with a DNA template, and the RNA product was a faithful copy of whatever DNA was used. Unfortunately, a young postdoc, particularly a woman, didn't stand much chance in the fierce competition for the discovery of RNA polymerase. The central dogma was falling into place, and Marshall was well aware of Audrey's experiments. But her role as one of the three independent discoverers of that enzyme is often overlooked.

Marshall's Rosetta Stone

Marshall needed a purer RNA for his protein synthesis experiments, and what could be a better source than an RNA

virus? So he went off to Heinz Fraenkel-Conrat's laboratory
at Berkeley, where he analyzed the protein derived from adding
tobacco mosaic virus RNA to his system. Heinrich had been left
to test two RNA polymers, each containing only one of the four
possible bases. The polymers had of course come from Heppel's
freezer. The first, poly(A), was a dud.* (Sometime later Severo Ochoa and his colleagues showed that poly(A) wasn't a
dud at all; but its artificial protein product, polylysine,
was soluble in the acid Marshall and Heinrich were using.)
Poly(U) worked the first time it was tried.** Shortly, it
was clear that the protein-synthesizing machinery translated
UUU—if the code was a triplet—to mean the amino acid phenylalanine.

Cracking the Code

There were two possible paths to follow. One was to make
mixed polynucleotides of each of the four bases in different
combinations. The other was to make polynucleotides in which
the first three bases were in some definite order (everyone was guessing the code was a triplet) and the rest simply
poly(U). The latter path would give more precise data. Marshall was inclined toward this approach, but needed help and
expertise in polynucleotide synthesis.

One of the leading experts on the enzyme used to make the
mixed polynucleotides was MAXINE SINGER, a former postdoctoral fellow of Heppel's. Now she was an independent investigator in his lab. Marshall went to Maxine to ask her to collaborate with him on the project. He laid out what he had,
most of which she and Leon already knew, having supplied Marshall and Heinrich with the original samples of poly(A) and
(U). [Later, also poly(C). Poly(G) of high molecular weight
is almost impossible to make.] Leon tried to persuade Maxine
to collaborate with Marshall, but she declined. She would help
him with anything he needed, but wouldn't take part directly
in the project. Marshall left disappointed.

"There goes your Nobel Prize," said Leon to Maxine. Maxine
didn't think so. The project, she explained, would always be
Marshall's baby no matter how much work and effort she put into it. If she were to make a name for herself, it would have
to be on something she had initiated.

---

*Poly(A): polyadenylic acid. A synthetic RNA in which the
base adenine repeats indefinitely.
**Poly(U): polyuradilic acid. Here the repeated nucleo-
tide is uracil. (Guanine, adenine, cytosine, and uracil form
RNA.)

In the spring of 1961 the Cold Spring Harbor Symposium came and went. Sidney Brenner waxed eloquent on messenger RNA and the messenger god, Hermes, until Erwin Chargaff pointed out that Hermes was also the god of liars and thieves. It must have been torture for the effusive Gordy Tomkins to sit through that meeting without mentioning Marshall's demonstration that poly(U) coded for polyphenylalanine and poly(C) for polyproline.

But long before Marshall and Heinrich's papers appeared in the *Proceedings of the National Academy of Sciences,* the rumors were flying. It was an open secret around NIH that Marshall was onto something BIG.

The International Symposium on Biochemistry was in Moscow that summer. Marshall presented his paper to a handful of participants in a small room. But Crick got wind of his work and graciously insisted that he repeat his presentation the next day at a major symposium. Crick, as chairman, added his own interpretation, and Marshall became an instant celebrity.

Married just before the meeting, Marshall joined his bride in Copenhagen and paused in Europe for a honeymoon before returning to Bethesda.

Photo Finish

I walked into Heppel's tiny lab library, where journals were kept. It was a Saturday afternoon in the Indian summer of 1961, and almost no one was around. Marshall was sitting alone at a table with his head bowed and his eyes glassy, obviously upset and depressed. He had just been to a meeting of the New York Academy of Sciences. After his presentation, Ochoa had announced his laboratory's confirmation of Marshall's work along with their own experiments using several mixed polynucleotides. How could Marshall and Heinrich keep up with a lab that had nearly 20 scientists? Marshall was desperate for help.

I tried my best to cheer him up and promised to lend a hand for a few months. A rather strange round-the-clock collaboration began. Maxine provided me with the enzyme and expertise, and I synthesized the polynucleotides. My wife was covering embassy parties for the *Washington Post* at the time—she called it the garbage run—so I worked her hours, from 2 or 3 p.m. till 1 a.m. Heinrich, who had a penchant for night work (when the radioactivity counters were more likely to be available), took the lobster shift from midnight to noon. He tested the polynucleotides for protein synthesis. Marshall, working from about 9 to 6 in the lab and the rest of the evening at home, analyzed the data. Although we were beaten for the first publication on mixed polynucleotides, we were in print with a large number of tentative code words by December of 1961.

Stetten and Tomkins were supportive, supplying Marshall with space and postdoctoral fellows. The race to make polynucleotides of defined sequences was on. I returned to my own work.

It is difficult to recreate the competitive atmosphere of the time. Perhaps the following example will serve. Several years later at a symposium at Cold Spring Harbor—Cold Spring Harbor always brings out the worst in people—a young postdoctoral fellow of Monod's, Michael Malamy, presented data suggesting that "frameshift mutants" (nucleic acid sequences whose message has been altered by nucleotide additions or deletions) were absolutely polar and abolished all gene expression beyond the mutation. Another young investigator presented data to the opposite effect—data that were considerably stronger. (As it turned out later, Malamy and Monod were looking at mutations arising from an exciting new genetic element, the transposon—not frameshift mutants at all.) But there was no way Malamy and Monod could gracefully retreat. Instead, Monod, in the front row, turned to a neighbor and started making loud comments to rattle the speaker.

We at NIH were terribly angry with Ochoa and his colleagues for jumping in on Marshall and Heinrich's discovery. But of course, they too were working on protein synthesis at the time. Peter Lengyel, Ochoa's director of operations, says they had planned those experiments before hearing of Marshall's work. I am sure he's right. In fact, the only truly surprising aspect of the entire discovery was that Tissières and Paul Doty—though they knew of the messenger theory, were thinking of the coding problem, and had the polynucleotides— had failed to put 2 and 2 together.

Marshall Nirenberg was certainly the first to crack the code, and his subsequent recognition by the Nobel committee was richly deserved. But there can be no question that the tide of science in the 1960s would have swept aside the coding problem without him, or that his discoveries would have been impossible without the input of many others—even the vendors who made radioactive amino acids readily available.

PHILIP LEDER, a college and medical school classmate of mine, stopped by the lab early in 1962. He had been awarded an NIH research fellowship that would start in six months, after he had finished a year of residency. He had pretty much decided to work with Marshall and wondered what I thought. I told Phil he was making an excellent choice.

A number of labs made important findings during the next few years, including Crick's proof that the code was a triplet; but the next major break came when Leder and Nirenberg showed that a complex could be formed among ribosomes, a particular nucleotide triplet, and a transfer RNA molecule tagged with its appropriate radioactive amino acid. A paper by Kaji and Kaji had demonstrated such a complex with ribosomes, poly(U), and phenylalanyl tRNA, but their method of analysis involved the time-consuming use of sucrose gradients. Leder and Nirenberg developed a filter binding technique that greatly simplified the work. Now it was only necessary to synthesize the 64 possible triplets and carry out the analyses.

Again the race was on. And again NIH came to Marshall's aid, this time with postdoctoral support—BILL JONES, SAM BARONDES, BILL SLY, Phil Leder—and Maxine Singer leading a cadre of collaborators. With many labs involved, the task was completed in a few years.

THE RNA GENETIC CODE

UUU ⎫
    ⎬ phenyl-
UUC ⎭ alanine
 	
UUA ⎫
    ⎬ leucine
UUG ⎭
	UCU ⎫
	UCC ⎬
	    ⎬ serine
	UCA ⎬
	UCG ⎭
		UAU ⎫
		    ⎬ tyrosine
		UAC ⎭
		
		UAA ⎫
		    ⎬ termination
		UAG ⎭
			UGU ⎫
			    ⎬ cysteine
			UGC ⎭
			
			UGA termination
			
			UGG tryptophan

CUU ⎫
CUC ⎬
    ⎬ leucine
CUA ⎬
CUG ⎭
	CCU ⎫
	CCC ⎬
	    ⎬ proline
	CCA ⎬
	CCG ⎭
		CAU ⎫
		    ⎬ histidine
		CAC ⎭
		
		CAA ⎫
		    ⎬ glutamine
		CAG ⎭
			CGU ⎫
			CGC ⎬
			    ⎬ arginine
			CGA ⎬
			CGG ⎭

AUU ⎫
    ⎬ isoleucine
AUC ⎬
AUA ⎭
 	
AUG   methionine
	ACU ⎫
	ACC ⎬
	    ⎬ threonine
	ACA ⎬
	ACG ⎭
		AAU ⎫
		    ⎬ asparagine
		AAC ⎭
		
		AAA ⎫
		    ⎬ lysine
		AAG ⎭
			AGU ⎫
			    ⎬ serine
			AGC ⎭
			
			AGA ⎫
			    ⎬ arginine
			AGG ⎭

GUU ⎫
GUC ⎬
    ⎬ valine
GUA ⎬
GUG ⎭
	GCU ⎫
	GCC ⎬
	    ⎬ alanine
	GCA ⎬
	GCG ⎭
		GAU ⎫
		    ⎬ aspartic
		GAC ⎭ acid
		
		GAA ⎫
		    ⎬ glutamic
		GAG ⎭ acid
			GGU ⎫
			GGC ⎬
			    ⎬ glycine
			GGA ⎬
			GGG ⎭

The nucleotide triplets of RNA (ribonucleic acid), at the left of each square, code for the amino acid(s) at the right: U=uracil, C=cytosine, A=adenine, G=guanine. The triplets UAA, UAG, and UGA code for the termination of protein synthesis.

Introduction

FROM THE GENETIC CODE
TO BETA THALASSEMIA

From the previous chapter, the reader will have learned something of the unraveling of the genetic code. It was established that each sequence of three nucleotides, variously termed a triplet or codon, in the enormously long DNA molecule codes for one of the 20 amino acids that are linked end to end in the process of protein synthesis. The next chapter carries the tale forward, revealing how the growing science of molecular biology increased our comprehension of a typical genetic disease: Cooley's anemia, or beta thalassemia.

To understand the nature of this disease, the reader must know that normal hemoglobin, the red pigment of human blood, contains four polypeptide chains. Two of these are of a type called alpha globin; the other two, beta globin. In Cooley's anemia the production of beta globin is deficient.

Why do the patient's blood-forming tissues fail to make beta globin? To answer this, it was necessary to extend observations made initially on simple microorganisms such as Escherichia coli to the far more complex human subject. Dr. Anderson recounts the quest for the reagents and reactions that control the rates of globin synthesis and the deviations from normal that result in production of abnormal hemoglobin molecules. Further, he shows that the genetic defect leading to thalassemia is demonstrable in messenger RNA derived from afflicted children. By many and difficult steps, the knowledge first acquired by molecular biologists from the study of microbial systems has been translated into an explanation of a serious human disease.

The ultimate goal, of course, is to find a way to correct the underlying defect so that the lives of victims can be prolonged and improved.

D. S.

15

FROM THE GENETIC CODE
TO BETA THALASSEMIA

W. French Anderson

My story begins where BOB MARTIN's interesting narrative ends. Interviewed by MARSHALL NIRENBERG in 1963, I accepted a position with him to start in July 1965. Marshall's interest in me stemmed from work I had just completed with Paul Doty. As a fourth-year Harvard Medical School student taking a six-month research elective, I had shared in a detailed study of the mechanism of action of polynucleotide phosphorylase, an enzyme important in the metabolism of RNA. The thesis brought me admission to what was probably the most exciting laboratory at the National Institutes of Health at that time.

Work deciphering the genetic code was moving rapidly toward completion when TOM CASKEY and I arrived. Space was so much in demand that for several months we had only a few feet of bench on which to work. We began with a training period of synthesizing and purifying oligonucleotides (nucleic acid segments with only a few nucleotide units) under the able supervision of MERT BERNFIELD. My desk was a slab of wood on a tin can. I erected it wherever I needed a writing surface. Mert was an excellent teacher, so Tom and I were soon making triplets (codons: three-unit segments of nucleic acid, coding for a specific amino acid). After $2\frac{1}{2}$ months PHIL LEDER left for Israel and I acquired his bench space.

I set up a research project with DOLPH HATFIELD to make oligonucleotides of defined sequence to study the mechanism of protein synthesis. But one evening in early December, Marshall came to me with evidence that GCG (the triplet guanine-cytosine-guanine) might be an ambiguous codon—might code for two different amino acids. It was possible, however, that the trinucleotide preparation being tested, since GCG was so hard to make and purify, was simply contaminated with another triplet. Marshall asked if I would make new GCG as soon as possible so that the specificity of the codon could be clarified.

W. FRENCH ANDERSON, M.D., Chief, Laboratory of Molecular Hematology, National Heart, Lung, and Blood Institute.

For the next 2½ weeks I hardly slept, working literally around the clock to synthesize GCG, verify that it was pure, and provide it to Marshall for testing. It coded for only one amino acid! No ambiguity. After this, Marshall had me synthesize all the triplets needed in the laboratory.

I was starting to get a little frustrated just making triplets when Marshall asked if I wanted to give the Federation* paper in April 1966. Of course, I was absolutely delighted. This turned out to be the first public presentation of the final genetic code. Since I would be speaking before thousands of scientists, Marshall wanted me to be ready. He groomed me to answer any possible question. But a week or so before the meeting, I answered one of his questions incorrectly. I was very concerned and spent the next several days and nights rereading everything written on the genetic code and rethinking all the data obtained in Marshall's lab over the previous three years. The talk went well, and not a single question was asked! Two months later Marshall himself presented the code at the 1966 Cold Spring Harbor meeting. Published in the Cold Spring Harbor volume, his talk remains a classic on the subject.

With the code deciphered, regulation of protein synthesis had to be explained next. Marshall suggested using poly(U) [see Martin chapter] and Phe-tRNA (phenylalanyl-transfer RNA) to test HARVEY ITANO's idea that a low level of a specific tRNA could be a mechanism for controlling the rate of protein synthesis. One fact to be taken into account was that AGA and AGG are poor codons for arginine in *Escherichia coli* but, as Tom Caskey was to show, good arginine codons in mammals. Perhaps this was due to low levels of Arg-tRNA (arginyl-transfer RNA) that recognizes AGA and AGG in the microorganism. Did AGA and AGG, then, serve as rate-limiting codons? I set up two in vitro polypeptide-synthesizing systems, one using poly(U) and Phe-tRNA and the other using poly(AG) and purified Arg-tRNA. The results demonstrated that tRNAs could indeed be rate-limiting in the biosynthesis of protein molecules.

I gave my manuscript on these findings to Marshall, but he was so backed up with others to publish that he kept putting off working on mine. After many months he asked me to publish it without his name. That was my first independent publication on the regulation of protein synthesis.

But even though protein synthesis in microorganisms was exciting, my training in pediatrics urged me to set up a human, or at least mammalian, system. Hemoglobin seemed the best bet, and I talked with ROBERT BERLINER, then the Scien-

*Federation of American Societies for Experimental Biology.

tific Director of the National Heart Institute, about letting
me establish an independent program to study protein synthesis
in humans and mammals. Marshall was to be out of the country
for two weeks. Bob Berliner said that he would approve my
program if Marshall did also, for I had planned to stay as a
section head with Marshall and, at his request, had taken
charge of renovating a wing of Building 10 for his newly
planned neurobiology group and my *E. coli* protein synthesis
section.

When Marshall heard my plan, he wanted me to continue
working until an orderly transition could be made without
disrupting the projects under way. So during the next year,
I spent half of my time working on *E. coli* and half on hemoglobin.

Why was (and is) hemoglobin such an obsession with me?
Three reasons. First, the reticulocyte, which is an immature
red blood cell, is unique among all the cells of the body
in that it has lost its nucleus and is essentially a bag of
protein-synthesizing machinery. All the complications that
would be presented by a nucleus are eliminated. (Rabbit reticulocytes had been shown by Richard Schweet and his colleagues to be an excellent protein-synthesizing system.) Second, the major product of red blood cells is hemoglobin, the
best studied of all proteins. And third, there are human
diseases of hemoglobin synthesis called thalassemias.

Beta thalassemia is an ideal genetic disease in which
to study the regulation of protein synthesis. "Thalassemia"
comes from the Greek *thalassa* (sea) because it was first observed in persons of Mediterranean origin. A molecule of
hemoglobin, the oxygen-transporting pigment of red cells,
is a protein containing four globin polypeptide chains. In
β-thalassemia, synthesis of the chain designated beta is diminished or absent, resulting in lack of hemoglobin A. Homo-
zygotes (persons inheriting the gene from both parents) are
severely anemic and can only live with frequent blood transfusions. The disease is also called Cooley's anemia, having been described by T. B. Cooley, an American pediatrician
(1871-1945).

NIH was the ideal place for carrying out a study on the
molecular basis of a genetic disease. Only at NIH (and a
few smaller research institutions like it) can one pursue
scientific goals unfettered by grant restrictions, such as
the requirement for prior approval of all major decisions.
Also, one can bring in patients specifically for research.
This latter opportunity is invaluable for carrying out long-
term clinical research projects.

I was in a rush to begin because I thought every scientist would want to work on hemoglobin. If I waited a year

or two, everything would be done. This was of course extremely naive. Nonetheless, as Bob Martin pointed out in
the previous chapter, science moves on steadily. In fact,
I believe that if two giants had remained in hemoglobin research, I would never have had the opportunity to discover
anything in that field. Richard Schweet was tragically killed
in a small plane crash in 1967, and PAUL MARKS (after classic
work on the molecular biology of β-thalassemia with ARTHUR
BANK) chose science administration over the bench. The departure of these two left a vacuum that pulled me in with
irresistible force.

Since SIDNEY UDENFRIEND and HERB WEISSBACH were moving to
New Jersey to found the Roche Institute for Molecular Biology,
I acquired space on the seventh floor of the Clinical Center
in July 1968. Equally important, a free-spirited young scientist, JEFF GILBERT, joined me, as did DAVID SHAFRITZ, JOHN
COMSTOCK, and PHILIP PRICHARD a year later. Our first job
was to get hemoglobin synthesis to occur de novo on rabbit
reticulocyte ribosomes. No one had yet accomplished this.

During our efforts a paper was published by Ronald Miller,
who had been a graduate student with Schweet. Ron was trying
to isolate "messenger RNA," an elusive molecule that had been
postulated but not yet found. He had not succeeded in demonstrating globin mRNA, but had reported a protein fraction from
rabbit reticulocytes that seemed to stimulate de novo synthesis of hemoglobin. This was very exciting, but we couldn't
get the Miller-Schweet protein fraction to work as Ron had
described. And neither, it seemed, could the "big" labs (Har-
desty, Moldave, Lipmann, etc.). So I called Ron and, after
talking with him extensively, concluded that his work was
valid but that the fraction must be very unstable and tem-
peramental. Our group started over again to try to set up
a cell-free system for synthesizing protein, using our own
approaches as well as Ron Miller's helpful advice.

One day Jeff Gilbert, in absolute frustration after trying every imaginable combination for magnesium ions and other
salts, just left out the magnesium entirely--a move that was
certain, I thought, to destroy the ribosomes in the reaction.
Instead, we got our first glimmer of activity!

After several more months of work, we finally obtained
from rabbit reticulocytes a stable, active cell-free system
that could initiate new hemoglobin chains. There were two
"tricks." First, leaving out magnesium. We later learned
that the active protein fraction already had large amounts
of this ion bound to it; thus additional amounts markedly
inhibited the initiation reaction. Second, a critical ratio
of ribosomes to protein fraction was essential. This ratio,
as luck would have it, called for the ribosomes to be present

in very small quantity. The addition of a large number of ribosomes in an effort to get activity results in inhibition.

Over the next year we isolated three separate initiation factors from this protein fraction and showed their overall roles in protein (hemoglobin) synthesis. With great excitement we prepared an abstract for the national Federation meeting to be held in April 1970. To our total dismay, it was rejected. Apparently, the selection committee simply did not believe that this unknown bunch of junior scientists could really have what they claimed to have. My branch chief at that time was DONALD FREDRICKSON. Don assured us that life was not over because of a rejected abstract. He suggested sending one to the Clinical meetings* to be held a month after the Federation meeting. We did so, and our abstract was accepted for presentation at the plenary session—a great honor.

Unfortunately this honor had one negative fallout. A ruling then, and now, is that any paper to be presented at the plenary session cannot be published or presented at a national meeting ahead of time. We immediately requested *Nature* and the *Journal of Biological Chemistry* to hold our papers until after the May meetings. In addition, I said nothing at the Federation meetings about our findings. At the Clinical meetings, the press was very interested in the work, in part because of its application to human genetic disease. I foolishly granted interview after interview to reporters. Articles appeared in the *New York Times,* the *Washington Post, Newsweek,* etc. Imagine my nonmedical colleagues' feelings at reading about the discovery of initiation factors in the newspaper when I had said nothing at the Federation meeting just one month before. It was a number of years before some of them forgave me.

Concurrent with our basic research studies on protein synthesis, we began to study patients with β-thalassemia. In 1968 I admitted a brother and sister with this disease: Nick and Judy Lambis.** They were the first two patients for what would soon become an active hematology service in the Heart Institute. In fact, through the development of this intramural hematology program and the acquisition of additional extramural responsibilities in this area, the National Heart Institute ultimately became known as the National Heart, Lung, and Blood Institute (NHLBI).

---

*American Federation for Clinical Research; American Society for Clinical Investigation; American Association of Physicians.

**Use of actual names has been approved by the family.

Nick and Judy, delightful, enthusiastic young people who constantly encouraged us in our research efforts, remained our patients for the rest of their lives, another 11-12 years. They provided the blood and bone marrow that resulted in several important advances. Most significant was the discovery, isolation, and characterization of human mRNA. One of my Clinical Associates, ARTHUR NIENHUIS (now Chief of the Clinical Hematology Branch in NHLBI), succeeded in isolating mRNA from patients with β-thalassemia (specifically, Nick and Judy), from patients with sickle cell anemia, and from normal persons. We showed that normal human hemoglobin was made when mRNA from normal reticulocytes was translated on rabbit ribosomes, using our rabbit initiation factors. When mRNA from β-thalassemic reticulocytes was used, the rabbit cell-free system produced the same abnormal ratio of α- to β-globin that was observed in the patient's own blood. Similarly, mRNA from sickle cell anemia patients produced human sickle hemoglobin.

Thus, by mid 1971 we were able to reproduce in a test tube the exact genetic abnormality demonstrated in the patient's blood, just by adding mRNA from such blood to our rabbit cell-free system. RON CRYSTAL, now Chief of the Pulmonary Branch in NHLBI, was able to show that the entire translational machinery in β-thalassemic reticulocytes is normal. In the subsequent 12 years, work in many laboratories as well as our own has helped to establish the exact molecular defect at the DNA, RNA, and protein levels in many different types of thalassemia and other genetic anemias.

The past 18 years at NIH have been exciting. The intellectual environment here is ideal for allowing interactions among scientists and physicians so that biological and medical questions can be studied optimally. And the excitement of research and discovery never seems to end. Since our ultimate goal is to try to cure lethal genetic diseases, our major objective has been gene therapy—treatment by providing normal genes to the patient. Progress along this line has been dramatic, as most readers will know. At present, we are trying to get a functional mouse β-globin gene into the cells of a β-thalassemic mouse—that is, a mouse that has the equivalent of the human disease. We do not know when we, or someone else, will succeed in this, if at all. But the effort to help patients (like Nick and Judy) who suffer tragic genetic diseases will go on.

Selected References

Anderson, W.F.   The effect of tRNA concentration on the rate
    of protein synthesis.   Proc Natl Acad Sci USA 62:566–573,
    1969.

Anderson, W.F., and E.G. Diacumakos.   Genetic engineering in
    mammalian cells.   Sci Am 245:106–121, 1981.

Nienhuis, A.W., and W.F. Anderson.   Isolation and translation
    of hemoglobin messenger RNA from thalassemia, sickle cell
    anemia, and normal human reticulocytes.   J Clin Invest 50:
    2458–2460, 1971.

Prichard, P.M., et al.   Factors for the initiation of haemo-
    globin synthesis by rabbit reticulocyte ribosomes.   Nature
    226:511–514, 1970.

Introduction

GENETIC DISEASES

The information that cells require to synthesize proteins is stored in the genes. In general, damage to a gene leads to aberrance in its product, the corresponding protein. If this sequence of events is followed by pathologic signs and symptoms, as it often is, we have a genetic disease. Elucidation of the biochemical defects that underlie a variety of such diseases has been a major objective in several Institutes of NIH.

Often the protein in question is an enzyme. If the enzyme is absent, then the reaction catalyzed by that enzyme will not occur, the anticipated product will not be formed, and the precursor of the reaction may accumulate in the body. If the product is essential to the body economy or the precursor is toxic, then signs and symptoms of disease may develop. Examples of toxic precursors that accumulate will be found in the following sections on galactosemia, the lipodystrophies, and mucopolysaccharide diseases.

The defective gene product, the protein, need not be an enzyme. Examples of genetic diseases of this type are presented in the section on hemoglobinopathies. Here will be found a variety of diseases related to abnormal production of globins.

Sickle cell disease is perhaps the most studied of all genetic diseases, and indeed we know a great deal about its chemical characteristics. It was the first so-called molecular disease, an apt term introduced by Linus Pauling. It was Pauling, in collaboration with HARVEY ITANO and others, who first demonstrated the Mendelian distribution of hemoglobin S, the abnormal globin in sickle cell disease characterized by its peculiar electrophoretic behavior.

Many of the genetic diseases are quite rare. However, the number of known diseases in this category increases monthly, and the total count today is approaching 3000. For this reason, the genetic diseases taken together have a considerable impact on the public health, and have been estimated to account for approximately a quarter of all pediatric admissions to hospitals.

305

The mere fact that a disease is rare does not, and should not, discourage the investigator. History has shown repeatedly that the study of a rare event can yield important results. For example, the sections to follow will reveal that the most convincing proof of the so-called "Lyon hypothesis," a fundamental doctrine of genetics today, has come from the study of Lesch-Nyhan syndrome, a relatively rare disease. It might be pointed out that isolation and study of radium, a rare substance in the earth's crust, sparked revolutionary changes in our understanding of matter and provided valuable tools to the biologist and the physician.

Furthermore, not all genetic defects are rare. Some are very common—indeed, apparently universal in the species Homo sapiens. Consider for a moment the nutritional disease scurvy. This is a disease peculiar to guinea pigs and to primates, including man. Somewhere early in their phylogeny, a mutation occurred that resulted in loss of an enzyme abundantly present in tissues of other animals—the enzyme catalyzing the conversion of gulonolactone into ascorbic acid. In the dog and the cat, for example, ascorbic acid is synthesized in this manner, and therefore scurvy, which results from ascorbic acid deficiency, cannot occur. In man, on the other hand, ascorbic acid must be ingested to prevent scurvy, a fatal disease if untreated.

In effect, we all have scurvy. Our species has lost, on a genetic basis, the capacity to synthesize ascorbic acid. It has become an essential nutrient (vitamin C). Happily, most of us have an appetite for fresh fruits and vegetables wherein this vital nutrient abounds, and thus we compensate for our enzyme deficiency by ingesting what in other species is a normal product of metabolism. The fact that scurvy can be prevented in man by a readily available nutritional supplement in no way negates the universal distribution of the genetic defect. Analyses of other "nutritional" diseases could doubtless be evoked to emphasize their underlying genetic nature.

D. S.

16

GENETIC DISEASES

I. Galactosemia: An Enzymological Approach

Herman M. Kalckar

Galactosemia is a genetic disorder marked by an inability of cells to convert dietary galactose, a component of lactose (milk sugar), into glucose. A London mother's complaint "Me milk don't do me baby good" is an accurate though understated description of the disease. In the galactosemic infant, mother's milk, rich in lactose, causes vomiting, diarrhea, and jaundice after a day or two. Later, there is loss of weight, first due to dehydration, then to lack of nutrients. In short, a hazardous state of affairs. If the child survives without a proper diet, chronic effects ensue, such as cataracts and moderate to severe mental retardation.

Early recognition of galactosemia, once called galactose diabetes, is essential. The condition must not be confused with diabetes mellitus, since insulin treatment can be fatal for the galactosemic infant. As one example, a general practitioner who found sugar in the urine of his newborn infant hastened to inject insulin. He nearly lost his son. The sugar was not glucose but galactose, and the condition turned out to be galactosemia. With high levels of galactose in the blood, glucose levels tend to be low, and insulin injections would aggravate the disturbed balance.

Correct therapy in galactosemia is strictly dietary. Vegetable milk, usually in soybean formulas, must be substituted for milk and milk products. Dietary therapy has been known for about 50 years, thanks to simple assays using baker's or brewer's yeast to distinguish galactose from glucose in the urine. Today's highly sensitive methods can reveal galactose and its phosphate derivative in a drop or two of blood.

HERMAN M. KALCKAR, M.D., Ph.D., Research Professor of Biochemistry, Boston University, College of Liberal Arts. Formerly Visiting Scientist, Biochemistry Laboratory, National Institute of Arthritis and Metabolic Diseases.

In a galactosemic newborn or child, enzymatic analysis of a drop of blood would disclose a breach of the galactose-free diet.

At first the device of instituting such a diet as early as possible after birth may have seemed simplistic in view of the continuing deposition of galactose compounds in the central nervous system. The normal brain is rich in galactolipids and galactoproteins. A major question was whether the developing brain of a galactosemic child on a strict galactose-free diet would become deficient in these lipids and proteins despite an improved state of health. I believe that our enzyme research on galactosemic children has provided a biochemical basis for the dietary therapy.

Background

Our NIH project on the biochemistry of galactosemia may be said to have begun in Copenhagen in 1950 through the influence of Luis Leloir in Buenos Aires.

Leloir's group had discovered that the conversion of glucose 1-phosphate to galactose 1-phosphate requires a cofactor, uridine diphosphate (UDP)-galactose. Leloir had also postulated a sequence of reactions leading to the formation of UDP-galactose: Galactose 1-phosphate (discovered in 1943 by H. W. Kosterlitz) might react with UDP-glucose, and this would be converted to UDP-galactose by an enzyme discovered in galactose-adapted yeast. The enzyme was called galactowaldenase.

My brain trust in Copenhagen included two young Danish biochemists, Hans Klenow and Agnete Munch-Petersen. We found that crude enzyme preparations from galactose-adapted yeast catalyzed a reaction between uridine triphosphate (UTP) and glucose 1-phosphate, forming a mixture of UDP-glucose and UDP-galactose.

At the kind invitation of BERNARD HORECKER, Chief of the Biochemistry Laboratory, I came to NIH in September 1954, prepared for adventures in the biochemistry of mammalian organisms. My excellent co-workers were ELIZABETH P. ANDERSON, JULIUS AXELROD, KURT J. ISSELBACHER, ELIZABETH S. MAXWELL, and JACK L. STROMINGER.

We discovered an enzyme in rat liver, UDP-glucose dehydrogenase, which brings about a two-step dehydrogenation of UDP-glucose to UDP-glucuronic acid and simultaneously reduces two moles of nicotinamide adenine dinucleotide (NAD) to reduced NAD (NADH). This highly specific enzyme turned out to be of great value in studying the formation of glucuronide complexes (1).

UDP-glucose dehydrogenase interested me particularly as a sensitive indicator for the enzymatic formation or disappearance of UDP-glucose. In early 1955 I undertook to demonstrate such reactions in human hemolysates (broken red blood cells), including my own. I soon found that the reversible reaction galactose 1-phosphate + UDP-glucose $\rightleftharpoons$ glucose 1-phosphate + UDP-galactose readily occurred. In fact, within 10 minutes of incubation at 37°, with a two- to threefold excess of galactose 1-phosphate, more than 80 percent of the UDP-glucose had been converted to UDP-galactose.

Fortunately, the hemolysate did not interconvert UDP-glucose and UDP-galactose by the galactowaldenase reaction, for this would have interfered with our measurements. The absence of such interconversion will be explained later.

The Biomedical Approach

During 1955 I came in closer contact with the Clinical Center. One of my friends, DeWITT (Hans) STETTEN, a scholarly M.D., had been appointed Director of Research at the National Institute of Arthritis and Metabolic Diseases (NIAMD). Hans brought to NIH a galaxy of highly talented young physicians with the ability to engage in sophisticated research.

Among them were Kurt Isselbacher and GORDON TOMKINS, and I was fortunate to become a friend of both. About that time, I was captivated by some articles on galactosemia. A group of British pediatricians in Manchester, led by A. Holzel and G. M. Komrower, had initiated family studies; and later they enlisted two biochemists, V. Schwartz and L. Goldberg. In 1955 they disclosed that red blood cells from galactosemic infants subjected to a galactose tolerance test accumulated large amounts of galactose 1-phosphate as well as galactose. Moreover, erythrocytes incubated with ^{14}C-labeled galactose accumulated radioactive galactose 1-phosphate. The British group deduced that galactosemics have a defect in galactose 1-phosphate metabolism, and they turned the spotlight on galactowaldenase.

Their view seemed to conflict with clinical observations. One of the more subtle but chronic effects of untreated galactosemia is mental retardation. This complication is usually averted if the condition is discovered early and the infants are placed on a strict galactose-free diet. Yet J. Folch-Pi's studies had shown that a large fraction of the galactolipids are deposited after birth, during the development of the mammalian brain.

Combine these biochemical observations with the known results of dietary therapy. The brain of a galactosemic infant who receives no lactose can still develop normally. Yet the galactowaldenase hypothesis would hold that galactosemic infants fed a galactose-free diet should make brain lipids lacking galactose. I was led by such reasoning to challenge the hypothesis. Drawing upon my Copenhagen experience and NIH findings, I proposed the following sequence:

(a)   galactose + ATP* → galactose 1-phosphate + ADP**

This is the well-known reaction catalyzed by galacto-kinase in mammalian liver.

(b)   galactose 1-phosphate + UDP-glucose ⇌ glucose 1-phosphate + UDP galactose

A reaction we demonstrated in hemolysates from non-galactosemic subjects. We named the enzyme galactose 1-phosphate uridyl transferase.

(c)   UDP-galactose ⇌ UDP-glucose

Demonstrated by us in mammalian liver. The enzyme, previously known as galactowaldenase, is now called UDP-galactose 4-epimerase. It requires NAD for activity, as described below.

(d)   UDP-glucose + pyrophosphate ⇌ UTP + glucose 1-phosphate

Demonstrated in yeast by our Copenhagen team in 1950; catalyzed by the enzyme UDP-glucose pyrophosphorylase.

The galactosemic infants in the British study were reported to have plenty of galactokinase, ruling out (a) as the metabolic error. I proposed that the specific error was not a lack of galactowaldenase (step c) but of the enzyme galactose 1-phosphate uridyl transferase, needed to catalyze step b.

I asked Kurt Isselbacher to consider whether it would be possible and advisable to bring to the Clinical Center, where we had just been relocated, enough galactosemic patients to prove the hypothesis. He thought the proposal had merit and lent his help and skill to the new study. Thanks to his ef-

---

*ATP: adenosine triphosphate, hydrolysis of which releases energy for cellular activity.

**ADP: adenosine diphosphate, an intermediate in energy production from ATP.

forts and those of JOSEPHINE KETY and others, more than a
dozen galactosemic subjects ranging from infants to adults
were assembled at NIH. The nationwide search netted, among
others, mentally retarded children and persons with more or
less severe blindness. In galactosemia a type of blindness
due to gradually developing cataracts must be ascribed to
accumulation of galactose and its reduction product galac-
titol (2).

The enzyme test I had designed (the "UDP-glucose consumption test," using UDP-glucose dehydrogenase) showed that the
galactose 1-phosphate uridyl transferase in hemolysates from
the galactosemic patients was very low—on the order of 1 percent or less of the levels from nongalactosemics (2,3).

Our first report appeared in February 1956. The Surgeon
General, in announcing our venture into human genetics, duly
assured the press that our attack on this rare disease in no
way threatened the profits of milk companies.

When HENRY KIRKMAN joined our unit in 1957, he developed
methods for accurate measurement of the uridyl transferase
reaction rate. It soon became clear that the enzyme was low
in several siblings of the galactosemics. These were presumed
to be carriers of the disease.

UDP-Galactose 4-Epimerase Requires NAD

I should like to comment on one additional discovery of
our NIH lab unit. Elizabeth Maxwell had been on our team in
1954 when we purified UDP-glucose dehydrogenase and had
stored appreciable amounts of it. Now she was engaged in
purifying UDP-galactose 4-epimerase—the enzyme of step c—
from rabbit and calf liver. The availability of these active
preparations enabled us to double-check our enzymatic assays
of UDP-glucose and -galactose.

Liz used our dehydrogenase test to assay for UDP-glucose.
She soon found that the epimerase needed a cofactor for its
activity—NAD—and that NADH was a powerful inhibitor (4).
This latter fact explained why the human hemolysates we had
tested did not interconvert UDP-glucose and -galactose: The
NADH present arrested any activity of the enzyme. When we
added excess NAD to the hemolysates, epimerase activity appeared. It also appeared in galactosemic hemolysates, re-
affirming that the specific defect was not a lack of epimerase but of galactose 1-phosphate uridyl transferase. Assays
on small liver biopsies corroborated these findings.

Biochemical Basis of the Dietary Strategy

Pinpointing the genetic defect in galactosemia as a deficiency of the enzyme galactose 1-phosphate uridyl transferase was important in terms of clinical and nutritional strategies. The enzymologic tests on liver biopsies and on broken red blood cells from galactosemics showed that complex galactose compounds were still formed from glucose by the endogenous pathway—that is, via UDP-galactose 4-epimerase. Had a lack of epimerase been responsible for galactosemia, as stated in the older literature, elimination of galactose or lactose from the patient's diet would be risky, for glucose metabolites would not be able to form the complex galactose compounds crucial for development of the central nervous system. Our resolution of the inborn errors shaped a reassuring basis for the unreserved nutritional strategy—the strict withholding of lactose and galactose from the diet.

In this connection, it has been reported that a galactosemic mother on a galactose-free diet provided her (nongalactosemic) infant with milk containing lactose (2).

In further explanation of the dietary therapy, it should be emphasized that the galactosemic symptoms arise as a consequence of a metabolic "traffic jam" in the galactose metabolic pathway and not as a consequence of deprivation. The conversion of dietary glucose to galactose compounds is not interrupted. It depends on the enzyme UDP-glucose 4-epimerase, which catalyzes a critical step in the conversion of glucose to galactose. We have found that patients with the classical form of galactosemia possess as much epimerase as normal persons.*

---

*There are other, very rare types of galactosemia. An infant with a deficiency of UDP-galactose 4-epimerase was described in 1981 by R. Gitzelman, a Swiss pediatrician. This patient cannot make UDP-galactose from glucose and therefore requires some dietary galactose (or lactose) for synthesis of galactolipids or galactoproteins. But the intake of galactose must be controlled very carefully, as any excess of the sugar brings on acute symptoms of galactosemia.

Another form of galactosemia is caused by a deficiency of galactokinase (reaction a). Patients with this enzyme defect, like those with a deficiency of galactose 1-phosphate uridyl transferase, respond well to a galactose-free diet.

Continuing Research

NIH investigators continue to study galactosemia with a view to improving diagnosis and therapy. In 1957 KIYOSHI KURAHASHI and I disclosed the existence of some bacterial mutants of UDP-galactose metabolism that opened up intriguing aspects of cell-surface antigenic patterns (2). ROBERT KROOTH and ARNOLD WEINBERG found in 1960 that fibroblast cultures from galactosemic infants showed a defect in galactose 1-phosphate uridyl transferase. In 1971 CARL MERRILL and co-workers reported that a bacterial virus, lambda gal, contains genes that could complement the synthesis of the missing or defective enzyme (2).

In our work at NIH, Hans Stetten shared our aspirations and enlightenment. He has lent his strong support to continued research on genetic aberrations in man and microorganisms.

References

1. Kalckar, H.M., and E.S. Maxwell. Biosynthesis and metabolic function of uridine diphosphoglucose in mammalian organisms and its relevance to certain inborn errors. Physiol Rev 38:77, 1958.
2. Kalckar, H.M., J.H. Kinoshita, and G.N. Donnell. Galactosemia, biochemistry, genetics, pathophysiology and developmental aspects. Biology of Brain Dysfunction 1:31-88, G.E. Gaull (ed.). New York, London: Plenum Press, 1973.
3. Kalckar, H.M. The enzymatic deficiency in congenital galactosemia and its heterozygous carriers. Mod Probl Paediatr (Basel) 6:409-419, 1959.
4. Gabriel, O., H.M. Kalckar, and R.A. Darrow. Uridine diphospho-galactose-4-epimerase, Chap. 3 of Subunit Enzymes Biochemistry and Functions, K.E. Ebner (ed.). In Enzymology 2:85-135. New York: Marcel Dekker, 1975.

GENETIC DISEASES

II. Gout and Lesch–Nyhan Disease

J. Edwin Seegmiller

Perhaps my interest in Lesch-Nyhan disease really began with my adolescent love affair with chemistry. I always thought I wanted to be a chemist until I was sent to NIH in 1943 by the National Defense Research Committee at Northwestern University, where I was working during World War II. At NIH I tested equipment we had developed to supply a chemical source of oxygen in high-altitude aviation. There I met physicians investigating chemical causes of disease—much more interesting problems than I had yet encountered. I soon decided to seek a degree in medicine.

Upon discharge from the Army I entered medical school with a long-range view to doing biochemical research. Following my internship at Johns Hopkins, I joined a newly formed group under ARTHUR KORNBERG in the old Experimental Biology and Medicine Institute at NIH and worked directly with BERNARD HORECKER. I suppose I was one of the first of what would be called Research Associates after EBMI evolved into the National Institute of Arthritis and Metabolic Diseases. Our work on the oxidative pathway of glucose metabolism and my demonstration of the cyclic nature of the oxidative pathway of glucose was my basic training.

I then did some clinical work on hepatic coma at Boston City Hospital with Charles Davidson, who was slated to be our Institute's clinical director. When Harvard gave him tenure, I joined DeWITT (Hans) STETTEN at the Public Health Research Institute of the City of New York. Hans kindled my interest in gouty arthritis. First described by Hippocrates, the disease results from high blood levels of a waste

J. EDWIN SEEGMILLER, M.D., Professor of Medicine, University of California, San Diego. Formerly Chief, Human Biochemical Genetics Section, National Institute of Arthritis and Metabolic Diseases.

NIH: AN ACCOUNT OF RESEARCH
IN ITS LABORATORIES AND CLINICS

ISBN 0-12-667980-0

product, urate, and the deposition of needle-shaped crystals of monosodium urate in and about the joints. After a year and a half, Hans and I went to the NIH Clinical Center in July 1954. There, through tracer studies with LEONARD LASTER, we proved genetic heterogeneity* in gout patients.

In studies with RODNEY HOWELL, PAUL ALEPA, and JAMES KLINENBERG, we demonstrated both an increased production of uric acid and a diminished ability of the kidney to excrete it in two patients with early onset of gout associated with a primary defect of carbohydrate metabolism, glycogen storage disease type I. This is caused by a genetic deficiency of an enzyme in the liver, glucose-6-phosphatase, responsible for generating blood sugar. In other studies with STEPHEN MALAWISTA and Rod Howell, we succeeded in inducing acute gouty arthritis by injecting monosodium urate crystals into the knee joint space of gouty volunteers. The crystals produced an inflammation and, in both induced and spontaneous episodes of acute gout, were attacked and engulfed by white cells. An obvious rational approach to control of the disease was to lower the plasma urate concentration to the normal range. Patients with a normal production rate but diminished renal secretion of uric acid need the drug probenecid, and those who overproduce uric acid need allopurinol.

My First Experience with Lesch–Nyhan Disease

In 1962, while Rod Howell was working with me, his wife was on the house staff in pediatric psychiatry at The Johns Hopkins Hospital. Through her he learned of the curious case of a child that William L. Nyhan was studying. This was a boy with cerebral palsy, a bizarre penchant for self-mutilation, and uric acid excretion so high that no one believed it. Rod suggested we verify the uric acid production with our highly specific enzymatic procedure. We did, all very informally. It seemed that further study of a disorder marked by uric acid overproduction even more severe than that seen in gouty arthritis might throw new light on the latter disease.

In 1964 I passed up an opportunity to observe a boy in New Hampshire with this same disorder and extensive destruction of the mouth and tongue. I wanted very much to study the child, but was just preparing to take a year's "sabbat-

---

*The principle that a single disease may be caused by various genetic defects. This generally occurs because each gene affects metabolism in such a way as to produce the same final effect—e.g., elevated serum urate concentrations in the case of gouty arthritis.

ical" with Charles Dent at University College Hospital in London. There I planned to learn more about human genetics from Charles Penrose, who was in his last year of directing the Galton Laboratory across the street.

Tissue Culture

While in London I developed some skill at growing human fibroblasts, though no one in the laboratory had ever done tissue culture and the facilities were completely inadequate. When my cultures kept getting infections, Professor Dent decided that his office was the cleanest place around and offered to let me use it in the mornings for my feeding of cells and transfers. This worked out quite well with the use of a small Plexiglas shield that we devised. We used our technique to demonstrate the enzyme defect in fibroblasts cultured from a patient with maple syrup urine disease—a little girl who became the first child in the world to be treated with a semi-synthetic diet meeting the minimal requirements for branched-chain amino acids. Roland Westall, the chemist who developed the diet, spent most of a morning every two weeks weighing out the patient's dietary components.

Another Lesch-Nyhan Case

One day Professor Dent asked me to accompany him to Hammersmith Hospital to see a boy who had a strange disease associated with hyperuricemia (an abnormally high level of uric acid in the blood). The child's hands were tied to his crib. When I untied them to examine his fingers for self-mutilation, he began to cry. His mother said, "He's afraid you'll let go of his hands and he'll bite them." This was my first direct encounter with the Lesch-Nyhan syndrome (named after Nyhan and MICHAEL LESCH, a medical student). The child was severely impaired neurologically, with uncontrolled movements and unintelligible speech. Fortunately, I had just attended Alexander Gutman's symposium in Princeton, New Jersey, where I heard Nyhan give a superb description of the disease. The overproduction of uric acid in Dent's patient was confirmed in London.

After returning to NIH in 1965, I set up our tissue culture unit, the Human Biochemical Genetics Section, with two Clinical Associates, FREDERICK ROSENBLOOM and JERRY SCHNEIDER. I was convinced that tissue culture could contribute substantially to our understanding of human hereditary diseases.

Differentiating Gout from Lesch-Nyhan Disease

About this time I learned that Leif Sorensen, at the University of Chicago, had studied two children with some of the clinical features of Lesch-Nyhan disease. He had reported earlier that azathioprine, a synthetic purine analog, would reduce uric acid production in gout. In the two children, however, uric acid synthesis continued despite the agent. A questionable diagnosis (in the absence of self-mutilation) prompted us to repeat the studies in gouty adults and eventually in children with well-defined Lesch-Nyhan disease. About this time we were joined by WILLIAM KELLEY, who was eager to become involved in our clinical investigations. By May 1966 we had found some Lesch-Nyhan children to study, and we soon confirmed their difference from most gout patients in that azathioprine failed to decrease their excessive uric acid production. Despite the manifest similarity of the two disorders, they were not metabolically identical.

We Investigate the Enzyme Defect

At the same time we began to study the biosynthesis of purines in skin fibroblasts from these children, using the cells' incorporation of radioactive formate into a purine precursor as an index of rate. We hypothesized a fault in the regulation of the synthetic process—initially, a defect in feedback regulation of the first enzyme in purine synthesis, phosphoribosylpyrophosphate glutamine amidotransferase. Hence, we tested the cells' response to a variety of known feedback regulators of that enzyme, including hypoxanthine, 6-mercaptopurine, and 6-methylmercaptopurine riboside. Only the riboside slowed purine synthesis in the children's cells.

Why was that compound effective but not the closely related 6-mercaptopurine? The answer might lie in the fact that neither compound regulates as such, but must first be converted to a corresponding nucleotide (a basic unit of nucleic acid and other vital products). Conversion of the riboside would only require addition of phosphate, which could be catalyzed by an enzyme known as a kinase, whereas 6-mercaptopurine or hypoxanthine would require the enzyme hypoxanthine-guanine phosphoribosyltransferase (HGPRT). This experiment pointed to HGPRT as a likely candidate for the enzyme defect in Lesch-Nyhan disease. But we had no Lesch-Nyhan patients to study at that time.

An Assay for the Missing Enzyme

Following a trip out of town to obtain skin biopsies and blood samples from other children suspected of having the disease, I arrived back at the laboratory rather late one evening. I had conceived of a simple assay for HGPRT. Since I wasn't sure the enzyme would hold up on storage of the blood samples, I decided to work that night. I incubated a lysate of washed erythrocytes (red blood cells) from normal and Lesch-Nyhan subjects with phosphoribosylpyrophosphate (PRPP) and hypoxanthine. In the lysate of normal cells, the disappearance of hypoxanthine could be monitored (by reaction with xanthine oxidase) as metabolism proceeded. The abnormal cell lysate, on the other hand, should be incapable of utilizing the hypoxanthine and yielding the nucleotide, in this case inosinic acid. As usual, working out the new assay took much longer than I had expected, but by early morning I was satisfied that erythrocytes from the affected child contained neither HGPRT nor an inhibitor that could account for the inactivity.

A week later, in early December 1966, FRANK HENDERSON arrived to spend a most productive three-month sabbatical. We developed a more sensitive radiochemical assay for HGPRT, using high-voltage electrophoresis to separate the products. As expected, we were able to demonstrate very little activity in the red cells of children with Lesch-Nyhan disease.

Testing for the Defect in Patients with Gout

About a month later we decided to see if any of our gout patients who produced excessive quantities of uric acid might have the same enzyme defect, for the elusive biochemical similarity between gouty arthritis and Lesch-Nyhan disease continued to intrigue us. Three brothers had been highly cooperative in many of our clinical studies, including those on acute gouty arthritis produced by injection of monosodium urate crystals into the joint. Bill Kelley had been checking HGPRT activity in these three patients. One morning I arrived at the laboratory around 6 a.m. and found that he had been working all night. "I'm so glad to see you!" he exclaimed. "Look what I found this morning in the three brothers. I know it will soon be in all the textbooks, but for the past three hours I've been the only one in the world who knew it!" To see a young person in the exuberance of discovery makes all the painstaking work of research seem worthwhile.

The brothers had shown a slightly less severe deficiency of HGPRT—around 1 percent of the normal level. Yet this small amount of remaining HGPRT activity was important in attenuating the severe clinical symptoms of Lesch-Nyhan disease. None of the brothers had neurological problems, but only an excessive uric acid production. We continued the search for evidence of the enzyme deficit in gouty patients. Eventually we found about 0.5 percent of the normal activity in two brothers from another family, both with severe gout and excessive uric acid synthesis. Unlike the three brothers mentioned above, they had a mild neurologic disorder—spinocerebellar syndrome —but this was quite different from the problems of Lesch-Nyhan patients. The enzyme deficit, however, clearly indicated that their condition was related to Lesch-Nyhan disease.

Genetic Basis

One aspect of the disease that we were interested in exploring was its apparent occurrence as a sex-linked recessive transmitted by the mother and manifest only in sons. Did the gene for HGPRT really reside on the X chromosome? We reasoned that we could prove X linkage if we could develop a test for detecting the presence or absence of HGPRT enzyme in individual cells of the mothers. This test would be based on the Lyon hypothesis of X chromosome inactivation in the female.* To detect HGPRT activity in individual cultured fibroblasts, Fred Rosenbloom developed a radioautographic method based on the incorporation of tagged (tritiated) hypoxanthine into nucleic acids. Normal cells showed an abundant uptake, while cells from affected children showed virtually none. According to the Lyon hypothesis, the mothers should show both normal and HGPRT-deficient cells in their body. You can imagine our excitement when we found both normal and abnormal cells in fibroblasts cultured from a skin biopsy from the apparently normal mother of a Lesch-Nyhan child, thus proving X linkage. In subsequent work it remained a useful test for female family members carrying the gene (heterozygotes).

---

*Formulated in 1962 by Mary Lyon of Oxford University, this "hypothesis" (with some modifications) is now accepted as one of the well-established rules of mammalian genetics. It states that only one of the two X chromosomes in the female cell (one derived from each parent) is active. In some cells the maternal X chromosome is functional; in others, the paternal. This determination is made at random (roughly 50-50) in the early embryo, and the commitment is perpetuated by some mechanism not yet understood. The inactivated X chromosome forms the "Barr body," characteristic of female cells.

Some Clinical Applications

By now it was late June 1967 and Kelley's and Rosenbloom's appointments had ended. But three very able and enthusiastic clinical associates arrived, WILFRED FUJIMOTO, MARTIN GREENE, and THEODORE FRIEDMANN, a pediatrician, and we soon had the laboratory in full operation again.

In clinical research settings, one is always under pressure to apply esoteric findings—as the Lyon hypothesis seemed at the time—to the solution of practical problems. About this time I learned, in talking to the mother of one of the Lesch-Nyhan children, that her sister's daughter was pregnant in New England. I knew I was the only person worried about the possibility of her carrying a fetus destined to have Lesch-Nyhan disease. Her obstetrician, learning of my concern, agreed to send me a skin biopsy in the sterile culture media we sent to him. It arrived in due time, and our test for heterozygosity revealed that the prospective mother was indeed a carrier. Within 24 hours we had a very frightened young lady in the Clinical Center who had never before left her hometown and was beside herself at the prospect of bearing a child who would need round-the-clock nursing care like her cousin.

Cecil Jacobsen, a colleague at George Washington University, was developing amniocentesis. He had accumulated evidence assuring that cells in the amniotic fluid surrounding the fetus were from the fetus rather than the mother. We arranged for him to remove a small amount (around 15 ml) of amniotic fluid from this young lady on the day of her admission to our Clinical Center. The amniotic cells showed the Barr bodies and two X chromosomes characteristic of a female fetus. So we told her she had nothing to worry about—that she was going to have a daughter, who would not be affected—and sent her home. Never having engaged before in prophecy, I must confess to some relief five months later when she did indeed deliver a baby girl.

Back in our laboratory, we cultured the cells and applied our radiographic procedure. We found normal and abnormal populations of both epithelial and fibroblast-type amniotic cells, showing that the fetus was a carrier of Lesch-Nyhan disease. The results, moreover, indicated that we should be able to diagnose an affected male fetus, thus demonstrating for the first time the utility of biochemistry in disclosing an X-linked disorder in utero.

Using the same method of radioautography with Ted Friedmann in my laboratory the following year, we asked the simple question whether DNA extracted from normal cells could correct the HGPRT deficiency of fibroblasts cultured from children with Lesch-Nyhan disease. When normal DNA was added along with a diamine, we found a partial correction of the enzyme deficit in 1-in-10^4 to 1-in-10^5 cells, while DNA from affected children showed no such evidence of correction. Unfortunately, we could never clone out the genetically corrected cells under conditions of selective growth that readily permitted the isolation of the corresponding number of normal cells added to mutant cells. We therefore concluded that we were achieving an abortive rather than a permanent genetic transformation.

These studies provided the impetus for the establishment of a human biochemical genetics program when I moved to the University of California (San Diego) in 1969. In the last 14 years, we have monitored 29 pregnancies at risk for Lesch-Nyhan disease and have found 8 affected fetuses. In each case the prenatal diagnosis was sufficiently early for the parents to have the pregnancies terminated. More important to me are the 21 nonaffected children, many of whom are here today because this technology was available to prompt the pregnancy in the first place.

Phosphoribosylpyrophosphate (PRPP) Synthetase Overproduction

After moving to San Diego I persuaded MICHAEL BECKER, one of GORDON TOMKINS' research associates, to become my first trainee in rheumatology. I also arranged to bring from the Washington area one of my former patients for clinical study, a man who produced excessive quantities of uric acid but had no HGPRT deficiency.

At a World Health Organization meeting in Bangkok, André DeVries and I had discussed an interesting family with purine overproduction. He had traced this to an elevated precursor in the red cells—PRPP—and then to hyperactivity of the enzyme PRPP synthetase. I persuaded Becker to check this enzyme in our patient. He found two to three times the normal activity in both red cells and cultured fibroblasts.

After working awhile in Henry Harris's laboratory at Oxford (1975), I came back with a library of Steven Goss's human-hamster hybrid cells containing various fragments of the human X chromosome. Hybridization experiments enabled Becker to demonstrate that the gene for PRPP synthetase is X linked and resides near the gene for HGPRT.

Further Opportunities in Goutlike Disorders

There are still other enzyme defects to be identified in goutlike conditions. Recently our present rheumatology fellow, Harry Gruber, produced evidence of a possible additional mutation in purine metabolism that may well be associated with excessive rates of purine synthesis in some of our patients.

The HGPRT enzyme defect has proved of great practical value to basic studies of cell biology and genetics as a result of the development of methods for selecting for growth either the normal or HGPRT-deficient cells. This property has allowed the HGPRT gene to be a favorite for studies of cell biology and molecular genetics. It has helped substantially in the recent development of the cloned HGPRT gene, first of mice by TOM CASKEY in Houston and, shortly afterwards, of the human gene by Douglas Jolly and associates working here in La Jolla in Ted Friedmann's laboratory, a few doors from mine. This group has now achieved a stable genetic transformation of HGPRT-deficient fibroblasts. In recent collaborative work with my laboratory, we have achieved a similar, relatively stable correction of a permanent lymphoblast line from an affected child.

Thus, gout research continues to be a most revealing pursuit, shedding light on the whole field of metabolic diseases. Of great interest at present are genetic errors of purine metabolism related to defects in the immune system. And gout has been on the forefront of new concept development. The principle of genetic heterogeneity, for instance, is certainly one of the major underlying themes to have emerged over the past few decades. As a physician I am also gratified by the marked improvement in therapy that has accompanied the explosion of basic knowledge. Hardly anyone today need suffer acute gout's recurrent, excruciating attacks, and the chronic problems are readily preventable.

Other Genetic Diseases

My years at NIH presented opportunities for numerous other explorations of genetic diseases which space does not permit me to describe here. One was the demonstration, with BERT LaDU, Leonard Laster, and VINCE ZANNONI, of the genetically determined enzyme defect in tyrosine metabolism in alkaptonuria, which can lead to severe, disabling "ochronotic" arthritis in adult life. Other demonstrations were the enzyme defect in the world's second known case of histidemia, with LaDu, Howell, Zannoni, and G. A. Jacoby, and the enzyme defect in xanthinuria, with Klinenberg, KARL ENGLEMAN, and AL SJOERDSMA.

With Jerry Schneider and Kay Bradley, we found the first biochemical abnormality associated with another crystal deposition disease, cystinosis. This claims young lives as a high intracellular concentration of cystine in fibroblasts and leukocytes. Its location in lysosomes was reported with Kay Bradley and Joe Schulman. With Schulman and Tom Lustberg, a medical student, we also described a new variant of maple syrup urine disease, in collaboration with J. L. Kennedy and M. Museles of the National Naval Medical Center. These are only a few of the fascinating scientific and clinical problems we investigated during my 20 years at NIH.

Selected References

Seegmiller, J.E., F.M. Rosenbloom, and W.N. Kelley. Enzyme defect associated with a sex-linked human neurological disorder and excessive purine synthesis. Science 155:1682-1684, 1967.

Kelley, W.N., et al. A specific enzyme defect in gout associated with overproduction of uric acid. Proc Natl Acad Sci USA 57:1735-1739, 1967.

Rosenbloom, F.M., et al. Biochemical bases of accelerated purine bio-synthesis de novo in human fibroblasts lacking hypoxanthine-guanine phosphoribosyltransferase. J Biol Chem 243:1166-1173, 1968.

Fujimoto, W.Y., et al. Biochemical diagnosis of an X-linked disease in utero. Lancet 2:511-512, 1968.

Becker, M.A., et al. Purine overproduction in man associated with increased phosphoribosyl-pyrophosphate synthetase activity. Science 179:1123-1126, 1973.

Willis, R.C., et al. Partial phenotypic correction of human Lesch-Nyhan (HPRT-deficient) lymphoblasts with a transmissible retroviral vector. J Biol Chem, in press.

GENETIC DISEASES

III. The Lipodystrophies

Roscoe O. Brady

My interest in lipid disorders dates from my first year at Harvard Medical School. While studying biochemistry, I began to investigate with Professor W. W. Westerfeld whether rats habituated to alcohol (a precursor of lipids) could be influenced in level of consumption by a newly reported "vitamin N." The experiments were finally completed during my fourth year. I learned from this experience that research can require much more devotion and stamina than I had anticipated. Another discovery was that I might be able to cope with such challenges.

In my third and fourth years of medical school, I became deeply involved with some of my patients. It was during World War II, when most of the functions of scarce hospital personnel were performed by medical students. Two heart disease patients in particular stand out. One was a young woman with small children, the other a man in his early fifties. Both died in the hospital, leaving me with a feeling that medicine should try to find ways to help these people.

After interning, I received a National Research Council fellowship in the medical sciences and, with Samuel Gurin at the University of Pennsylvania School of Medicine, undertook to examine the biosynthesis of long-chain fatty acids and cholesterol. We were strongly advised to develop an appropriate enzyme system. After many difficulties and delays, toward the end of my third postdoctoral year, I began to obtain consistently active preparations and to examine the requirements for lipogenesis. Shortly thereafter, however, I was ordered to active duty in the medical corps of the Navy. I am sure every investigator can understand my disappointment

ROSCOE O. BRADY, M.D., Chief, Developmental and Metabolic Neurology Branch, National Institute of Neurological and Communicative Disorders and Stroke.

ISBN 0-12-667980-0

when, having finally opened the door to this field, I had to leave it so abruptly and with so much to be learned. But off I went to the National Naval Medical Center, across the street from NIH. In order to continue some experimentation, I worked in EARL STADTMAN's laboratory in the National Heart Institute evenings and weekends.

Introduction to the Lipid Storage Disorders

As my tour of duty in the Navy drew to a close, SEYMOUR S. KETY was establishing a basic research program under the combined aegis of the Neurology and Mental Health Institutes. He chose me to head a section on the metabolism of lipids, to be studied because of their involvement in brain development and their potential role in demyelinating disorders. In 1954 I began to study the biosynthesis of sphingolipids, which appeared to be particularly important in the nervous system. Work centered on enzymes that catalyzed the synthesis of these lipids in the neonatal period, when their formation was most active.

I was constantly mindful of the sphingolipidoses, a group of heritable lipid storage disorders. At that time nothing was known about the etiology except that pathologic quantities of sphingolipids accumulated in the organs and tissues of patients. Gaucher's disease is the most frequently encountered disorder of this type. Patients have enlarged spleens and livers, low blood platelets, bone damage, and occasionally brain damage. The lipid that accumulates injuriously is glucocerebroside.

It seemed to me that three likely explanations for this accumulation might be explored. The first was an abnormality of carbohydrate metabolism resulting in the formation of glucocerebroside rather than galactocerebroside, known as a major brain lipid since the beginning of the century. Using ^{14}C-labeled glucose and galactose, I examined this possibility by investigating cerebroside synthesis in surviving slices of spleen tissue from Gaucher patients who had undergone splenectomy because of thrombocytopenia. The observation that both labeled hexoses were used in the synthesis of glucocerebroside and galactocerebroside was evidence for normal operation of those metabolic pathways.

The second possibility was overproduction of glucocerebroside, normally a minor tissue component. I was also able to exclude this alternative. Glucocerebroside formation from labeled precursors such as ^{14}C-glucose, -galactose, or -acetate occurred no more rapidly in spleen slices from Gaucher patients than in those from controls.

This left the third possibility; and thus I postulated the metabolic defect to be a deficiency of a catabolic enzyme required for glucocerebroside disposal.

Exploration of Glucocerebroside Metabolism

After a number of unsuccessful attempts to follow the metabolism of unlabeled glucocerebroside, I concluded that the best way to examine its fate would be to introduce a radioactive tracer into specific portions of the molecule. Attempts at biosynthesis, however, did not provide lipid with sufficient radioactivity to carry out these experiments. Accordingly, JULIAN KANFER and I, in collaboration with David Shapiro of the Weizmann Institute of Science, synthesized glucocerebroside chemically in two preparations—one with ^{14}C in the glucose portion of the molecule, the other with ^{14}C in the fatty acid portion.

An enzyme, glucocerebrosidase, was found to catalyze the cleavage of glucose from glucocerebroside in all mammalian tissues studied. We isolated glucocerebrosidase from normal human spleen and determined the optimal conditions for its activity. With this information in hand, we were able, in 1964, to assay the enzyme in tissue samples from normal humans and from patients with Gaucher's disease. The patients' tissues showed a striking decrease in the activity, thus establishing the metabolic defect.

Inborn Errors Established in Ten Lipodystrophies

The following year, in a similar series of investigations with ^{14}C-sphingomyelin, we demonstrated a deficiency of sphingomyelinase in patients with Niemann-Pick disease. These findings permitted correct predictions of the enzymatic defects in other lipid storage disorders, including Fabry's disease, Tay-Sachs disease, and generalized gangliosidosis. My co-workers and I documented the defect in Fabry's disease in 1967. In 1969 EDWIN KOLODNY and I, working with Bruno Volk at the Kingsbrook Jewish Hospital in Brooklyn, demonstrated that patients with Tay-Sachs disease were deficient in the enzyme hexosaminidase, which catalyzes the cleavage of N-acetylgalactosamine from the accumulating ganglioside G_{M2}. Eventually, through efforts in many laboratories, the metabolic lesions in all 10 of the sphingolipid storage disorders were demonstrated. In each instance the defect was a deficiency of a lipid-catabolizing enzyme required for the initial step in degradation of the accumulating substance.

Diagnosis

Shortly after the metabolic defects in the lipid storage disorders were identified, my attention turned to the development of practical diagnostic tests. In 1967 my associates and I demonstrated that leukocytes from a small sample of venous blood afforded reliable assays. These cells are now widely employed in the diagnosis of metabolic disorders.

The usefulness of cultured skin fibroblasts for diagnosis of the sphingolipidoses was soon established. Fibroblasts have high levels of sphingolipid hydrolytic activity. And they can be transported frozen from remote points of collection to an appropriate facility for measurement of enzyme activity.

Prevention

Next came the demonstration that leukocytes and cultured skin fibroblasts could also be used to identify carriers of lipid storage disorders. These findings provided the necessary background for accurate genetic counseling. Except for Fabry's disease, all of the lipid storage diseases are transmitted as autosomal recessive disorders. This simply means that only if both parents are carriers can the child be affected and that such couples have a 25 percent chance with each pregnancy that the fetus will be abnormal. Fabry's disease is an X chromosome-linked recessive disorder in which only the female need be a carrier to produce an affected male child.

Tests were developed to monitor pregnancies occurring when both parents are heterozygotes or when the mother is a carrier of Fabry's disease. These tests are enzyme assays using extracts of cultured amniotic cells obtained during the second trimester. The reliability of such assays for the prenatal diagnosis of Gaucher's disease, Niemann-Pick disease, and Fabry's disease was established in my laboratory. Investigators at the Jewish Chronic Diseases Hospital in Brooklyn and the University of California (San Diego) documented the validity of prenatal diagnosis for Tay-Sachs disease. Thus, couples at risk for any of these disorders may now have normal children.

Current Approaches to Therapy

My current research is primarily concerned with the development of effective therapy for patients with hereditary metabolic defects. A number of young patients with Gaucher's disease appear to have benefited from infusions of purified glucocerebrosidase obtained from human placental tissue. Although we find this highly encouraging, I believe the treatment can be improved by augmenting delivery of the requisite enzymes to lipid-storing cells. Promising results in targeting these enzymes have been obtained.

Another, perhaps more difficult undertaking is the delivery of enzymes to the brains of patients with central nervous system damage. Indications that this approach may be feasible are beginning to emerge. It is quite apparent, however, that enzyme replacement for patients with brain involvement is an enormous task, and it is difficult to predict when such therapy will become available.

I have concentrated on the main thrust of my work in the lipid storage diseases and have tried to convey a sense of the devotion that went into these efforts. There were also a number of pleasurable discursions into related fields, such as neurophysiology with ICHIJI TASAKI, neuroanatomy with WAYNE ALBERS, neuropharmacology with JULIUS AXELROD, and glycolipid metabolism in neoplastic tissues with a host of co-workers in NCI. Currently under way in my branch are studies on the function of glycolipids as membrane transducers of environmental signals and on the role of glycoproteins in myelination. One hopes that these investigations will in time yield practical applications for the treatment of neoplastic diseases and of demyelinating conditions such as multiple sclerosis.

Selected References

Trams, E.G., and R.O. Brady. Cerebroside synthesis in Gaucher's disease. J Clin Invest 39:1546-1550, 1960.

Brady, R.O., J.N. Kanfer, and D. Shapiro. Metabolism of glucocerebrosides. II. Evidence of an enzymatic deficiency in Gaucher's disease. Biochem Biophys Res Commun 18:221-225, 1965.

Brady, R.O., et al. Demonstration of a deficiency of glucocerebroside-cleaving enzyme in Gaucher's disease. J Clin Invest 45:1112-1115, 1966.

Brady, R.O., et al. The metabolism of sphingomyelin. II. Evidence of an enzymatic deficiency in Niemann-Pick disease. Proc Natl Acad Sci USA 55:366-369, 1966.

Brady, R.O., et al. Enzymatic defect in Fabry's disease. Ceramidetrihexosidase deficiency. N Engl J Med 276:1163-1167, 1967.

Kampine, J.P., et al. The diagnosis of Gaucher's disease and Niemann-Pick disease using small samples of venous blood. Science 155:86-88, 1967.

Kolodny, E.H., R.O. Brady, and B.W. Volk. Demonstration of an alteration of ganglioside metabolism in Tay-Sachs disease. Biochem Biophys Res Commun 37:526-531, 1969.

Cumar, F.A., et al. Enzymatic block in the synthesis of gangliosides in DNA virus-transformed tumorigenic mouse cell lines. Proc Natl Acad Sci USA 67:757-764, 1970.

Brady, R.O., W.G. Johnson, and B.W. Uhlendorf. Identification of heterozygous carriers of lipid storage diseases. Am J Med 51:423-431, 1971.

Epstein, C.J., et al. In utero diagnosis of Niemann-Pick disease. Am J Hum Genet 23:533-535, 1971.

Tallman, J.F., W.G. Johnson, and R.O. Brady. The metabolism of Tay-Sachs ganglioside: Catabolic studies with lysosomal enzymes from normal and Tay-Sachs brain tissue. J Clin Invest 51:2339-2345, 1972.

Brady, R.O., et al. Replacement therapy for inherited enzyme deficiency: Use of purified ceramidetrihexosidase in Fabry's disease. N Engl J Med 289:9-14, 1973.

Brady, R.O., et al. Replacement therapy for inherited enzyme deficiency: Use of purified glucocerebrosidase in Gaucher's disease. N Engl J Med 291:989-993, 1974.

Barranger, J.A., et al. Modification of the blood-brain barrier: Increased concentration and fate of enzymes entering the brain. Proc Natl Acad Sci USA 76:481-485, 1979.

Ginns, E.I., et al. Mutations of glucocerebrosidase: Discrimination of neurologic and nonneurologic phenotypes of Gaucher's disease. Proc Natl Acad Sci USA 79:5607-5610, 1982.

GENETIC DISEASES

IV. Mucopolysaccharide Storage Diseases

Elizabeth F. Neufeld

I started to work on the Hurler syndrome in 1967. This fatal genetic disease—which affects all organs, but particularly the brain, heart, and skeletal system—was thought at the time to result from overproduction of mucopolysaccharides. These cell products, comprising amino sugars and uronic acid units, accumulate in tissues and spill in the urine. During my postdoctoral training as a biochemist, I had studied the biosynthesis of plant cell-wall polymers, some of which, containing uronic acids, resemble mucopolysaccharides of animal origin. Thus I knew something of the metabolism of the uronic acid derivatives—called sugar nucleotides—that are precursors of mucopolysaccharides. It was reasonable to think that the regulation of such precursors had gone astray in Hurler patients.

This idea, tested on fibroblasts cultured from a patient's skin, proved to be wrong. However, the six-month experiment was not a total loss. It taught me something about the culture of skin fibroblasts, a technique that had been introduced in the study of genetic diseases. Also, I was hooked on the problem. If deranged regulation of sugar nucleotides was not the basis of the Hurler syndrome, then what was?

Tracking the Biochemical Defect

In the fall of that year, JOSEPH FRATANTONI and I decided to examine the prevailing assumption that the Hurler syndrome was due to overproduction of mucopolysaccharides. We fed medium containing radioactive sulfate to fibroblasts from

ELIZABETH F. NEUFELD, Ph.D., Chief, Genetics and Biochemistry Branch, National Institute of Arthritis, Diabetes, and Digestive and Kidney Diseases.

ISBN 0-12-667980-0

patients and normal persons, thus tagging the mucopolysaccharides.* The rate of incorporation of the radioisotope indicated that synthesis of the mucopolysaccharides in Hurler
cells was not impaired, but that their degradation was abnormally slow. The material not yet degraded was stored in the
lysosomes—organelles that had been implicated in 1964 by Bel-
gian investigators (Hers, Van Hoof, and colleagues), who had
also introduced the concept of lysosomal storage disease.

The experiments were extended to cells from patients with
mucopolysaccharide storage diseases, such as the Hunter and
Sanfilippo syndromes, which were clinically related to Hurler's. Fratantoni and I became intrigued by a new publication of Danes and Bearn (1967) showing that fibroblasts cultured from mothers of Hunter patients obeyed the Lyon hypothesis of X-chromosome inactivation. This states that the
genetic information from only one of the two X chromosomes in
female cells is actively expressed in any one cell. The
Hunter syndrome is transmitted on the X chromosome.** Thus
mothers of Hunter patients should have a mosaic constitution,
with some cells that are genetically normal and others that
have the Hunter gene, like those of their affected sons.

Logically, we would have expected these women—Hunter
syndrome carriers—to exhibit at least a mild form of the disease. But they were reported to be clinically normal. Perhaps, we reasoned, their normal cells assist the abnormal ones
in disposing of the mucopolysaccharide. We had no access at
that time to fibroblasts from mothers of Hunter patients, but
thought that a mixture of cells from a Hunter patient and a
normal male might, in light of the Lyon hypothesis, be a close
approximation. We planned to study the pattern of radioactive
sulfate incorporation in such a mixture.

The experiment was relegated to the back burner, perhaps
because it seemed a bit odd. But a few weeks later Fratantoni
emerged from the culture room saying he had inadvertently
mixed cells from a Hurler and a Hunter patient. Since we had
talked of mixing cells, we took advantage of this mishap. The
result was dramatic: the mixture was almost biochemically
normal.

A little more work established that cells from one patient
were aided by macromolecular substances transmitted from cells

---

*For application of tissue culture to genetic research,
see references to ROBERT S. KROOTH in papers by Eagle and
Kalckar. Others who contributed to the technique were Danes
and Bearn at Rockefeller University and J. E. SEEGMILLER (see
Section II of this chapter).

**See footnote in Seegmiller section for an explanation
of the Lyon hypothesis.

of the other patient through the culture medium. Patients could be sorted into groups according to their cells' ability to correct the defect in other cells. Normal cells corrected all the groups. By and large the groups followed Victor McKusick's classification of the storage diseases, though with some interesting discrepancies. ULRICH WIESMANN, a Visiting Scientist from Switzerland, found that Sanfilippo patients could be subdivided into two cross-correcting groups, whereas patients with the relatively benign Scheie syndrome could not be distinguished from severely affected Hurler patients by the test.

Corrective Factors and Degradative Enzymes

We realized that further study of the macromolecular sub-stances, which we called corrective factors, might lead to precise identification of the metabolic defects in this group of disorders. The years 1969–1971 were devoted to the purifi-cation of the corrective factors. ROBERT BARTON, MICHAEL CANTZ, and HANS KRESSE, respectively, undertook to purify those that were corrective for Hurler and Hunter cells and for one of the Sanfilippo subtypes. We guessed that these factors might be enzymes and developed the purification procedures accordingly. The procedures were monitored by laborious tests on cultured cells. With heroic effort, one person could assay 60 samples a week.

Eventually the three factors were purified—if not com-pletely, at least sufficiently to show that they were not identical to known enzymes. Our suspicion that they must be degradative enzymes, however, was reinforced when we found an enzyme deficiency in a new patient with a mucopolysaccharide storage disease. Cells from this child had been sent to us by W. S. SLY (Washington University, St. Louis) for diagnosis by our cross-correction tests. When none of the familiar muco-polysaccharide storage diseases could be identified, CLARA HALL assayed a number of lysosomal enzymes. The cells turned out to be deficient in one of these, β-glucuronidase; and bo-vine β-glucuronidase proved as corrective as our purified fac-tors had been for cells of the Hurler, Hunter, and Sanfilippo patients. Furthermore, we could determine that during the correction process, the enzyme entered the deficient cells.

We did not realize at the time just how fortunate we were to have received the sample. In 10 years, only a dozen new cases of β-glucuronidase deficiency have been found worldwide, making this probably the rarest in a group of rare diseases.

With clean factors at hand, GIDEON BACH, a postdoctoral fellow from Israel, started to study their function. If a corrective factor was an enzyme, then its substrate must be some specific group in the mucopolysaccharide that accumulated in the corresponding deficiency disease. Indeed, the substrate for the Hunter corrective factor—the block causing mucopolysaccharide to accumulate in cells of Hunter patients —turned out to be sulfated iduronic acid residues; and the substance that we had purified as the corrective factor was the enzyme, iduronate sulfatase.

In identifying the Hurler corrective factor, we received invaluable help from Bernard Weissmann of the University of Illinois, who provided us with a compound that one of his graduate students had synthesized—phenyliduronide. This allowed us to identify the Hurler factor as the enzyme α-L-iduronidase. Soon other laboratories, sometimes using similar, sometimes quite different strategies, had classified most of the known mucopolysaccharide storage diseases by their enzyme deficiency. More biochemical defects underlying mucopolysaccharide storage were added later, making a total of 10 in 1981. Major contributors to the field were Albert Dorfman and Reuben Matalon (University of Chicago) and John O'Brien (University of California).

Recognition Marker and Receptor

Corrective factors, so much harder to assay and study than enzymes, might have become a thing of the past, except for a new surprise. Factors and enzymes turned out to be not exactly identical. Only some forms of lysosomal enzymes were corrective, and those were the forms that would enter into the cells in a very efficient manner. We suggested that the enzyme's entry into cells was not a function of its usual working end (catalytic site)—that it had to be "recognized" by some specific chemical structure.

That structure was shown by LARRY SHAPIRO and SCOT HICKMAN in 1974 to be a carbohydrate linked to the enzyme protein, analogous but not identical to the galactose signal previously shown by GILBERT ASHWELL to be required for selective entry of circulating glycoproteins into liver cells. The precise structure of the recognition marker eluded us for several years. Finally, in 1977, the problem was solved in an unexpected way by A. Kaplan (St. Louis University) and Sly, who showed the marker to be mannose 6-phosphate groups on the enzyme. Such a structure had not been observed before in mammalian cells.

That the lysosomal enzymes bore a recognition marker implied the presence of a complementary molecule—a receptor—on the cell surface. A receptor would bind the enzymes and

ensure their entry into the cell and eventually into lysosomes. One that specifically interacts with lysosomal enzymes was first described by GLORIA SANDO and LEONARD ROME in
my laboratory and was purified by Sahagian and Jourdian (University of Michigan). GARY SAHAGIAN subsequently came to us,
bringing his expertise in this area.

We might not have understood the significance of the
marker/receptor system if not for another genetic disorder.
In I-cell disease, which is even more severe than the Hurler
syndrome, many lysosomal enzymes (including some we had been
studying, such as α-L-iduronidase, iduronate sulfatase, and
β-glucuronidase) are abnormally low within cultured fibroblasts but abnormally high in the culture medium and in
patients' blood and urine. In other words, the enzymes are
in the wrong place—outside the cell rather than inside the
lysosomes. Hickman in 1972, ANDREJ HASILIK while with us in
1977-1979 and later, and investigators in other laboratories
showed that enzymes made by I-cell disease patients did not
have the mannose 6-phosphate recognition marker. Thus the
real function of the marker (which we had discovered in the
context of correction) must be to guide the cell's enzymes
to their normal lysosome destination.

Diagnosis and Treatment

The early days of research into the mucopolysaccharide
storage diseases were exciting, not only because we were un-
covering new information and developing new concepts but also
because of the very real opportunity to help afflicted families. The diagnostic services based on the correction tests
and later on enzyme assays have been invaluable for management and counseling.

Prenatal diagnosis of these disorders was greeted with
enthusiasm as a way for heterozygous couples to have normal
children and avoid the potential tragedy of another affected
child in the family. It is regrettable that pressure of the
antiabortion movement has probably diminished the positive
aspects of this service while imposing an additional burden
of guilt on families wishing to avail themselves of it.

The correction experiments raised the hope that if fibroblasts could be cured of their biochemical deficiency, so
could affected children. It did not take long to appreciate
the technical and biological difficulties: the need for large
quantities of highly purified enzymes of human origin, with
the appropriate recognition markers to target them to cells
where storage occurs. These problems have led some clinical
investigators to attempt shortcuts to enzyme replacement by

administration of plasma, leukocytes, or fibroblasts; but such procedures have not brought significant long-term improvement. Bone marrow transplantation has been tested, particularly in England, as a way to provide a constant supply of circulating cells that secrete lysosomal enzymes. Unfortunately, the risk of the procedure greatly outweighs its potential benefit. Transplantation of amnion has been proposed, also by English investigators, as a safe alternative, and we are currently evaluating its possible efficacy at NIH in collaboration with JOSEPH MUENZER and MICHAEL ZASLOFF of the National Institute of Child Health and Human Development (see figure).

The rapid advances in molecular biology have given new impetus to the field. It will soon be possible to extend our understanding of these disorders to the level of the gene. And the problem of limited enzyme supply may yield to the new technology for synthesis of human proteins in microorganisms.

Selected References

Fratantoni, J.C., C.W. Hall, and E.F. Neufeld. The defect in Hurler's and Hunter's syndromes: Faulty degradation of mucopolysaccharide. Proc Natl Acad Sci USA 60:699-706, 1968.

Fratantoni, J.C., C.W. Hall, and E.F. Neufeld. Hurler and Hunter syndromes: Mutual correction of the defect in cultured fibroblasts. Science 162:570-572, 1968.

Bach, G., et al. The defect in the Hurler and Scheie syndromes: Deficiency of α-L-iduronidase. Proc Natl Acad Sci USA 69:2048-2051, 1972.

Hickman, S., and E.F. Neufeld. A hypothesis for I-cell diseases: Defective hydrolases that do not enter lysosomes. Biochem Biophys Res Commun 49:992-999, 1972.

Bach, G., et al. The defect in the Hunter syndrome: Deficiency of sulfoiduronate sulfatase. Proc Natl Acad Sci USA 70:2134-2138, 1973.

Hickman, S., L.J. Shapiro, and E.F. Neufeld. A recognition marker required for uptake of a lysosomal enzyme by cultured fibroblasts. Biochem Biophys Res Commun 57:55-61, 1974.

Rome, L.H., B. Weissmann, and E.F. Neufeld. Direct demonstration of binding of a lysosomal enzyme, α-L-iduronidase, to receptors on cultured fibroblasts. Proc Natl Acad Sci USA 75:2331-2334, 1979.

Neufeld, E.F. Lessons from genetic disorders of lysosomes. Harvey Lectures 1979-1980. New York: Academic Press, 1981.

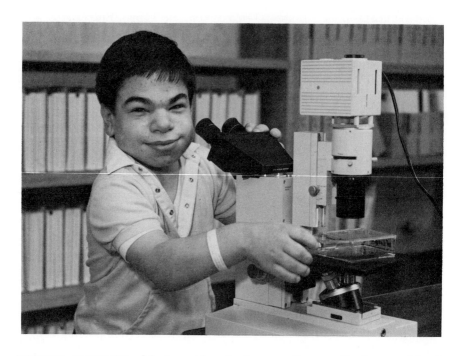

MICHAEL SOCHACKI, 14, has the Hunter syndrome. He is a patient in the Clinical Center, enrolled in a program to evaluate amnion transplantation in the treatment of mucopolysaccharide storage diseases. An eager ninth grader with a burgeoning interest in science, Michael was delighted to visit a biochemical laboratory and view cultured fibroblasts under the microscope. He has a form of the Hunter syndrome in which physical development is markedly affected but the intellect is not impaired. Many patients with mucopolysaccharide storage disorders are not so fortunate, the brain being severely affected. To understand in molecular terms how an apparently identical enzyme deficiency can cause mental retardation in some patients but not in others is one of our research goals.

GENETIC DISEASES

V. Sickle Cell Disease

Alan N. Schechter

William A. Eaton

The initiation of research at NIH in sickle cell disease and later in the other hemoglobinopathies and the thalassemia syndromes can be traced directly to the classical work that started in Linus Pauling's laboratory at the California Institute of Technology in 1946.

HARVEY ITANO was born in California of Japanese ancestry. He graduated from the University of California (Berkeley) and, after internment during the war, from the St. Louis University School of Medicine. In 1946 he went to Pauling's laboratory and began to investigate the molecular basis of sickle cell anemia. The project, inspired by a conversation between Pauling and William Castle of Harvard on an overnight train trip, culminated in the identification of an electrophoretically abnormal hemoglobin in patients with sickle cell anemia. Pauling, Itano, Singer, and Wells reported the work in *Science* in 1949 under the title "Sickle Cell Anemia, a Molecular Disease." This classic paper not only initiated the modern era of sickle cell disease research, but provided the basic paradigm for much of the study of disease at the molecular level.

Itano joined the National Cancer Institute as a Public Health Service Officer in 1950. Assigned at first to Caltech, he moved to Bethesda in 1954 when the Clinical Center was completed. He later wrote to one of the authors:

ALAN N. SCHECHTER, M.D., Chief, Laboratory of Chemical Biology, National Institute of Arthritis, Diabetes, and Digestive and Kidney Diseases. WILLIAM A. EATON, M.D., Ph.D., Chief, Macromolecular Biophysics Section, Laboratory of Chemical Physics, NIADDK.

ISBN 0-12-667980-0

You asked to what extent explaining sickle cell anemia and/or thalassemia served as the goal of my work. That and working out the genetics of the hemo-globinopathies were the major goals. In the *Science* paper, we postulated a mechanism for sickling which is substantially the same as that accepted today. With respect to thalassemia, my colleagues and I recognized that Hb A was produced by some thalassemia genes, but not by others, from our studies on Hb S-thalassemia and Hb E-thalassemia patients.

We also were interested in the variability in the severity of sickle cell disease. Some of the varia-tions in severity were explained by heterozygosity with Hb C, Hb D, and thalassemia. We observed varia-tions in the severity of thalassemia major and re-ported several cases of "intermediate" Cooley's ane-mia. I studied the trimodal distribution of A/S ratios in sickle cell trait. These subjects were dis-cussed in my review in *Advances in Protein Chemistry* in 1957 which I wrote early in my Bethesda years. This review introduced the concept of the evolution of hemoglobin and myoglobin genes by duplications of an ancestral gene and postulated that the thalassemia genes were allelic with the abnormal hemoglobin genes.

I observed that mixtures of Hb S and C were less soluble than mixtures of Hb S and A with the same per-centage of S and postulated a greater stabilizing interaction in S-C aggregates than in A-S aggregates. I presented this work at a symposium in Washington, D.C., in 1955. Subsequently, I studied the hybridiza-tion of hemoglobin molecules and used this technique to show that the α-chains and β-chains were controlled by independent genes.

At about the time of these studies by Itano at NIH, MAKIO MURAYAMA, a biochemist from California, was doing postdoctoral work in Linus Pauling's laboratory. In 1958 he came to NIH and began a long career of investigating sickle cell anemia. He characterized the effects of temperature, solvents, and gases on the solubility of sickle hemoglobin, thus effectively doing the first studies on a possible chemical approach to therapy. Murayama obtained some of the earliest electron micrographs of the sickle hemoglobin polymer, initiating in-tensive studies on the macromolecular structure of the gel formed inside sickle erythrocytes, a major field of research today. He also devised the first models for the structure of the polymer.

In the early 1960s SHERMAN WEISSMAN, a physician trained

at Harvard, began an independent research program at NIH devoted to exploring the control of globin gene expression. He has written:

> I began working in hemoglobinopathies with the specific idea in mind that it would be interesting to study thalassemia as an example of a disease in which there might be a mutant affecting the rate of production of an animal cell protein without affecting the structure of the protein, and that this might give some insight into quantitative regulation of gene expression in animal cells. In my earliest work I began first with Dr. DAVID HEYWOOD, then with Dr. BERNARD FORGET when he joined as a Research Associate, doing chain-labeling studies with cells from thalassemia patients. This was initiated independently by several groups using what were not very satisfactory methods, but we were able to get mostly correct results showing that the thalassemias had nonproduction of beta as compared with alpha chains and therefore confirming the early genetic deductions.
>
> Early on, we also began the studies on sequencing of globin mRNA. These studies, completed in my first years at Yale, did give an almost complete sequence for the beta chain in the days prior to message cloning and prior to the modern technology for DNA sequencing and, in addition, demonstrated the single-base substitutions in sickle cell disease, providing the first confirmation at the nucleotide level of a single base mutation producing a disease.
>
> In my days at NIH I did some clinical work; Dr. Forget and I managed several thalassemia patients with the question of understanding thalassemia as a disease as one part of the motivation for the work, although an equally important goal was the hope to study aspects of gene regulation in general. I began this work simply because it seemed that most problems that were accessible to this detailed investigation could possibly uncover new principles of gene structure and function that would be of general interest.

It should be mentioned that at this time another group at NIH was involved in the study of hemoglobin biosynthesis. MARCO RABINOVITZ, a biochemist in the National Cancer Institute, and his colleagues, investigating the actions of amino acid analogs on protein synthesis in rabbit reticulocytes, had noted the accumulation of globin chains bound to polyribosomes when certain analogs were used. With M. FREEDMAN, G. HONIG,

H. WAXMAN, and others, Rabinovitz systematically followed up these observations and eventually discovered a hemin-controlled translational repressor—a specific protein kinase that phosphorylates the initiation factors for hemoglobin translation.

The relevance of this and related work to understanding the thalassemia syndromes is taken up in the Anderson chapter. Here we follow further two aspects of the work in hemoglobin chemistry related to sickle cell anemia. First we trace physicochemical studies characterizing the kinetics and thermodynamics of sickle hemoglobin polymerization which opened up a new approach to understanding the disease. Then we trace studies that started as biochemical attempts to inhibit the polymerization process and led to fundamental insights into the resultant cellular and clinical pathophysiology.

Hemoglobin S Polymerization and Its Relation to Disease

The explosion of knowledge in the 1970s concerning the mechanism of hemoglobin S polymerization and its relation to sickle cell disease was initiated by a group of scientists in the National Institute of Arthritis, Metabolism and Digestive Diseases. The principal workers involved in the initial investigations—all trained in physical chemistry—were WILLIAM A. EATON, JAMES HOFRICHTER, PHILIP D. ROSS, and ALLEN P. MINTON.

William Eaton came to the Laboratory of Physical Biology in 1968 as a Commissioned Officer immediately after receiving his doctoral degrees from the University of Pennsylvania. In 1968-1969 he collaborated with ELLIOT CHARNEY in an investigation of the near-infrared circular dichroism* of heme proteins. He then renewed an interest in single crystal spectroscopy and constructed a microspectrophotometer, using mostly spare parts from the laboratory of FREDERICK S. BRACKETT, who had retired from experimental work. In the course of building the instrument, Eaton had many conversations with RODNEY A. OLSON, a physiologist investigating the polarized absorption of chlorophyll protein crystals. Olson told him about photographs of deoxygenated sickle cells in polarized light that he and WILLIAM H. JENNINGS, Jr., had taken in collaboration with Murayama. Interpretation of the linear dichroism observed in these photographs depended on knowledge of the electronic spectroscopy of the heme chromophore, one of the subjects of

---

*For more on circular dichroism, see section entitled "The Study of Chiroptical Phenomena" in Becker-Sharpless chapter.

Eaton's Ph.D. thesis. Thus Eaton became interested in sickle cell disease.

His experimental work began with the arrival of DAVID G. HENDRICKER, an inorganic chemist who came to Eaton's laboratory in 1971 on sabbatical leave to learn about the application of crystal spectroscopy to biological systems. In 1972 Eaton and Hendricker demonstrated that it was possible to measure in a single sickled cell the optical density of the polymerized hemoglobin S molecules in polarized light. Systematic work did not begin, however, until Eaton and James Hofrichter had learned of unpublished electron microscope studies in which John T. Finch and Max F. Perutz from the Medical Research Council Laboratory of Molecular Biology in Cambridge, England, proposed a structure for the hemoglobin S polymer. Hofrichter had arrived at NIH about six months earlier to work as a Staff Fellow with Charney on the linear dichroism of DNA. Eaton and Hofrichter were excited by the Finch-Perutz results, realizing that an accurate determination of the polarized absorption properties of the polymer could provide crucial tests of the structures being postulated. Hofrichter, with the generous encouragement of Charney, decided to put aside his DNA project to work with Eaton on sickle cells. The atmosphere of freedom of inquiry in the Arthritis Institute encouraged such scientific adventures.

Beginning a fruitful collaboration that continues today, Hofrichter and Eaton investigated the polarized absorption properties of deoxygenated single sickle cells. They were able to place important constraints on the possible orientations of the hemoglobin S molecule within the polymer. Their results ruled out the molecular orientation proposed by Murayama; and subsequent model-building studies, aided by RICHARD J. FELDMANN's newly developed molecular graphics system [see Pratt chapter], argued strongly against the Finch-Perutz structure. Since that time Hofrichter and Eaton's optical study has played a central role in the continuously evolving description of the sickle cell polymer.

The model-building studies during the summer of 1973 raised immediately relevant questions about the energetics of polymer formation. In the fall of that year Philip Ross of the Laboratory of Molecular Biology expressed to Eaton an interest in research on sickle cell hemoglobin. Ross, who had come to NIH in 1960, had been doing calorimetric studies on model biochemical systems and platelet aggregation. Eaton, Hofrichter, and Ross decided to collaborate on the calorimetric determination of the heat of gelation and began to work full time on the project about January 1974.

Their combined backgrounds and expertise brought rapid progress and with it the excitement of discovery. They soon observed the unusual kinetics of polymerization with a delay time enormously sensitive (30th power) to the hemoglobin S concentration. This finding led to several fundamentally new concepts. First, it resulted in the development of a nucleation mechanism for the assembly of hemoglobin S molecules into polymers, which explains a wide variety of solution and cellular phenomena. Second, it introduced the role of the dynamics of events in the microcirculation to the pathophysiology of sickle cell disease. The probability that intracellular polymerization would take place in the microcirculation could not be determined from equilibrium considerations, but required knowing the rate of polymerization relative to the time of transit through the microcirculation. The tremendous sensitivity of the delay time to physiological variables provided a natural explanation for their relation to clinical severity.

These ideas rationalized a number of clinical observations about sickle cell disease and provided a framework for thinking about therapeutic approaches. The kinetic formulation of the pathophysiology suggested that complete inhibition of polymerization would not be needed to obtain a therapeutic effect, but that amelioration could result from lengthening the delay time so that more cells could escape the microcirculation before polymerization began. The finding of the enormous concentration dependence of the delay time focused attention on the critical role of intracellular hemoglobin concentration in determining disease severity. The new strategy for therapy suggested by the kinetic studies was to decrease the intracellular hemoglobin S concentration, either by increasing the red cell volume or decreasing hemoglobin biosynthesis. This has become a major thrust in current research on drug development in sickle cell disease.

Along with the kinetic studies, Hofrichter, Ross, and Eaton also carried out a series of experiments on the thermodynamics of polymerization. This work was motivated by their finding that the kinetics and thermodynamics were closely related. It profited considerably from theoretical studies being carried out by Allen Minton in the Arthritis Institute's Laboratory of Biophysical Chemistry. Minton had come to NIH as a Staff Fellow to work with HARRY A. SAROFF on the problem of cooperativity in hemoglobin. He then turned his attention to hemoglobin S and carried out an important series of theoretical studies that became the foundation for analyzing equilibrium data on polymerization. These included the first quantitative thermodynamic model for gelation, and the development of the theoretical framework for analyzing the effects of partial oxygenation and non-S hemoglobins on polymerization.

In 1976 Minton, Ross, Hofrichter, and Eaton became interested in the large nonideality present in the concentrated hemoglobin solutions found in red cells, recognizing it as a vital component in the kinetic and thermodynamic description of polymerization. Minton and Ross found that it could be completely accounted for in a simple way from hard-sphere excluded-volume effects. Meanwhile, Hofrichter and Eaton pursued a thorough investigation of the kinetics of polymerization, both experimentally and theoretically. With postdoctoral fellows FRANK A. FERRONE and MASSIMO COLETTA, they developed a laser-photolysis light-scattering technique to measure the kinetics of polymerization in solution and in single cells. The solution study led to the development of a novel dual nucleation mechanism that could explain both the existence of a sharp delay and the sensitivity of the delay time to solution conditions. The cell study made the important point that the mechanism of polymerization in cells is the same as that observed in purified solutions.

Another postdoctoral fellow, HELEN R. SUNSHINE, working with Eaton and Hofrichter, carried out the first comprehensive thermodynamic study on polymerization in hemoglobin mixtures and on the control of polymerization by oxygen. The study on the effect of oxygen, together with the distribution of intracellular hemoglobin S concentrations obtained from the single-cell kinetic experiments, provided the data for explaining the results of a variety of classic experiments on sickle blood at various oxygen pressures. The mixture study showed a clear correlation between the rate and extent of polymerization and the clinical severity of various sickle cell syndromes. It formed the basis for a quantitative analysis of the problem of inhibiting polymerization in patients and established criteria for judging the potential efficacy of therapeutic agents that are widely used in drug development.

The overall impact of the work of Eaton, Hofrichter, Ross, and Minton has been to introduce the quantitative techniques and concepts of physical chemistry into the understanding of sickle cell disease. As a result, a comprehensive thermodynamic and kinetic description of the polymerization of sickle cell hemoglobin and its relation to the pathophysiology and therapy of the disease is now available. In fact, these studies may be viewed as among the first successful applications of physical chemistry to human disease.

Pharmacological, Cellular, and Clinical Studies

In early 1975 Alan N. Schechter, a physician in the Arthritis Institute, became interested in the sickle cell. He had trained at Cornell and Columbia Universities and had worked for a number of years at NIH with CHRISTIAN B. ANFINSEN on fundamental problems of protein folding [see the chapter "Studies on Proteins"].

Schechter and his colleagues had just developed new ways to study the folding of native and chemically synthesized peptides and proteins using monospecific antibodies. These methods, devised to study the folding of staphylococcal nuclease, were being applied to human hemoglobins. In particular, Schechter, J. CURD, N. YOUNG, and A. EASTLAKE-DEAN sought to obtain antibodies specific for each of the major human hemoglobins by synthesizing peptides corresponding to regions where the hemoglobin of interest differed significantly from related ones. The peptides were applied through affinity chromatography to purify monospecific antibodies (in the era before monoclonal antibodies), and these were used to quantitate the hemoglobins and study their conformation. The group had just prepared antibodies specific to sickle hemoglobin in this way, using a synthetic fragment corresponding to the first 13 residues of the β^S chain.

In 1974 Schechter's friends William Eaton and JOHN HERCULES had drawn him into the recently initiated Sickle Cell Disease program of the National Heart and Lung Institute as a consultant. He then realized that some of the hemoglobin peptides that his group had been synthesizing might act as stereospecific inhibitors of the polymerization of deoxy sickle hemoglobin. With CONSTANCE T. NOGUCHI, a physicist who had just joined his group, Schechter began a systematic study of the effects of peptides on the solubility of sickle hemoglobin. The work was aided greatly by the studies and advice of their colleagues in the Arthritis Institute, Eaton, Hofrichter, Ross, and Minton.

Schechter and Noguchi showed that aromatic amino acids and short peptides containing them were effective inhibitors of the molecular aggregation of sickle hemoglobin. However, longer peptides designed with the aid of the molecular graphics facility at NIH to maximize their potential binding to sites of intermolecular interactions had limited efficacy due to nonideality effects and to intrinsic problems of solubility and transport into the red cell. Thus, these peptides, which are very effective on hemoglobin solutions, cannot yet be used clinically. However, a large number of laboratories throughout the world are attempting to develop a chemical therapy by this approach. In an effort to solve the problems of solubility and permeability, Noguchi and Schechter have arranged with Max Perutz to use X-ray crystallography to identify the exact site at which the short peptides are bound to hemoglobin. This information is being applied to design peptide analogs that may be more potent and permeable and thus useful in the treatment of sickle cell disease.

At the same time, Philip Ross and S. SUBRAMANIAN, a Research Associate, carried out in NIADDK an extensive investigation of inhibitors of sickle hemoglobin gelation. They found that the most efficient organic noncovalent inhibitors of gelation had an aromatic residue with a pendant side chain having hydrogen-bonding capability. They explained this in terms of a simple mechanism of binding, based upon the location of the reported intermolecular contacts between β chains in polymerized sickle cell hemoglobin. This model can account for the action of most noncovalent inhibitors found to date.

One effect of these pharmacological studies was to persuade Schechter of the need to develop a method for measuring the aggregation of hemoglobin inside sickle erythrocytes. With J.W.H. SUTHERLAND, a postdoctoral fellow, and DENNIS TORCHIA, a physicist in the Dental Institute, he developed a method using NMR (nuclear magnetic resonance) spectroscopy with natural-abundance carbon-13 to observe the physical state of hemoglobin inside the red cell. Noguchi used concentrated sickle hemoglobin solutions to show that the new method gave accurate and precise results, and then demonstrated, to general surprise, that sickle hemoglobin polymer could be detected inside sickle erythrocytes at very high oxygen saturation values. Indeed, she demonstrated polymer where cell sickling was not evident. She further showed that the thermodynamic analyses of Eaton, Hofrichter, and Ross and the nonideality analyses of Minton could largely predict the results that were being obtained with the NMR measurements.

Later Noguchi and Schechter, using newly developed cell fractionation techniques to separate sickle erythrocytes by density, showed that when both cell heterogeneity and new analyses of solvent nonideality were explicitly considered, the NMR measurements could be even more closely determined on the basis of the theory that had been developed for sickle hemoglobin solutions. In summary, these studies demonstrated that intracellular polymerization could be predicted from measurements of the hemoglobin concentration and composition in individuals with sickle cell anemia.

These findings have led to comprehensive attempts to determine a quantitative pathophysiology for the disease and its related sickling syndromes in terms of intracellular polymerization. With H. F. BUNN, a Fogarty Scholar from Harvard University, a team comprising Noguchi, Schechter, Eaton, Hofrichter, and Geraldine P. Schechter (of the Washington Veterans Administration Medical Center) studied hemoglobin SC disease by kinetic and thermodynamic analyses of the polymerization of hemoglobin S and C mixtures and by cell fractionation and NMR studies of SC cells. They explained why hemoglobin SC is a disease while sickle trait (AS) is not, attributing the syndrome primarily to the high percentage of hemoglobin S in SC cells and the presence of SC cells of very high density, a reflection of high total intracellular hemoglobin concentration. The changes in solubility of the mixtures, observed 20 years earlier by Itano and others, have a lesser effect. In collaboration with G. Brittenham of Western Reserve University, Noguchi and Schechter also showed that the severity of the sickle syndromes, especially in terms of anemia, correlated precisely with average intracellular polymer content.

These studies have resulted in new emphasis on the importance of continuous changes in the flexibility of the sickle erythrocyte—changes due to the formation of intracellular S hemoglobin polymer. Primary consideration of a discrete morphological event of "sickling" no longer prevails. A corollary is that problems of impaired flow through the microcirculation may well occur at the precapillary sphincters, rather than in the capillaries and venules, as the conventional wisdom held. If true, this view has important implications for therapeutic approaches to sickle cell anemia, specifically the possible use of vasodilators of the precapillary arterioles.

With the idea of testing this hypothesis concerning the microcirculatory mechanisms, as well as developing general noninvasive methods of evaluating disease severity, GRIFFIN RODGERS, a Medical Staff Fellow in Schechter's group, has worked during the last several years with investigators throughout the Clinical Center. They are using new methods—laser-Doppler velocimetry, PET scans, NMR imaging, etc.—to evaluate blood flow in various tissues and organs of sickle cell patients.

In addition, Schechter and Noguchi have collaborated with ARTHUR NIENHUIS and TIMOTHY LEY of the Clinical Hematology Branch, National Heart, Lung, and Blood Institute, in evaluating the effects of administering 5-azacytidine to sickle cell disease patients. Nienhuis and Ley had shown that this agent increases fetal hemoglobin synthesis in thalassemia, and it is now known to have a similar effect on sickle cell disease. Whether this effect is large enough to be therapeutically beneficial, and whether the potential long-term toxicity of the drug is acceptable, must yet be established. Other drugs that affect fetal hemoglobin synthesis and may be less toxic are also being tried on sickle cell and thalassemia patients.

This work represents the first attempt to use pharmacological agents to manipulate the expression of a human gene in a way that may be therapeutically beneficial, and has been a focus of interest not only throughout NIH but also nationally and internationally. It is noteworthy that these studies reunite sickle cell and thalassemia research, two areas that started together at NIH in the laboratory of Harvey Itano 30 years ago.

It should also be noted that in all of this work on sickle cell disease, the intellectual freedom and scientific cooperation that characterize NIH are very significant denominators. The scientists had complete support to follow promising leads into new areas of investigation. They easily found colleagues, and even collaborators, who had the knowledge, theory, or equipment to help in imaginative and sophisticated ways. These attributes—freedom and cooperation—have been as important as any in allowing the NIH scientific enterprise to flourish.

Selected References

Coletta, M., et al. Kinetics of sickle hemoglobin polymerization in single red cells. Nature 300:194-197, 1982.

Dean, J., and A.N. Schechter. Sickle cell anemia: Molecular and cellular bases of therapeutic approaches. N Engl J Med 299:752-763, 804-811, and 863-870, 1978.

Eaton, W.A., J. Hofrichter, and P.D. Ross. Delay time of gelation: A possible determinant of clinical severity in sickle cell disease. Blood J Hematol 47:621-627, 1976.

Ferrone, F.A., et al. Kinetic studies on photolysis induced gelation of sickle cell hemoglobin suggest a new mechanism. Biophys J 32:361-377. 1980.

Furie, B., et al. An immunological approach to the conformational equilibria of staphylococcal nuclease. J Mol Biol 92:497-506, 1975.

Hofrichter, J., D.G. Hendricker, and W.A. Eaton. Structure of hemoglobin S fibers: Optical determination of the molecular orientation in sickled red cells. Proc Natl Acad Sci USA 70:3604-3608, 1973.

Hofrichter, J., P.D. Ross, and W.A. Eaton. Kinetics and mechanism of deoxyhemoglobin S gelation. A new approach to understanding sickle cell disease. Proc Natl Acad Sci USA 71:4864-4868, 1974.

Ley, T.J., et al. 5-Azacytidine selectively increases γ globulin synthesis in patients with sickle cell anemia and β^+ thalassemia. Blood 62:370-380, 1983.

Minton, A.P. A thermodynamic model for gelation of sickle-cell hemoglobin. J Mol Biol 82:483-498, 1974.

Minton, A.P. Relations between oxygen saturation and aggregation of sickle-cell hemoglobin. J Mol Biol 100:519-542, 1976.

Noguchi, C., and A.N. Schechter. Inhibition of sickle hemo-
    globin gelation by amino acids and their analogues. Bio-
    chemistry 17:5455-5459, 1978.
Noguchi, C.T., D.A. Torchia, and A.N. Schechter. Determination
    of deoxyhemoglobin S polymer in sickle erythrocytes upon
    deoxygenation. Proc Natl Acad Sci USA 77:5487-5491, 1980.
Noguchi, C.T., and A.N. Schechter. The intracellular poly-
    merization of sickle hemoglobin and its relevance to
    sickle cell disease. Blood 58:1057-1068, 1981.
Noguchi, C.T., D.A. Torchia, and A.N. Schechter. The intra-
    cellular polymerization of sickle hemoglobin: Effects of
    cell heterogeneity. J Clin Invest 72:836-852, 1983.
Ross, P.D., and A.P. Minton. Analysis of non-ideal behavior
    in concentrated hemoglobin solutions. J Mol Biol 112:
    437-452, 1977.
Sunshine, H.R., J. Hofrichter, and W.A. Eaton. Requirements
    for therapeutic inhibition of sickle hemoglobin gelation.
    Nature 275:238-240, 1978.
Sunshine, H.R., et al. Oxygen binding by sickle cell hemo-
    globin polymers. J Mol Biol 158:251-273, 1982.
Young, N.S., et al. Isolation of antibodies specific to sickle
    hemoglobin by affinity chromatography using a synthetic
    peptide. Proc Natl Acad Sci USA 72:4759-4763, 1975.

Introduction

VIRAL ONCOLOGY

This chapter traces the understanding of cancer as it proceeded from "a disease of unknown etiology" to "a disease of
possible viral etiology." The importance of the work described
herein is self-evident. One effect of the persistent interest
in the mechanism of cancer causation has been a vigorous stimulation of such fields as virology, immunology (both humoral
and cellular), and molecular biology.

The quest for a cancer virus started with the simplistic
notion that cancer was like a number of other viral diseases
in being the result of a specific infection by a specific
agent. Indeed, a number of animal models supported this view.
Beginning early in this century, identification of viruses as
tumorigenic agents in a wide variety of animals led to expectations of an ultimate isolation of "the virus of human
cancer." In preparation for this event, NIH constructed a
suitable edifice to house the formidable organism. Building
41, completed in 1969, included sophisticated devices for
viral containment. But the virus of human cancer has not been
found. Building 41 is occupied by worthy scientists who perform other worthy experiments. Some of its features were put
to explicit use when the development of recombinant DNA technology called for high-containment conditions.

With the passage of time, other etiologies of cancer have
come to the fore. Many human cancers are attributable to non-
living environmental agents such as cigarette smoke, asbestos,
sunlight, ionizing radiation, and a number of well-identified
organic molecules. While these have seized center stage, one
glimpses in the wings still other suspects, including dietary
and genetic factors. One of these, mentioned in the following
pages and expounded in the chapter by EDWARD M. SCOLNICK, is
the oncogene, a factor conceived as a gene of viral origin—
perhaps the elusive "common denominator" of cancer causation.
The study of viruses will continue to play an important role
in cancer etiology.

D. S.

17

VIRAL ONCOLOGY

Frank J. Rauscher, Jr.

Michael B. Shimkin

In biomedical science the last quarter of the nineteenth century belongs to Louis Pasteur and Robert Koch, who laid the groundwork for the field of microbiology. Their discoveries led to the conquest of many infectious diseases, probably the greatest victory of science over human afflictions. Pasteur's vision extended beyond bacterial pathogens. In 1882 he concluded that rabies—a disease that was to represent one of his triumphs—was not due to a bacterium but to an "ultramicroscopic agent." A decade later D. V. Ivanovski of Russia and, independently, M. W. Beijerinck of Holland reported that tobacco mosaic disease could be transmitted by something that passed through a porcelain filter impassable for bacteria. Thus "filterable viruses" joined the ranks of infectious microorganisms.

During the heyday of bacteriology, many attempts were made to find a microbial cause of cancer. Bacteria, fungi, and other microorganisms, often named after their discoverer, were isolated and proposed as candidates. But none of the claims withstood the rigorous criteria of bacterial causation enunciated by Koch.

Filterable viruses were suggested as the cause of cancer by several investigators at the turn of the twentieth century, most persuasively by Amédée Borrel of France. In 1908 two Danish veterinarians, Vilhelm Ellermann and Oluf Bang, reported their studies on leukemia in chickens. They had succeeded in transmitting the disease by cell-free filtrates.

FRANK J. RAUSCHER, Jr., Ph.D., Senior Vice President for Research, American Cancer Society. Formerly Director, National Cancer Institute. MICHAEL B. SHIMKIN, M.D., Professor Emeritus of Community Medicine and Oncology, University of California (San Diego). Formerly Associate Director for Field Studies, NCI.

NIH: AN ACCOUNT OF RESEARCH
IN ITS LABORATORIES AND CLINICS

350

ISBN 0-12-667980-0

At that time, however, leukemia was not considered to be a
neoplasm, but a separate disease of the blood.

Another line of investigation is even older. Experimental cancer research became possible when investigators
succeeded in transplanting cancers from one animal to another
of the same species. M. A. Novinsky, a Russian veterinarian,
transplanted two cancers in dogs in 1877, but the work was
forgotten. In 1903 a Danish veterinarian, Carl O. Jensen,
reported tumor transplantation in mice. His work attracted
immediate attention because mice in which the transplants
grew and then regressed were found to be immune to further
transplants. Jensen also reported preliminary data suggest-
ting that serum from immunized rabbits endowed rabbits with
tumor immunity, but the finding did not survive more rigorous
experimentation.

In the first decade of the twentieth century, transplanted
tumors in mice and rats became the major experimental material
in the few laboratories interested in cancer. Morphologists
became convinced that the mouse tumors, most often mammary,
were similar to those of humans. Biologists established that
such tumors could only be successfully transplanted if viable
tumor cells were used, and that the cells multiplied by mi-
totic division, retained characteristics of the donor, and
acquired their blood supply from the host.

These basic observations on rodent tumors became dogma
in cancer research. When Peyton Rous, a young investigator
at the newly established Rockefeller Research Institute in
New York, reported in 1911 that he had transmitted a sarcoma
in chickens by cell-free extracts, the discovery came at the
wrong time. The infectious etiology of cancer seemed to have
been thoroughly disproved; tumor transmission was believed to
require viable cells. Rous's result must have been an exception limited to chickens, or the tumor was an infectious gran-
uloma mimicking a true neoplasm. Rous retreated into other
research for over two decades, but in 1966 was finally rewarded for his discovery with a Nobel Prize.

NIH Becomes Involved

By 1910 the enigma of cancer had attracted the attention
of the Hygienic Laboratory, the predecessor of the National
Institutes of Health. GEORGE W. McCOY, later director of
the Laboratory (1915-1937), reported the occurrence of tumors
in rats and ground squirrels caught on the West Coast in a
plague prevention program. The report of the Surgeon General
for the year 1910 included a section on cancer, probably written by McCoy. It suggested studies on immunity to cancer that

could be carried out in connection with work on vaccines, serums, and toxins.

The first budget requests to include cancer among the concerns of the Hygienic Laboratory were denied. Cancer research in the Public Health Service can be dated from 1922. The Division of Pharmacology, under CARL VOEGTLIN at the Hygienic Laboratory in Washington, began studies on the effects of metals on transplantable cancer in rodents. At the same time, a PHS-funded field station on cancer was established at the Harvard School of Medicine in Boston under Assistant Surgeon General J. W. SCHERESCHEWSKY.

The Division conducted its investigations along biochemcal lines, but later a tissue culture expert was added to the staff. The Boston station also expanded its staff after a Surgeon General's advisory conference in 1927 recommended greater emphasis on cancer research. Study of viruses was not among the recommendations, for the viral etiology of cancer was then in disrepute despite some doughty proponents.

A virologist, however, was the first addition to the Boston staff—HOWARD B. ANDERVONT, from Johns Hopkins, who had published several articles on chicken tumor viruses. Upon his transfer to Boston, Andervont shifted his attention to mice. He started several lines of inbred mice and studied the effect of heredity on the growth of transplantable tumors.

Along another line of research, chemical carcinogens—polycyclic aromatic hydrocarbons—had been isolated in London in 1930. At Harvard Louis F. Fieser synthesized analogs to the carcinogens, which were being tested by another member of Schereschewsky's group, MURRAY J. SHEAR. Following up on their work, Andervont began a series of investigations into the tumor response of inbred mice to pure chemical carcinogens. His involvement in viral oncology was broadened when John J. Bittner, at the Jackson Laboratory, reported in 1935 that mammary tumors in mice were transmitted by an agent in the mother's milk. Andervont repeated and extended Bittner's observations and established several sublines of homozygous mice, some carrying the milk agent and some not.

The case for a viral origin of mammalian cancer gained further support in 1935 when Rous and Joseph W. Beard, working with Richard E. Shope at the Rockefeller Institute, demonstrated that a virus isolated by Shope from a papilloma of the wild rabbit would induce carcinomas in domestic rabbits.

National Cancer Institute, 1937–1950

Virus research in cancer was relegated to a subordinate position by the advisory report that set the tone for the 1937

Act creating the National Cancer Institute, the first cate-
gorical Institute of NIH. The advisory group concluded: "The
very exhaustive study of mammalian cancer has disclosed a
complete lack of evidence of its infectious origin." This
revealed the prejudices of the participants. They seemed to
ignore Bittner's mammary tumor in mice and Shope's tumors in
rabbits.

NCI took shape through amalgamation of the Washington and
Boston activities. Its staff was expanded by research fellows
authorized under the new Act, including W. RAY BRYAN, trained
in virology, and MICHAEL B. SHIMKIN, an internist whose interests turned to laboratory cancer research. Both were placed
administratively in Andervont's biology group.

Bryan had become a proponent of the viral etiology of
cancer through his work on chicken oncogenic viruses at Duke
University. At NCI he applied statistical methods to bioassay determinations of the concentration of the Rous virus.
He found to his disappointment that virus research was in
disfavor at NCI, despite Andervont's classic studies on the
milk factor in mice. Another outlet for Bryan's biometric
interests was an extension of quantitative studies on carcinogenic polycyclic hydrocarbons, initiated earlier by Shimkin
in Boston.

As soon as Andervont, Bryan, and Shimkin had settled down
in NIH's new Building 6 at Bethesda, they decided to focus
their attention on the substance in mouse milk that was involved in the genesis of mammary tumors. Andervont undertook
the genetic aspects, Shimkin the hormonal, and Bryan the isolation of the agent. The three workers met almost daily and
cooperated closely.

Their work was supplemented by that of others, especially
HERBERT KAHLER, a biophysicist, and THELMA B. DUNN, a pathologist. In 1945 the collaboration culminated in the first NCI
monograph, *Mammary Tumors in Mice.* Several scientific advances
were stimulated by the report. One area of investigation
yielded physical and chemical techniques suitable for quantitative studies on the milk factor. Another demonstrated that
sera from rabbits injected with agent-rich tissues and mouse
milk could protect mice against agent-induced mammary cancer.
This established the possibility of antitumor immunization in
mammals. A third advance was the previously mentioned development of mouse substrains, some negative for the milk factor
and some positive. These allowed dissociation of genetic from
milk-factor influences.

Inbred strains of mice—the first established by C. C.
Little in 1909—had become an important tool of cancer re-
search. In the mid 1940s WALTER E. HESTON, a geneticist at
NCI, worked out the role of heredity in mammary tumor devel-

opment in the mouse. He showed that the genes operate through hormonal stimulation of the mammary tissue and propagation and transmission of the milk agent.

It is revealing of the conservatism then prevalent that while the milk agent was recognized by 1945 as being, most probably, a filterable virus, the NCI monograph concluded with the statement "It should be emphasized that the virus nature of the milk influence is not established." This, of course, was before the electron microscope had revealed virus particles and before the use of tissue culture in viral oncology.

Work on the milk agent faced two major experimental obstacles. To identify the agent required, first, adequate supplies of the tissue of origin and, second, ability to measure the concentration of the agent. The first obstacle was overcome by the establishment of a mouse dairy at NCI, where mice were milked with a specially constructed device. The second obstacle proved to be more of a problem. Bioassays to quantify the agent required the appearance of mammary tumors, and thus each step took up to a year to complete.

Biochemists were not interested in collaborating in research that moved at so slow a pace. The cancer researchers decided that use of models other than the mouse mammary tumor would be more rapid and productive. The tumors evoked in chickens by the Rous agent were proposed.

Voegtlin, NCI Director, and R. R. SPENCER, his successor, were persuaded to authorize a change of direction. The Rous sarcoma agent could be viewed as a chemical carcinogen and studied by statistical methods that had been demonstrated on polycyclic aromatic hydrocarbons. Thus Bryan returned to his favorite field of research. A chicken colony was started in the attic of Building 6, and Bryan's basement laboratory was modestly expanded in size and technical personnel.

Bryan proceeded with his meticulous experiments on the Rous sarcoma virus and published a half-dozen papers during the mid 1950s. A particularly intriguing result was that Rous sarcomas induced with minimal amounts of the agent initially failed to yield recoverable virus. Using the Rous virus in chicks, Bryan showed that the amount of virus recoverable from tumors was directly related to the amount needed to induce them. In contrast, other RNA viruses, such as those of influenza, measles, mumps, and Newcastle disease, are recovered at the highest and purest yield when limited doses of virus are used. Bryan's observation, unique in virology at the time, was later confirmed by FRANK J. RAUSCHER, Jr., and Vincent Groupé, using Rous sarcoma virus in different systems. It suggests that failure to recover virus from a human tumor does not necessarily mean that the tumor was not virus induced.

This discovery was made in the days when scientists were looking predominantly for a possible "infectious" virus, well before it became known that whole or partial genomes of RNA
viruses could be incorporated into host cells.

A viral etiology for neoplasia had been gaining the attention of more investigators. In 1949 Groupé at the Rutgers
Institute of Microbiology became interested in the Rous sarcoma agent and contacted Bryan for samples. A flourishing
collaboration evolved, with Bryan appointed Visiting Professor
at Rutgers, and Rutgers graduate students and research fellows
indoctrinated with a commitment to viral oncology and biometric design. Some of the research fellows were appointed to
NCI, among them Rauscher, who would serve as Director from
1972 to 1976.

The Rutgers-NCI collaboration included the work of Groupé
and ROBERT MANAKER, one of the Rutgers fellows who came to NCI.
In 1956 they reported that infection of chick embryo cells in
vitro with Rous sarcoma virus resulted in discrete foci of altered cells. In vitro procedures at once replaced the longer,
more cumbersome in vivo assays in many laboratories.

It should be emphasized that the advances in bioassay
methods were based on developments in cell culture over previous decades, some performed for aims other than their application to oncology. For example, WILTON R. EARLE's group
at NCI produced the first sizable tissue cultures of cancer
cells, and KATHERINE K. SANFORD of that group developed the
first clone from an isolated cancer cell. Their procedures
were later simplified for wider applicability. HARRY EAGLE,
NCI's first Scientific Director, modified tissue culture procedures and developed media that could be prepared and distributed on a commercial basis.* The use of tissue culture
methods in targeted research on poliomyelitis also accelerated their evolution. As can be demonstrated by many other
examples, separation of basic and applied research is largely
artificial, and often advances in one line of investigation
have major influence on another line seemingly unrelated.

Viral oncology acquired a new dimension when the minute
particles became visible through the electron microscope. Leon
Dmochowski, of Houston, early applied electron microscopy to
oncologic problems. At NCI ALBERT J. DALTON became an expert
electron microscopist, helping to develop classifications of
oncogenic viruses.

Progress in viral oncology, as well as in other research,
was strengthened at NCI by extensive, detailed studies on the
histomorphology of animal tumors. This essential aspect of

---

*See sections by Evans and Sanford and by Eagle in chapter
entitled "Tissue Culture."

cancer research was in the hands of HAROLD L. STEWART and Dunn, who developed pathologic criteria for lymphomas and other cancers in mice.

Collaborations and consultations with pathologists, tissue culture experts, geneticists, bioengineers, and others of the expanding "critical mass" of scientists at NCI not only facilitated research in viral oncology but accelerated its acceptance by a wider audience among professional groups.

Viruses Against Cancer

During the 1950s there arose another application of virology to cancer: the use of viruses as possible therapeutic agents in advanced cancer by exploiting their lytic (destructive) effect on cells.

At the Memorial Hospital in New York, Chester Southam and Alice E. Moore explored the use of neurotropic (nerve-seeking) viruses against cancer.

At the Laboratory of Experimental Oncology, an NCI branch in San Francisco, scientists observed remarkable temporary remission of acute leukemia in children who had developed chickenpox or other acute infections. Attempts to reproduce this occurrence by inoculating patients with chickenpox and cat pancytopenia viruses were unsuccessful.

At the newly opened NIH Clinical Center, ROBERT R. SMITH, NCI's chief surgeon, injected adenovirus into advanced cervical cancers in an attempt to produce lysis. The adenoviruses had been isolated and identified under ROBERT J. HUEBNER of the National Institute of Allergy and Infectious Diseases (NIAID). The work was discontinued because immunity against the viruses developed, negating the limited cytolytic (cell-destroying) effects, and because of ethical complications. Nevertheless, research may yet return to this interesting application of virology to neoplasia. The current exploration of interferons—antiviral proteins produced by cells—may be traced to a hypothesis that would link antiviral and antineoplastic activity.

Gross and Stewart, 1952–1960

The events that opened the next chapter of viral oncology occurred in the Veterans Administration Hospital in the Bronx, New York, and at the Public Health Service Hospital in Baltimore. The protagonists were Ludwik Gross and SARAH E. STEWART. Although these immortals of viral oncology were at first ignored, their stubborn convictions prevailed.

Gross, an expatriate Pole who served in the U.S. Army, had failed to secure a position at NCI. He joined the staff of the VA hospital with the understanding that he could use an unoccupied room in the basement and devote one afternoon a week to his research. Stewart, trained in virology and employed by the NIH Division of Infectious Diseases, was denied NCI appointment for lack of full qualifications. After attaining an M.D. degree, she was assigned to an NCI unit at the Baltimore hospital. Later she transferred to the main campus in Bethesda.

Gross and Stewart were convinced that cancer was caused by a virus, and both resolved to prove it. History records that Gross had a clear lead in demonstrating the transmission of leukemia in mice by cell-free filtrates. He astutely used newborn mice as recipients and chose a genetically susceptible cross. He also observed that the filtrates evoked parotid tumors as well as leukemia, and proved that these two reactions were due to different viruses.

Stewart, repeating Gross's work, also encountered the parotid tumor response. Her chief contribution was made in collaboration with BERNICE E. EDDY, a long-time friend at the NIH Division of Biologics Standards. They grew the parotid tumor virus in tissue culture and found that it gained in potency and spectrum of activity. After cultivation, the agent produced a wide variety of tumors in rats, rabbits, and hamsters. It was named the "polyoma virus," reflecting Stewart and Eddy's important advance—their demonstration that the range of this virus could be extended by appropriate techniques to induce a variety of tumors in several species.

It was years before these brilliant investigations became widely accepted. They were reviewed and rereviewed by expert pathologists. Questions were raised regarding the filtration processes. Only after several false starts were the findings reproduced by scientists known for their conservative, careful work. LLOYD W. LAW of NCI was one of the prime contributors to the verification and extension of Stewart and Eddy's results. Gross later received long-overdue accolades for his achievements, but Sarah Stewart died before her contributions were accorded the honors she richly deserved.

After Gross's isolation of the mouse leukemia virus, investigators throughout the world sought to demonstrate a viral causation for many tumors of mice. Among the early successes were those of Charlotte Friend of New York (1956), who isolated a virus from the Ehrlich carcinoma, and A. Graffi of Berlin (1957), who isolated a virus from sarcoma 37. NCI investigators contributed two potent strains of mouse leukemia virus, one from sarcoma 37 and the other from a leukemia induced in Swiss mice. These two strains acquired the customary eponymic designations—the Moloney virus (1960) and the Rauscher virus (1962).

Gross, in the 1970 edition of his book, records at least 10 other leukemogenic viruses recovered from tumors or tissues of mice, some following treatment of the animals with X-rays or carcinogenic chemicals. Many strains of leukemogenic and sarcogenic viruses show interesting differences in effect. The question has been raised whether all or most of these RNA-type viruses represent closely related variants of the same basic entity.

Rebirth of Viral Oncology, 1950–1959

By the latter part of the 1950s, viral oncology was again accepted by the scientific community as a promising research activity to be directed toward solution of the cancer problem. Compelling scientific evidence was provided by an increasing number of investigators in the United States and Europe. The new findings destroyed the dogma that oncogenic viruses are invariably specific as to host species and tumor type.

Actually, as early as 1942, Francisco Duran-Reynals of Yale had shown that the Rous tumor virus could be transferred from chickens to other fowls if inoculated early in life. Lev Zilber, founder of the Russian school of viral oncology, reported the induction of sarcoma in rats injected with large doses of the Rous chicken agent (published in 1965). His work eventually overcame the skepticism of American scientists.

The few investigators interested in cancer viruses gathered in August 1944 at Gibson Island, Maryland. It was at this meeting, a precursor of the Gordon Research Conferences on Cancer, that the NCI group reported an antibody against the mouse milk factor. A section on viral oncology at the Gordon Research Conference of 1955 attests to the steady growth of the field during the next decade.

The position for research in viral oncology was forcefully stated by Wendell M. Stanley, who had shared the 1946 Nobel Prize in chemistry for his isolation of tobacco mosaic virus. In his address before the Third National Cancer Conference of 1956, Stanley concluded: "The experimental evidence now available is consistent with the idea that viruses are etiologic agents of most, if not all, cancer including cancer in man. Acceptance of this idea as a working hypothesis is urged because it will result in the doing of experiments that might otherwise be left undone. . . ."

In 1957 a symposium on viral oncology at the M. D. Anderson Hospital in Houston was attended by a group of distinguished American investigators. They included Stanley, Ernest Goodpasture, Albert Sabin, and J. T. Syverton, as well as Duran-Reynals, Gross, Bryan, and Andervont. Interest in the oncologic aspects of virology was mounting rapidly.

It must be pointed out that this scientific interest in viral oncology was related to a victory of biomedical science —the conquest of poliomyelitis. Many of the investigators who had contributed to this intensive research effort now turned their sights on the intriguing problem of neoplasia.

At the National Cancer Institute, 1959–1964

The scientific ferment over viral oncology was reflected in greater appropriations for NCI and in the expansion of intramural as well as grant-supported research. Two events that furthered the administrative and budgetary developments were reports of possible oncogenic viral contamination of polio vaccine, and a report that particles morphologically resembling oncoviruses had been found in cow's milk. In 1959 NCI announced that $1 million was to be set aside for research grants in viral oncology. This undoubtedly accelerated the growth of the field.

From the Laboratory of Biology at NCI was created a Laboratory of Viral Oncology under Bryan, grouping Manaker, MARY FINK, JOHN MOLONEY, Rauscher, Sarah Stewart, and Dalton. These scientists, who had all contributed to the study of avian and murine tumor viruses, formed the administrative nucleus for the management of the coordinated program that evolved from the Acute Leukemia Task Force in 1962 to the Special Virus Cancer Program in 1964. Andervont and Bryan were reluctant administrators, devoted to self-directed research. They maintained close relationships with their staff on an informal basis and took pride in the development of younger associates. Many of the group remember with pleasure the weekly staff luncheons.

Involvement of investigators from other NIH Institutes has already been noted. Bernice Eddy, of the Division of Biologics Standards, who had collaborated with Sarah Stewart, discovered in 1961 that cultures from rhesus monkey kidney contained an agent that produced sarcomas in hamsters—the agent identified in Maurice R. Hilleman's laboratory as simian virus 40 (SV40). This important story, told in more detail in the section by Kirschstein, involved NCI when JOSEPH F. FRAUMENI, Jr., and others conducted epidemiologic inquiries into the effect of using monkey kidney cultures for poliomyelitis vaccine. Fortunately, no adverse effects of this contamination have been encountered in the human population.

Epidemiologic research on leukemia was also stimulated by the report of a small cluster of leukemic children in Niles, Illinois. This was investigated by W. Clark Heath of the Communicable Disease Center (now Centers for Disease Control), a Public Health Service facility at Atlanta, Georgia. No etiologic agents were uncovered. Other subsequently reported clusters were analyzed by NATHAN MANTEL, but again no statistical evidence of transmission could be adduced.

An important associate of NCI was the infectious disease laboratory of the National Institute of Allergy and Infectious Diseases (NIAID), with Huebner and WALLACE P. ROWE as the protagonists. This group had descended from distinguished predecessors such as Charles Armstrong, known for his classical work on St. Louis encephalitis and lymphocytic choriomeningitis in the 1930s. Huebner had pioneered in research on Coxsackie viruses and adenoviruses during the early 1950s. He had provided the adenovirus 12 that John J. Trentin, in Houston, used to induce sarcoma at the site of injection in hamsters—the first human virus to prove oncogenic (though showing no evidence of such action in man, its natural host). Huebner explored the occurrence of polyoma virus in wild mice and found that it was widely distributed among mouse populations both urban and rural. He transferred to NCI in 1968 but continued to interact closely with the NIAID group.

Virus Cancer Program, 1964–1980

During the 1960s the intensity and support of viral oncology were increased in anticipation of translating the findings on mice and other animals to man. The many virus-induced and virus-associated neoplasms in frogs, rodents, cats, dogs, and cattle, now firmly established, indicated that man was not likely to be exempt. The target of the research was to find viruses in human tumors, relate them etiologically to cancer, and develop means of blocking their effects.

A national program of targeted, managerially guided research on viral oncology began in 1964. The Congress, supported by testimony from scientists, provided a special appropriation to NCI for intensified research on the posited viral origin of leukemia. By this time NCI had had a decade of experience with a targeted program in cancer chemotherapy, which had used the contract method of research support. The method involved management of the contracts by NIH scientists and administrators. Thus the heads of intramural laboratories acquired responsibilities in the program, while input from many virology and other experts continued through advisory and review mechanisms.

In 1968 other cancers were added to leukemia in the search for viral etiologic agents. Rauscher headed the program, now in NCI's Division of Cancer Cause and Prevention.

By 1970 the virus program had 88 contracts, totaling $17 million. The program became part of the National Cancer Plan of 1971, which increased the funds available for all activities, including viral oncology. The growth and the method of funding raised questions from the scientific community, and the National Academy of Sciences was asked to examine the program. A committee chaired by Norton D. Zinder was critical of the size of the program and the use of contract funds for extensions of work by a few NCI investigators. The committee also criticized the competitions between basic and applied research and between research on cancer and other health problems.

Involvement in the National Cancer Plan increased, with a shift in the method of funding research from contracts to grants. By 1976 the viral oncology program allocations were at $98 million, or 16.5 percent of NCI's total research budget. When Rauscher became Director of the Institute, the virus program came under Moloney and included five laboratories under Huebner, Manaker, GEORGE J. TODARO, and EDWARD M. SCOLNICK.

Some Achievements of the Virus Cancer Program

In retrospect, the Virus Cancer Program is seen to be a seminal, productive investment that has led to many advances beyond its targeted goals. It stimulated molecular biology, which is certainly as basic as biological research can be at present. And though the "human cancer virus" has not been found—and probably does not exist in any conventional sense —the interaction of viruses with some specific neoplasms has been demonstrated.

The progress achieved is best gauged by comparing the status of knowledge over three decades. In 1942 Engelbreth-Holm published the book *Spontaneous and Experimental Leukemia in Animals.* At that time the only leukemias established to be of viral origin were in fowl. In 1978 the leukemia-lymphoma-sarcoma complex, as described in Theilin and Madewell's *Veterinary Cancer Medicine,* was firmly established as a viral disease widely distributed over the animal kingdom, and protective vaccines were available for cats and chickens. It would seem reasonable to expect the human species to be added eventually to the list, though the "virus" concerned may be more intimately hidden in the genome recesses of the cell.

Laboratory research on animals added more and more information on virus-cell interaction, the role of genetics, and control mechanisms. For basic questions in molecular biology, oncogenic viruses provide an excellent model.

Detection of antigens produced by a virus may be used to ascertain its presence. Sensitive tests for antigens have revealed that viruses of a type associated with carcinogenesis —type-C RNA viruses*—are highly prevalent in mice of all strains and in hamsters, chickens, and cats. Prenatal presence of virus has been demonstrated by immunologic techniques. A cocarcinogenic effect is suggested by the fact that cells replicating such viruses were highly susceptible to malignant transformation by the DNA simian virus 40, adenoviruses, and carcinogenic chemicals. Host genes had a profound effect on the replication of these viruses and their malignant expression.

Different strains of type-C virus can exist in the same species. In the hamster, mouse sarcoma virus activated four strains that shared antigens with one another but not with the viruses of the mouse, chicken, or cat. These observations led Huebner and Todaro to propose that all vertebrates possess type-C virus genomes transmitted as part of normal inheritance and controlled by host regulator genes and repressors. Genetic defects, mutations, carcinogens, and aging could act to decrease repression of such endogenous agents. This was the "oncogenic theory" of cancer, viewing the disease as a biological event triggered by spontaneous or induced activation of universal, specific viral "oncogenes."

Rowe and others reported Mendelian genetic studies showing that the expressions of endogenous RNA tumor viruses were controlled by identifiable dominant and recessive host genes. The intimate link between viruses and cell components made terms and concepts developed for infectious diseases inapplicable. As Rowe stated, the causal factor could be termed either a genetic infection or an infectious gene.

A cocarcinogenic relationship between type-C virus and chemicals was established, in that cultured rat, mouse, and hamster cells, exposed simultaneously to murine leukemia virus and carcinogenic hydrocarbons, were transformed within a month. Either agent alone had no observable effect. Moreover, there was no effect if the chemical was introduced be-

---

*Type-C virus: in electron microscopy, an RNA tumor virus classified morphologically. Type B, also an RNA tumor virus, is mentioned later. These two types are distinguishable by location of the center, budding characteristics, etc.

fore the virus, suggesting that virus initiation of scheduled intracellular events is requisite to carcinogenesis.

Particulates resembling RNA viruses were observed in human milk, in leukemia cells and serum, and in some tumors; but further attempts to correlate these particles with cancer in man, or indeed to prove that they are viruses, were unavailing at the current state of the art. Innovative techniques of nucleic acid templates and cell hybridization have opened new approaches to the problem. One of the limitations, of course, is the need to establish that human cells are transformed without using human subjects. Nude, athymic mice, as well as ever-improving tissue culture methods, may provide additional insights. For the latter, there is need for better definition of the nutritional requirements of human cells in vitro.

The Virus Cancer Program grouped interested scientists throughout the world and led to the augmented support of their research proposals. Participants came from the Soviet Union, Japan, Germany, and other European countries. Funds were allocated through either the grant or the contract mechanism, each having its proponents and opponents. The intimate participation of intramural scientists in the contract-supported research was criticized as self-serving. But by this time intra- and extramural scientists were more closely related in many programs, and the story of their combined achievements was becoming the story of biomedical science rather than of viral oncology.

The Virus Cancer Program, in addition to supporting national and multinational research, developed many essential services available to research workers. Since its inception in 1964, the program has

- Produced and distributed highly purified and characterized virus preparations.

- Produced, characterized, and distributed a large series of antibody and antigen preparations.

- Produced many different cell lines, developed methods for preservation and revival, and distributed characterized lines.

- Developed a computerized banking system for tissues, sera, and cell lines. The system has the capability to correlate data on these materials with information on clinical history and various other characteristics and to maintain quality control.

● Conducted developmental research that led to large-scale production of primates as needed for the program and other activities.

● Developed safety procedures for the handling of potentially dangerous biologic materials, including the design of special facilities. A building was designed and erected at NIH for the containment of viruses of possible danger to man.

● Developed several special animal species for laboratory studies.

● Developed an information system for cancer virology activities, including distribution of key abstracts.

Several NCI scientists have made important contributions to viral oncology since the program began.

About 1970 Todaro and colleagues showed that viral genes can be incorporated into the cellular genetic information of a distantly related species. In a series of comprehensive studies, it was demonstrated that retrovirus* genes could be conserved in the new host to alter its genetic information. The work provides a mechanism for the movement of genes from one species to another.

By way of contrast, PETER M. HOWLEY showed recently that papilloma virus DNA remains extrachromosomal—that the malignant transformation induced by this virus may therefore be mediated by nonintegrated viral genetic information.

STUART AARONSON, JOHN R. STEPHENSON, and colleagues described the spontaneous or inducible release of endogenous infective leukemia viruses (type-C retroviruses) of mice. Different classes of endogenous viruses became distinguishable, and the expression of each was found to be under separate control by host cells. Later, endogenous viruses were found in the cellular DNA of all mouse strains. By the early 1970s all cells of chickens and mice had been shown to have RNA tumor virus information in their genomes. This knowledge had broad biological significance as regards the regulation of virus expression in normal and abnormal cells, stimulating studies on the role of these viruses in other cellular functions.

PETER J. FISCHINGER and others found that the highly oncogenic avian, murine, feline, and primate RNA tumor viruses arose by recombination of replicating leukemia virus with either host cellular sequences or endogenous xenotropic (host-

---

*Retrovirus: see introduction to Scolnick chapter.

seeking) viral genes. These studies helped to generate the concept that certain sequences of RNA tumor viruses appear to be of cellular origin.

Many NCI scientists have participated in isolating products of mammalian transforming viruses. Assays for the structural proteins and antigens of type-C and -B viruses were developed at NCI and elsewhere.

The information has provided understanding of the genetic structure of this group of mammalian tumor-causing viruses. A classic example is the murine sarcoma virus, an agent that can transform cells but cannot, itself, replicate. Scolnick and his colleagues, using sarcoma virus strains in which most of the genes coding for viral structural proteins were deleted, demonstrated that certain sequences of mouse type-C virus represent a conserved rat gene responsible for the virus's transforming ability. The rat gene, in turn, codes for a protein required for maintenance of the transformed state.

Recapitulation and Analysis

Viral oncology at the National Institutes of Health has shared in the growth and development of the institution. The role of NIH funds and intramural NIH scientists may be gauged from the following statistics. In 1974 Tooze and Sambrook edited a collection of 109 articles on tumor virology, emphasizing the molecular biology aspects. Nineteen papers were from foreign sources. Of the 90 reports from American institutions, 20 were from NIH. NIH grant support is acknowledged in 59 papers and contract support in 13. Grant or contract support is mentioned in some papers involving intramural NIH investigators.

Both the scientific and administrative roles of NCI viral oncologists are well attested by a 1980 book on viral oncology edited by George Klein of Sweden. The book comprises 20 chapters, of which 4 were contributed by members of separate NCI laboratories: ROBERT C. GALLO, Howley, Scolnick, and Todaro. No other institution in the world is so well represented. This indicates the overwhelming importance of NIH support of viral oncology both within and outside the United States. The commanding role of the intramural NIH scientists who were at the heart of the program is evident.

It has been disappointing that the goal of discovering a human cancer virus and a vaccine against it has not been reached during two decades of programmatic accentuation and ever-increasing support. This goal remains the central theme of viral oncology. The tactics, however, have shifted from direct approaches gleaned from studies on infectious viruses to more subtle investigation that may point to new directions rather than replace the objective.

Increasing concern with the role of environmental chemicals in human cancer has also led to a reassessment of the scientific orientation of the virus cancer program. While the search for a definitive human cancer virus has not been abandoned, it is evident that cancer results from a complex interaction of factors. Detection of a virus would not be the complete answer, for a number of factors that interact with viruses to control their expression have been identified. They include host factors (genetics, hormones, and immune responses) and environmental factors (chemicals, X-rays, and ultraviolet irradiation).

A reassessment of goals during the late 1970s, with greater realization of the multifactorial nature of the neoplastic reaction, was certainly appropriate. Not so, however, is the pessimism expressed by some critics. Cancer, as pointed out since the earliest years of its scientific study, represents an extensive group of diseases; to approach it as a single entity may be an error.

An impressive demonstration that viral oncology remains of great concern in the study of human cancer was the isolation of Epstein–Barr DNA virus from the African lymphoma described by Denis P. Burkitt and its role in cancer of the nasopharynx and in the self-limiting acute mononucleosis. More recently the discovery of a growth factor, interleukin 2, and the isolation of human T cell leukemia virus by Robert Gallo and associates, as confirmed in Japan and at Duke University, may well represent the attainment of one of the major original goals of NCI's viral oncology program. Add to this the more tenuous relations of the hepatitis B virus to liver cancer and of herpes simplex virus (type 2) or human papilloma viruses to cervical carcinoma, and the conclusion of controlled optimism is reinforced.

We predict that viruses will be found to be the key to some of the neoplastic diseases of man. For the RNA viruses, the lymphoma-leukemia complex in man is probably related to similar states in chickens, mice, cats, and cattle, and there may well be subtle transmission routes between the species. Human breast cancer also, as in the animal models, may well have a viral etiologic component. We are less sanguine about other cancers, especially those of the epithelial surfaces.

The shortest route to testing these predictions is research. Periodic assessments and reassessments of the goals as well as the methods are essential. But pessimism is not justified, for indeed man, through scientific research as a way of thinking and doing, will eventually overcome the malignant crab.

Acknowledgments

The authors are grateful to LOUIS R. SIBAL, Office of Extramural Research and Training, NIH, and W. EMMETT BARKLEY, Office of Research Services, NIH, for providing information on the Special Virus Leukemia Program and the Special Virus Containment Facility (Bldg. 41), respectively. We also appreciate remembrances from CARL G. BAKER, Joseph W. Beard, KENNETH M. ENDICOTT, William Feller, MARY A. FINK, Ludwik Gross, Vincent Groupé, and C. GORDON ZUBROD.

Selected References

Gross, L. Oncogenic Viruses, ed. 2. New York: Pergamon Press, 1970. A scholarly history and authoritative text on viral oncology.

Hahon, N. Selected Papers on Virology. Englewood Cliffs, N.J.: Prentice-Hall, 1964. A historical collection that includes translations of Pasteur's 1884 paper on rabies and Beijerinck's 1898 paper on tobacco mosaic.

Hiatt, H.H., J.D. Watson, and J.A. Winsten, eds. Origins of Human Cancer, 3 vols. (Coldspring Harbor Lab., 1977). Volume C contains sections on DNA and RNA viruses, pp 957–1306.

Klein, G., ed. Viral Oncology. New York: Raven Press, 1980 (842 pp).

1976 NCI Fact Book. DHEW Publication No. (NIH) 77-512. Revised 1977.

Shimkin, M.B. Contrary to Nature. Washington: GPO, 1977 (498 pp). For sale by Superintendent of Documents, U.S. Govt. Printing Office, Washington, D.C. 20401.

Stewart, S.E., and B.E. Eddy. The polyoma virus, in Advances in Virus Research 7:61-102, 1960. Their account of the polyoma work. Compares to that of Ludwik Gross.

Tooze, J., and J. Sambrook. Selected Papers in Tumor Virology (Coldspring Harbor Lab., 1974).

The history of the National Cancer Institute, on its twentieth anniversary, is summarized in the J of NCI 19:133-349, 1957, and on its fortieth anniversary, in J of NCI 59: 545-765, 1977. Virology is described by R.J. Manaker, L.R. Sibal, and J.B. Moloney in the latter volume, pp. 623-631.

Introduction

VIROGENES TO ONCOGENES

Francis Crick enunciated the dogma that information in biological systems flowed from DNA to RNA to protein, and uniquely in that direction. This left unexplained the modus operandi of certain cancer-producing viruses, such as the Rous sarcoma virus, which contains no DNA. How was its information transmitted to the host cell?

An exciting series of events beginning about 1970 has gone far to clarify the role of the RNA tumor viruses. Howard Temin and David Baltimore simultaneously announced a key discovery that revealed an imperfection in Crick's dogma. They found that all RNA viruses contain an enzyme, reverse transcriptase, which catalyzes the assembly of DNA upon the RNA template. This came to be known as copy DNA, and the viruses as retroviruses.

Some retroviruses carry genes whose protein products are capable of transforming host cells. Oncogenes, as these tumor-causing genes are called, were found not only in the viral genome but, surprisingly, in the host genome as well. Research on these genes and on the products of their expression has constituted a major forward thrust in our understanding of the cancer process.

D. S.

18

VIROGENES TO ONCOGENES

Edward M. Scolnick

During the period 1970–1981 the National Cancer Institute enjoyed unprecedented growth in its various research programs concerned with the causes and treatment of cancer. Investigation of oncogenic, or tumor-causing, viruses at NCI and other institutions has led to a major intellectual change in the field of cancer biology. Some advances in viral oncology by intramural NCI scientists are reviewed in this chapter.

Viral Oncology in 1970

By the beginning of the decade, the scientific leadership of the Institute had decided to concentrate most of its intramural virology on RNA tumor viruses. As their name implies, these viruses contain ribonucleic acid (RNA), not deoxyribonucleic acid (DNA), as their genetic material. They had been found to infect cells and become stably associated with them. A variety of such viruses were known to produce naturally occurring tumors in chickens, mice, and rats, and it was clear that they could cause solid tumors or leukemias in the species of origin.

Several types of RNA tumor virus had been isolated. Most of these were self-replicating, or "helper-independent." Less common ones were highly oncogenic but replication-defective, requiring a helper virus to be infectious. Methods to increase the virus concentration of isolates in cell culture were being developed. Some highly oncogenic variants could be cultivated, and their oncogenic effects quantitated by assays on mouse cells.

A puzzling observation had been made by Howard M. Temin of the McArdle Laboratory for Cancer Research and JOHN P. BADER

EDWARD M. SCOLNICK, M.D., Senior Vice President, Research, Merck Sharp & Dohme Research Laboratories. Formerly Chief, Laboratory of Tumor Virus Genetics, Division of Cancer Cause and Prevention, National Cancer Institute.

of NCI. Inhibitors of DNA synthesis, and of DNA-dependent synthesis, interfered with the replication of RNA tumor viruses in vitro. This led the investigators to postulate a DNA intermediate in the virus life cycle—a mechanism by which genetic information could flow from RNA to DNA as well as vice versa. But clear evidence for such a model was lacking.

The field of viral oncology was plagued by many technical and intellectual problems. RNA tumor viruses grown in cell culture were generally of much lower concentration than were SV40, polyoma, or nontumor RNA viruses such as poliovirus or reovirus. The structure of viral RNAs was unclear, and their instability hampered molecular approaches. Above all, one was limited in framing incisive experiments without a clear understanding of how these viruses (lacking DNA) replicated.

Virogenes, or RNA Virus Replication Clarified

Then, in 1970, the entire field of tumor virology, and especially of RNA tumor viruses, received a major impetus from the discovery of reverse transcriptase. Working with avian and murine viruses, David Baltimore at MIT and Temin and Satoshi Mizutani at McArdle elucidated the enzymatic machinery for the synthesis of DNA within RNA tumor virions (whole virus particles). Once a DNA intermediate—a "virogene"—in the virus life cycle had been identified, plausible models for the cycle could be devised and the heritable nature of these infectious RNA viruses understood. Proof that the intermediate could integrate with the DNA of cells was obtained, and a much clearer picture of viral replication emerged. RNA-containing tumor viruses became known as retroviruses by virtue of the "backward" transcription of their RNA into DNA as a step in their propagation.

By means of reverse transcriptase, investigators were able to prepare radioactive "copy DNA" (cDNA) from viral RNA. This became a valuable tool for tracer studies on the retroviruses. These technical advances, combined with a liberal infusion of funds, fostered a major expansion in the field over the next few years.

Intramural NCI scientists now focused on the helper-independent retroviruses of mammals. Most extramural scientists were studying the Rous chicken tumor virus, which is indeed an excellent model for investigating cancer causation. In the intramural program, however, the mammalian retroviruses were deemed more likely to yield useful information about human cancers.

The Search for a Cancer Virus in Humans

The foremost goal of ROBERT J. HUEBNER's group was to isolate a human cancer virus. There had been a frequent association between the replication of retroviruses and the enhanced
prevalence of various leukemias in murine hosts, and the high-
incidence thymic leukemia system of the AKR mouse was considered a possible prototype for other leukemias. In the NCI
studies a major thrust was to develop ways to find and isolate
infectious retroviruses from leukemias of man. During the
period 1970-1975, intramural scientists made several important
discoveries in the course of this quest for a leukemia-causing
agent.

It seemed advantageous to develop and characterize permanent cell lines that might be used to study virus replication.
Earlier, at New York University, Howard Green and GEORGE J.
TODARO had developed contact-inhibited (i.e., nononcogenic)
cell lines from outbred Swiss mice. Between 1967 and 1970,
Todaro and his colleagues, by then at NCI, developed two such
lines from inbred Balb/c mice and NIH Swiss mice. A similar
type of cell was subsequently developed from C3H mice by
CHARLES HEIDELBERGER at McArdle to quantitate the effects of
chemical carcinogens in oncogenesis.

These new cell lines were also well suited for studies
on replication-defective retroviruses. The infectious complex of an oncogenic RNA virus (also called sarcoma virus)
and its virus helper was difficult to study, and a systematic
method for separating the sarcoma virus from the helper was
not available. Using the new cell lines, however, STUART
AARONSON and WALLACE P. ROWE succeeded in isolating helper-
free Moloney* and Kirsten sarcoma virus. And by a somewhat
different approach, PETER J. FISCHINGER and ROBERT H. BASSIN
achieved similar results with a Moloney virus strain.

Detection of Retrovirus Proteins

The protein structure of mammalian retroviruses was another major subject of investigation. In large part the main
thrust for this work was made by Huebner's colleagues Ray Gil-
den of Flow Laboratories, WADE PARKS of NCI, and the author.

Gel electrophoresis, used to separate proteins by size,
revealed a consistent pattern of protein bands associated with
mammalian retrovirus particles. Antisera to the purified proteins proved invaluable in demonstrating the widespread epidemiologic occurrence of retroviruses in mice and mouse embryos.

---

*JOHN B. MOLONEY was at NCI from 1947 to 1979.

One of these virion proteins, p30 (p = protein; 30 = MW of 30,000), was found to be a useful group-specific antigen of murine retroviruses and received the most attention. Sera prepared to p30 offered a broad set of immunologic reactions, and some even revealed immunologic determinants shared with retroviruses from other mammalian species. Many an NCI meeting was inspired by the depth and scope of Huebner's intellect in discussing p30 and its ramifications.

Sensitive radioimmunoassays devised for detecting retroviruses aided greatly in isolating new ones. Several classification schemes were developed, and retroviral proteins were purified to essential homogeneity. Aaronson and JOHN R. STEPHENSON found some proteins with type-specific determinants, enabling mammalian retroviruses to be classified with precision.

Retrovirus Isolation

Through improved methods of cell culture and virus classification, the number of retrovirus isolates began to mount. The work of isolation was much advanced by the introduction of halogenated pyrimidines as inducers. Rowe and his colleagues JANET W. HARTLEY, DOUGLAS R. LOWY, and NATALIE TEICH had noted the efficacy of IudR and BudR as inducers for AKR embryo cells. They showed that these compounds could convert barren cells to virus-producing cultures. As a result of this discovery, retroviruses carried silently in many other strains of mice were isolated—mice that normally express only low levels of infectious retrovirus throughout their lives.

A flurry of research was undertaken to isolate retroviruses from various mammalian species and to determine the prevalence of these agents known to be silently carried but potentially infectious. New facts and concepts as well as new isolates emerged. A given vertebrate species could harbor several distinct types of retrovirus. Retroviral sequences, as shown by ROBERT CALLAHAN and Todaro, could constitute up to 0.1 percent of the genomic DNA of mice. Viruses were isolated from baboons and apes, and a primate model for retrovirus-induced leukemia was recognized. Through molecular hybridization techniques, it was soon demonstrated that some retroviruses were transmitted horizontally and others genetically.

Meanwhile the quest for human retroviruses quickened. New cell lines that might be permissive to their replication were developed. DNA copies of retroviral genomes were used in molecular hybridization experiments to probe DNA from normal and cancerous human cells in the search for retrovirus footprints. Unfortunately, however, the zeal of the investigators was not rewarded with bona fide infectious isolates, and molecular approaches failed to detect a consistent pattern of viral antigens.

Several novel mammalian viruses were discovered during these intensive searches, and the oncogenic retroviruses are now used widely as investigative tools. Moreover, the groundwork had been laid for major advances relating to oncogenesis.

Enter the Oncogene

In the early part of the decade, little was known of the virus genome. Then genetic studies by Steven Martin at the University of California and Bader of NCI revealed that the Rous virus contains a gene, termed *src* (sarcoma), that codes for the transforming function. A similar type of gene was identified in the Kirsten sarcoma virus. Forthwith such oncogenic genes of tumor viruses became the subject of many investigations.

These genes have become known as oncogenes—i.e., genes that cause tumors. Like other genes, they are transcribed to messenger RNA (mRNA), which in turn is translated to protein. The protein products have been called oncogenic proteins, since their action causes neoplastic transformation of cells. A concept of oncogenes was first postulated by Huebner and Todaro in the 1960s.

The most highly oncogenic of the known mammalian retroviruses are replication-defective. As noted earlier, fewer of these than of the helper-independent type have been isolated. Despite the interest in their oncogenic property, these sarcoma viruses were largely ignored during the early part of the decade. They were considered interesting, but probably irrelevant to human cancer. Then SCOLNICK and colleagues, in 1973, published findings on the origin of the oncogenes of sarcoma retroviruses.

The work began with the study of the genetic composition of Kirsten sarcoma virus, which had derived from passage of a mouse retrovirus through a rat. By means of molecular hybridization, rat genetic sequences were detected in the Kirsten virus's genomic RNA. A model was postulated for acquisition of cellular "onc" genes by transduction, or transfer by a viral agent. Proof of the transduction hypothesis—the capture of cellular genes by retroviruses—comes not only from the work of these NCI scientists, but also from several extramural studies on Rous sarcoma virus and more recently from NCI studies by GEORGE F. VANDE WOUDE and Lowy.

Cellular onc genes have been detected in a wide variety of vertebrate species, including man. Recently, Robert Weinberg and his colleagues at MIT found them in *Drosophila,* confirming their prevalance if not ubiquity in eukaryotes.* From work on Moloney sarcoma virus (Vande Woude, Fischinger, DONALD G. BLAIR and LYNN W. ENQUIST) and on Harvey sarcoma virus (Scolnick, Lowy, and colleagues), it is now clear that these transduced "normal" host genes can transform cells. Using the powerful methods of recombinant DNA technology, each of these groups has cloned a normal host gene homologous to the transforming onc gene of a sarcomagenic retrovirus. The cloned genes, when reintroduced into NIH 3T3 cells, result in their malignant transformation.

The discovery that vertebrates carry diverse genes capable of inducing cancer was startling. It has ushered in a new era in cancer biology and will surely be viewed in the future as a turning point in the scientific approach to the cancer problem. We should note that the discovery was not an original targeted goal of the NCI Virus Cancer Program. Indeed, it occurred largely outside the more targeted areas of tumor virology research.

Oncogenic Proteins

After the discovery of onc genes and their identification by oligonucleotide** fingerprinting and molecular hybridization, investigators turned their attention to detection of the gene product. The first definitive identification of an oncogene-derived protein came in 1977 at the University of Colorado. Joan Brugge and Raymond L. Erikson developed rabbit antisera that recognized the radiolabeled p60 product of the Rous sarcoma gene.

Within NCI other classes of oncogenic proteins were identified between 1977 and 1979. The two most notable proteins were discovered by Stephenson, CHARLES J. SHERR, and Scolnick. Stephenson and Sherr described the protein p85, a product of the onc gene of a feline sarcoma virus. Scolnick and colleagues identified the onc protein p21, coded for by the Kirsten virus. Intensive biochemical studies on these proteins are designed to map the metabolic pathways involved in the malignant conversion of cells. The clear goal of the field is to identify the associated enzymes and to characterize their metabolic role.

---

*Organisms composed of cells with nuclei, in contrast to bacteria and viruses.

**Tantamount to a nucleic acid fragment.

Oncogenic Enzymes?

One such quarry appears to be tyrosine protein kinase, the p60 onc protein of the Rous virus. This product of the *src* gene proved to be an enzyme that adds phosphate ions to the tyrosine component of protein. Extensions of this work over the past two years have indicated that phosphorylation of tyrosine is a function of the onc proteins of five distinct RNA retroviruses.

With the realization that protein kinase activities are important in oncogenesis, attention has shifted to the search for cellular elements with which the onc proteins interact. Potential cellular targets for kinases are turning up almost as fast as new retroviruses did five years ago. Applying immuno-electron microscopy, MARK C. WILLINGHAM and IRA H. PASTAN, molecular biologists at NCI, located onc proteins of the Rous sarcoma and Kirsten viruses (p60 and p21) at the inner surface of the plasma membrane of cells.

Experiments by Stanley Cohen of Vanderbilt University School of Medicine and Anthony Hunter of the Salk Institute for Biological Studies suggest that the plasma membrane may also be the onc proteins' initial site of action. These workers showed that a normal stimulant of cell division, epidermal growth factor, apparently binds to the membrane through a process involving phosphorylation by tyrosine protein kinase. Thus the onc protein p60 may have a role in regulating normal cell growth. Analogies have emerged between the modus operandi of onc proteins and that of various polypeptide hormones, and an intellectual wedding of tumor virology and endocrinology seems to be occurring.

The New Biology

Attempts to isolate an infectious human virus are no longer proceeding with their former vigor. Many investigators feel that this goal is not so critical now that oncogenes have been discovered in the normal vertebrate genome. It should be noted, however, that ROBERT C. GALLO and his colleagues at NCI have recently isolated a promising new retrovirus from humans with an unusual (cutaneous T-cell) leukemia. This candidate human virus appears to be a novel isolate, and the possibility of an etiologic role is being explored.

It has also become clear that the discoveries arising in studies of tumor viruses are widely applicable to cell biology. Indeed, the impact of tumor virology on the broader field emphasizes the rather unexpected turns that basic research can take. For example, tumor virologists have greatly contributed to the study of eukaryotic genes, which has been an explosive field in the past decade.

The enzyme system reverse transcriptase, mentioned above, has been invaluable as a research tool. In the early 1970s, NCI scientists JEFFREY ROSS and Scolnick, in collaboration with PHILIP LEDER of the Child Health Institute, utilized DNA primers to prepare a cDNA from globin mRNA. This primer technique and variations are being used widely to obtain cDNA probes that serve as critical reagents in a broad range of molecular hybridization studies.

DNA sequencing experiments by RAVI DHAR in collaboration with Enquist, Vande Woude, and WILLIAM L. McCLEMENTS of NCI have helped confirm John Taylor's prediction that retroviruses would be found to share structural features with prokaryotic transposable elements—genes that change their chromosomal location in prokaryotic organisms.* A search for similar movable genes in eukaryotic cells is under way. Experiments by GEORGE KHOURY and Leder were among those that led to the discovery of introns—sequences between the genes in a DNA strand—and to the development of virus vectors for introducing genes into cells. One new and promising vector system, recently described by PETER M. HOWLEY, uses bovine papilloma virus. Such findings are already being applied in clinical genetic problems.

A growth factor for the long-term propagation of mature T cells—thymus cells cultured for their immunologic properties —was a by-product of studies by Gallo and FRANK RUSCETTI directed at the isolation of human retroviruses. The factor has allowed T cells to be cloned into various classes. Several groups of investigators are attempting to develop ways to treat human tumors with such differentiated T cell populations.

Studies on the mouse mammary tumor virus (Bittner) by Parks, Scolnick, and HOWARD H. YOUNG revealed its utility for investigating steroid hormone action. The investigators developed a tissue culture system for studying how glucocorticoids regulate transcription of Bittner virus cDNA to RNA. GORDON L. HAGER, extending these observations, identified a "promoter" for hormones of the glucocorticoid class. These findings will further our understanding of steroid action, both in gene regulation and therapeutic modalities.

It was stated earlier that the last decade has witnessed critical advances in the field of cancer biology. From a discipline that was based on phenomenology and dominated by empiricism, it has become one of the most rational and pro-

---

*Composed of a cell or cells lacking a true nucleus, such as bacteria.

ductive approaches to exploration of the eukaryotic cell. Clearly, the primary contributions to cancer biology have come from molecular biology in general and tumor virology in particular. The NCI intramural research program has richly contributed both concepts and techniques, and the coming decade should witness an even greater expansion of knowledge. It is a privilege to participate in a research field that is highly stimulating intellectually while fundamentally relevant to an important clinical problem.

Selected References

Aaronson, S.A., and W.P. Rowe. Nonproducer clones of murine sarcoma virus transformed BALB/3T3 cells. Virology 42:9-19, 1970.

Bishop, J.M. Retroviruses. Annu Rev Biochem 47:35-88, 1978.

Collett, M.S., and R.L. Erikson. Protein kinase activity associated with the avian sarcoma virus src gene product. Proc Natl Acad Sci USA 75:2021-2024, 1978.

DeFeo, D., et al. Analysis of two divergent restriction endonuclease fragments homologous to the p21 coding region of Harvey murine sarcoma virus. Proc Natl Acad Sci USA 78:3328-3332, 1981.

Dhar, R., et al. Nucleotide sequences of integrated Moloney sarcoma provirus long terminal repeats and their host and viral junctions. Proc Natl Acad Sci USA 77:3937-3941, 1980.

Gruss, P., and G. Khoury. Expression of simian virus 40-rat preproinsulin recombinants in monkey kidney cells: Use of preproinsulin RNA processing signals. Proc Natl Acad Sci USA 78:133-137, 1981.

Huebner, R.J., et al. Rescue of the defective genome of Moloney sarcoma virus from a non-infectious hamster tumor and the production of pseudotype sarcoma viruses with various murine leukemia viruses. Proc Natl Acad Sci USA 56:1164-1176, 1966.

Hunter, T., and B.M. Sefton. Transforming gene product of Rous sarcoma virus phosphorylates tyrosine. Proc Natl Acad Sci USA 77:1311-1315, 1980.

Jainchill, J.F., S.A. Aaronson, and G.J. Todaro. Murine sarcoma and leukemia viruses: Assay using clonal lines of contact inhibited mouse cells. J Virol 4:549-553, 1969.

Khan, A.S., D.N. Deobagkar, and J.R. Stephenson. Isolation and characterization of a feline sarcoma virus-coded precursor polyprotein. J Biol Chem 253:8894-8901, 1978.

Lowy, D.R., et al. Murine leukemia virus high-frequency acti-
    vation in vitro by 5-iododeoxyuridine and 5-bromodeoxy-
    uridine. Science 173:155-156, 1971.
Lowy, D.R., E. Rands, and E.M. Scolnick. Helper-independent
    transformation by unintegrated Harvey sarcoma virus DNA.
    J Virol 26:291-298, 1978.
Oskarsson, M., et al. Properties of a normal mouse cell DNA
    sequence (sarc) homologous to the src sequence of Moloney
    sarcoma virus. Science 297:1222-1223, 1980.
Rowe, W.P., W.E. Pugh, and J.W. Hartley. Plaque assay tech-
    niques for murine leukemia viruses. Virology 42:1136-
    1139, 1970.
Scolnick, E.M., et al. Studies on the nucleic acid sequences
    of Kirsten sarcoma virus: A model for formation of a mam-
    malian RNA-containing sarcoma virus. J Virol 12:458-463,
    1973.
Scolnick, E.M., A.G. Papageorge, and T.Y. Shih. Guanine
    nucleotide-binding activity as an assay for src protein of
    rat-derived murine sarcoma viruses. Proc Natl Acad Sci
    USA 76:5355-5359, 1979.
Sherr, C.J., et al. Pseudotypes of feline sarcoma virus con-
    tain an 85,000-dalton protein with feline oncornavirus-
    associated cell membrane antigen (FOCMA) activity. Proc
    Natl Acad Sci USA 75:1505-1509, 1978.
Willingham, M.C., et al. Localization of the src gene product
    of the Harvey strain of MSV to plasma membrane of trans-
    formed cells by electron microscopic immunocytochemistry.
    Cell 19:1005-1014, 1980.

Introduction

SV40

Occasionally an important area of science is opened as a result of an accident. In the 1850s William Perkin was stirring an organic mixture with a thermometer (a poor laboratory practice). The bulb of the thermometer broke, and the mercury released into the mixture proved to be the catalyst necessary for the desired reaction. History reveals that out of this accident and the resulting synthesis was born the vast aniline dye industry.

This chapter recounts an initially frightening accident investigated and interpreted at the National Institutes of Health. Early batches of poliomyelitis vaccine released to the public were found to contain a virus pathogenic in hamsters: simian vacuolating virus 40. Fortunately, the catastrophe that was envisioned with intense anxiety never materialized. As far as we know today, no one vaccinated with the contaminated material has suffered adverse effects.

The novel virus SV40 turned out to be an excellent model for a variety of studies. In the hands of many investigators, it has been a fruitful source of information about viruses in general, the nature of viral genetics, and some highly specialized areas of biology such as the extraordinary topology of virus genomes. It is used in recombinant DNA experiments to insert foreign genes into microorganisms. A number of laboratories, both at NIH and elsewhere, are still exploring the characteristics of this important virus.

D. S.

19

SV40

I. The Virus and Poliomyelitis Vaccine

Ruth L. Kirschstein

Poliomyelitis, or infantile paralysis (a misnomer), hard as it may be to believe today, was a devastating disease which occurred in epidemic proportions in the United States until the 1960s. The disease was shown to be caused by a virus in the early 1900s (1), and many years later, three distinctive types of poliovirus were identified. Despite early identification of the cause of this dread disease and continued scientific endeavors to understand the nature of the virus and its pathogenicity, progress was slow. This was so primarily because the virus could only be propagated in animals (essentially only in primates, at that) or in explants of primate central nervous system tissue. All this was to change in the late 1940s when John Enders and his associates (2) found that poliovirus grew in glass flasks in cultures of cells from humans and a number of different primates, including kidney cells from rhesus monkeys.

The significance of this finding, for which Enders, Thomas Weller, and Frederick Robbins were awarded the Nobel Prize in 1954, was immediately evident not only to virologists but also to the Director of Research of the National Foundation for Infantile Paralysis ("March of Dimes"), Harry Weaver. Here was a method for propagating large quantities of poliovirus which could then lead to the prevention of the disease, which he firmly believed was more promising than a cure. And so it was that the National Foundation, led by Weaver, upon the advice of most of the leading research virologists, embarked on a targeted effort to develop a successful vaccine to prevent "infantile paralysis."

It should be noted that two previous attempts to prevent "polio" by use of a vaccine had ended in disaster (3,4). Nev-

RUTH L. KIRSCHSTEIN, M.D., Director, National Institute of General Medical Sciences.

ISBN 0-12-667980-0

ertheless, Weaver was convinced that this time successful
vaccines could be developed.

Also noteworthy are the enormous contributions to poliomyelitis research of two early NIH intramural scientists,
CHARLES ARMSTRONG (5) and C. P. LI (6), both of whom found
that certain types of polioviruses could be adapted to grow
in animals other than primates, namely the cotton rat and the
mouse. The importance of these discoveries was, of course,
superseded by the ability to grow the virus in vitro, namely
in cell cultures.

Pursuit of a "poliovaccine" under sponsorship of the National Foundation became an obsession for two men, Jonas Salk
and Albert Sabin. Each, however, took a very different course.
Salk (7), modeling his vaccine after that for influenza, which
he had studied for many years, worked on the development of
an inactivated antigenic material which, after intramuscular injection, would be able to induce protective antibodies
against all three types of polioviruses. After long years
of research, including small-scale human experiments, a number of pharmaceutical manufacturers began to produce large
quantities of poliovirus in enormous flasks of primary rhesus
monkey kidney cell cultures covered by nutrient medium. The
replicating virus destroyed the cells, releasing into the
nutrient medium the poliovirus, cellular debris, and any other
passenger materials contained within the monkey kidney cells.
These fluids were then harvested and the poliovirus particles
concentrated into small volumes. The poliovirus harvests were
inactivated by formaldehyde, filtered, and prepared as final
vaccines. After a large-scale field trial of the experimental
"Salk vaccine," it was found to be effective and safe. On
April 12, 1955 (8,9), the National Institutes of Health, then
responsible for the regulation of biological products, announced the licensing of this new product for use by the general public, particularly children and young adults who had
no previous exposure to infantile paralysis. Despite a number
of serious problems confronting the regulation of this Salk
vaccine, it became widely used and the incidence of poliomyelitis dropped dramatically over the next several years.

Many scientists, however, of whom Albert Sabin (10) was
the most vocal, were concerned that the antibody levels induced by the Salk vaccine might not remain high enough to
assure protection over a lifetime. Indeed, Sabin, pursuing
the goal of permanent immunity, had been developing a "live
virus vaccine" (11) with support from the National Foundation
at the same time that Salk was developing his inactivated
vaccine. The tactics used by those researchers interested in
developing a live virus vaccine involved the attenuation (or
weakening) of the virulence of each of the three poliovirus

strains to the point where they could be ingested (the normal route of poliovirus infection), would replicate in the gastrointestinal tract, and would produce high levels of immunity but not cause paralytic disease. Sabin reasoned that such an infection with attenuated virus would produce not only circulating antibody but also permanent enteric immunity, thus preventing future infection with virulent, paralytogenic polioviruses. The methods used by Sabin to attenuate the virus involved repeated passage in monkey kidney cell cultures at various temperatures, along with passage in monkeys by inoculation of brains and spinal cords. The latter procedure served not only to adapt the virus to central nervous system tissue but to test its attenuation as well.

By about 1960, three different attenuated live virus vaccines, developed by Sabin and two other virologists, Herald Cox of Lederle Laboratories and Hilary Koprowski of the Wistar Institute, were ready for large-scale clinical trials. Furthermore, evidence of waning immunity in persons who had received the Salk vaccine several years earlier made the prospect of live virus vaccines most attractive. The extensive clinical trials conducted in South America by Lederle Laboratories, in Africa and Poland by Koprowski, and in Russia using Sabin vaccine led, in 1962, after much agonizing analysis of data, to approval by NIH of only the Sabin strains for use as Poliovirus Vaccine, Live, Oral (12).

It must be emphasized that both the Salk and Sabin vaccines initially were produced in primary *rhesus monkey* kidney cell cultures obtained by removing the kidneys of monkeys imported from India. These animals were deemed healthy by virtue of survival for a quarantine period after import and by evidence of lack of infection with tuberculosis. It was known, however, that monkey kidney cell cultures often degenerated "spontaneously," and a group of "simian" viruses were discovered in control cell cultures. Using various assays, manufacturers of either type of vaccine were required by the NIH regulatory body, the Division of Biologics Standards (DBS), to demonstrate that the production lots did not contain any of the known simian virus contaminants.

In 1960, at the Second Pan-American Conference on Live Poliovirus Vaccines, Benjamin Sweet and Maurice Hilleman (13) of the Merck Institute for Therapeutic Research shocked the conferees by presenting evidence that a new, hitherto unknown simian virus had been discovered in rhesus monkey kidney cells and that its presence could only be detected by testing fluids from rhesus kidney cells on vervet, or African green monkey, kidney cell cultures. Furthermore, Hilleman showed that the Sabin Live Poliovirus Vaccine strains, as well as the experimental lots used in clinical trials, contained large quantities of this newly discovered (but obviously long-existing) virus. The virus was called "vacuolating virus" because it caused a degeneration characterized by the production of cellular vacuoles in green monkey cells. It was renamed simian virus 40 (SV40), since it was the fortieth monkey virus discovered. Great concern was raised as to whether this passenger virus, contained in the vaccine, could infect man and cause any disease. Hilleman's further studies indicated that persons receiving the Salk, or inactivated, poliomyelitis vaccine had low levels of antibody to SV40 but that persons fed Sabin vaccine had none. There was no evidence of short-term harm from the SV40 virus, and Hilleman himself, late in 1960, described it as "just one more of the troublesome viruses to be conquered in the quest for vaccines which are safe and effective when used in man."

This statement proved not to be prophetic, for SV40 became not only an extremely important agent for study by molecular biologists but also a subject of great controversy and concern.

During the period from 1958-1960, when Sweet and Hilleman were studying vacuolating virus but had not yet reported its existence to the scientific community, BERNICE EDDY of DBS was devoting her studies to finding a virus in monkey kidney cells which might be oncogenic (that is, cause tumors). Eddy, along with SARAH STEWART of the National Cancer Institute (NCI), had already described a new mouse virus, the polyoma virus (14), which, when injected into newborn hamsters or mice, after a long incubation period, produced tumors different from any previously studied. Using this model system, Eddy injected extracts of rhesus monkey kidney cell cultures into newborn hamsters and waited patiently. After nine months, malignant subcutaneous and visceral tumors appeared (15a).

Excited by the fact that her prediction was true, that these monkey kidney extracts were indeed oncogenic, Eddy immediately prepared a paper for publication. However, her superiors, concerned that the tumors she described were similar to those induced by polyoma virus, thought that further evidence was needed that the rhesus monkey cell extracts she had injected were not contaminated by the mouse virus. Her manuscript was held up and not cleared for publication. The fact that there was a suspicion that cell cultures used to produce vaccines for human use might contain oncogenic viruses was kept within the confines of DBS and NIH for close to a year. But when Hilleman reported on the discovery of SV40, Eddy obtained this virus from the Merck Institute and quickly showed that it was the agent in the rhesus monkey kidney cells which was responsible for the induction of the hamster tumors. At that point, over a year after the discovery, the administration of DBS and NIH relented, and the first publication by Eddy and her colleagues of the fact that the cell cultures used to prepare vaccines for human use could cause malignant tumors in hamsters became available to the scientific community (15b).

Thereafter, studies relating to SV40 took several directions. Of most immediate importance were attempts (1) to elucidate the mechanism by which the virus induced tumors, (2) to determine if any of the millions of persons who had received poliovirus and adenovirus vaccines (the only ones then grown in monkey kidney cell cultures) had developed tumors, and (3) to produce these vaccines uncontaminated by the oncogenic virus. Other studies of SV40 used it primarily as a model of cell transformation and for elucidation of the molecular biology and biochemistry of DNA-containing viruses, of DNA-protein interactions, and of DNA as a chemical. These studies are described in Section II of this chapter.

Those who studied the mechanism of tumor induction by SV40 included some of the most illustrious names in modern-day virology: ROWE, HARTLEY, TAKEMOTO, HUEBNER, and HABEL of the National Institute of Allergy and Infectious Diseases; GERBER of DBS; Hsiung of Yale University; MELNICK and Rapp of Baylor University; and RABSON of NCI. The most crucial finding was that the tumor cells or cells that have undergone malignant transformation in vitro do not contain the whole virus but only the viral nucleic acid that becomes integrated into the DNA of each cell. This discovery opened up a whole new area of virology and led to the search for latent human oncogenic viruses, a search that continues today.

A long-range epidemiologic study was begun by JOSEPH FRAUMENI (16) of NCI to determine whether there was any evidence that SV40 was oncogenic in man. In 1960 a group of newborn infants had received large doses of inactivated poliomyelitis vaccine in an attempt to induce early and long-lasting immunity to polio. This vaccine was later shown to be contaminated with SV40. Since the study was designed to determine the long-term effects of the vaccine, followup was possible (17). From the careful epidemiology done on these children and other studies by Shah and Nathanson (18) at Johns Hopkins University, certain conclusions are now possible:

● Widespread introduction of SV40 into the human population through the use of contaminated inactivated and live poliovirus and adenovirus vaccines has not resulted in establishing this virus as part of the flora of human beings.

● The inadvertent inoculation of SV40 into children has not caused an increased incidence of cancer or other diseases.

Once the fact was accepted that SV40 was indeed a serious contaminant of both types of poliovirus vaccine, DBS set about establishing regulations to assure that this virus and other oncogenic materials were excluded from all biological products. Since SV40, latent and undetectable in rhesus monkey kidney cell cultures, could be tested for in cultures of African green monkey kidney cells and since polioviruses could grow just as well in such cultures, all poliovaccines were required to be grown in such cell systems. Furthermore, the seed strains of the attenuated live polioviruses which were badly contaminated with SV40 were cleared by repeated passage of the virus pools in green monkey kidney cell cultures in the presence of neutralizing antibodies to SV40. Although there was concern that the attenuated polioviruses would revert to virulence after removal of the SV40 contamination, this did not prove to be the case, and resumption of the manufacture of safe and effective poliovirus vaccines quickly followed. By the end of the 1960s, the incidence of poliomyelitis in the United States was at an all-time low. Since then, the public has been assured of immunity against this disease, and the horrors of life in iron lungs and of children with paralyzed limbs have vanished forever, not only in the United States but throughout most of the world.

References

1. Flexner, S., and P.A. Lewis. The transmission of poliomyelitis to monkeys. J Am Med Assoc 53:1639, 1909.
2. Robbins, F.C., J.F. Enders, and T.H. Weller. Cytopathogenic effect of poliomyelitis viruses in vitro on human embryonic tissues. Proc Soc Exp Biol Med 75:370, 1950.
3. Brodie, M., and W.H. Park. Active immunization against poliomyelitis. J Am Med Assoc 105:1089, 1935.
4. Kolmer, J.A.. Vaccination against acute anterior poliomyelitis. Am J Public Health 26:126, 1936.
5. Armstrong, C. The experimental transmission of poliomyelitis to the eastern cotton rat, *Sigmodon hispidus hispidus*. U.S. Public Health Reports 54:1719, 1939.
6. Li, C.P., and M. Shaeffer. Adaptation of type 1 poliomyelitis virus to mice. Proc Soc Exp Biol Med 82:477, 1953.

7. Salk, J.E. Principles of immunization as applied to poliomyelitis and influenza. Am J Public Health 43:1384, 1953.

8. Francis, T., Jr., et al. Evaluation of the 1954 field trial of poliomyelitis. Ann Arbor, Michigan: University of Michigan, 1957.

9. U.S. Department of Health, Education and Welfare; Public Health Service, Regulations for Poliomyelitis Vaccine, Part 73, Biologics Products, Federal Register, 1956.

10. Langmuir, A.D. Inactivated virus vaccines: protective efficacy, poliomyelitis. In Fifth International Poliomyelitis Conference, J.B. Lippincott Co., 1961, p. 105.

11. Sabin, A.B. Recent studies and field tests with a live, attenuated poliovirus vaccine. In Proc. First International Conference on Live Poliovirus Vaccines, Scientific Publication No. 44, p.14, Washington, D.C.: Pan-American Sanitary Bureau, 1959.

12. U.S. Department of Health, Education and Welfare, Public Health Service Regulations for Poliovirus Vaccine, Live, Oral, Part 73, Biologics Products, Federal Register, 1962.

13. (a) Sweet, B.H., and M.R. Hilleman. Detection of a non-detectable simian virus (vacuolating agent) present in rhesus and cynomologous monkey-kidney cell culture material. A Preliminary Report, in Proc. 2nd International Conference on Live Poliovirus Vaccines, Scientific Publication No. 45, p.79, Washington, D.C.: Pan American Health Organization and the World Health Organization, Pan-American Health Organization, 1960. (b) Sweet, B.H., and M.R. Hilleman. The vacuolating virus, SV40. Proc Soc Exp Biol and Med 105:420, 1960.

14. Stewart, S.E., B.E. Eddy, and N.G. Borgese. Neoplasms in mice inoculated with a tumor agent carried in tissue culture. J National Cancer Institute 20:747, 1958.

15. (a) Eddy, B.E., et al. Tumors induced in hamsters by injection of rhesus monkey kidney cell extracts. Proc Soc Exp Biol 107:191, 1961. (b) Eddy, B.E., et al. Identification of the oncogenic substance in rhesus monkey kidney cell culture as Simian Virus 40. Virology 17:65, 1962.

16. Fraumeni, J.F., Jr., F. Ederer, and R.W. Miller. An evaluaton of the carcinogenicity of Simian Virus 40 in man. J Am Med Assoc 185:713, 1963.

17. Fraumeni, J.F., Jr., et al. Simian virus 40 in polio vaccine: Follow-up of newborn recipients. Science 167:59, 1970.

18. Shah, K. and N. Nathanson. Human exposure to SV40: Review and comment. N Am J Epidem 103:1, 1976.

SV40

II. The Virus as a Model and Probe of Cellular Regulatory Processes

Norman P. Salzman

Molecular research with oncogenic (tumor-causing) viruses grew out of biochemical studies with lytic (cell-destroying) viruses, such as poliovirus. These earlier studies were begun when procedures for growing animal cells in culture became available.

At the National Institute of Allergy and Infectious Diseases (NIAID), HARRY EAGLE had described in 1955 a defined medium in which animal cells divided every 20 hours and in which each of the components was shown to be required for optimum growth [see Eagle in chapter "Tissue Culture"]. At about the same time, Theodore Puck demonstrated that a homogeneous population of cells could be derived from a single animal cell by means of simple technical procedures. Meanwhile, Renato Dulbecco was the major scientific figure who realized that it was time to apply to animal virology the elegant techniques being used in bacteriophage research. His work rested on the cell culture procedures developed in Eagle's laboratory. In these early studies, Dulbecco described the first plaque assay for poliovirus and measured the yield of viruses from single cells.

JAMES DARNELL, LEON LEVINTOW, and NORMAN SALZMAN, in Eagle's lab, started doing biochemical work with animal viruses in 1957. The following year Darnell and Eagle published their first virus paper, "Glucose and Glutamine in Poliovirus Production by HeLa Cells"; and in 1959 Salzman and ROYCE LOCKART published "Alteration in RNA Metabolism Resulting from Poliomyelitis Infection of HeLa Cells." During 1959 and 1960, Dulbecco organized three meetings—one in

---

NORMAN P. SALZMAN, Ph.D., Chief, Laboratory of Biology of Viruses, National Institute of Allergy and Infectious Diseases.

Berkeley and two at Cal Tech—for all those doing molecular studies with animal viruses. About 30 attended, including Eagle, Darnell, Levintow, and Salzman.

There were other virologists at NIH then, but their interests and approaches were separate from ours. They included ROBERT HUEBNER and his associates ROBERT CHANOCK and WALLACE ROWE. Others were KARL HABEL, SARAH STEWART, and BERNICE EDDY. Stewart and Eddy had succeeded in cultivating a virus, later called polyoma, that induced tumors at multiple sites in newborn animals.

A method for quantifying malignant cell transformation by tumor viruses in vitro, using a focus-forming assay, was described by ROBERT MANAKER and Vincent Groupé at Rutgers.

Dulbecco, drawing on the above observations and applying techniques from his work on lytic viruses, perceived that one of the most interesting biologic riddles, the transformation of normal to malignant cells, could be approached systematically as had been done with bacterial viruses. It was hoped that this would ultimately provide an understanding of the causes of human cancer. In the late 1950s Dulbecco began his studies on the transformation of cells, using two closely related oncogenic viruses, polyoma and SV40.

Depending on the species of cultured cells used, polyoma and SV40 can either cause cell transformation or undergo a lytic cycle of virus replication. Huebner, Rowe, and Habel had detected an antigen in transformed cells that was specified by the virus rather than the cell. When lytically infected cells were found to contain a protein with the same immunologic properties as one detected in transformed cells, lytic systems were critically examined to determine what role the product of the viral transforming gene might have in virus replication.

Studies of the past 20 years have shown that SV40 and polyoma are powerful probes and reliable models of cellular processes. They have provided valuable new information on virus-cell interaction.

The Lytic Cycle of Viral Replication

The work of Dulbecco, Roger Weil, and Jerome Vinograd showed that the DNA of SV40 and polyoma viruses is a double-stranded circular molecule of 3.4×10^6 daltons. The small amount of DNA in the virus particles indicated a limited number of virus-specified gene products. How many there were and how they functioned became clearer when JANICE CHOU and ROBERT MARTIN at NIAMD isolated temperature-sensitive mutants of SV40 and defined at least four groups based on complementation—capacity for functional interaction permitting defective viruses to replicate.

These studies and those of Walter Eckart at the Salk Institute, Peter Tegtmeyer at Case Western Reserve, and Giampiero DiMayorca in Naples, Italy, showed that three complementation groups defined regions of the viral genome that coded for synthesis of structural proteins. The fourth complementation group (A) coded for the tumor (T) antigen. Martin and others showed that transformation occurred when cells were infected with group-A mutants at the permissive temperature. It did not occur if cells were infected at a temperature where T antigen could not function normally.

Viral Infection in Lytically Infected Cells

There was an expectation that all of the DNA in viruses containing limited amounts of genetic information would be transcribed—would give rise to RNA that would either have a regulatory role or code for viral-specified proteins. MALCOLM MARTIN and GEORGE KHOURY showed that this was true. In infected cells, there were viral transcripts corresponding to almost the entire viral genome. In collaboration with Daniel Nathans at The Johns Hopkins University, these NIAID scientists mapped the transcripts and found that viral genes with coordinated expression were physically clustered. Specifically, this clustering on the viral genome reflected production of proteins early or late in the infectious cycle. These studies rested on Nathans' work with restriction enzymes. They powerfully demonstrated the use of these enzymes in assigning biologic function to specific DNA fragments.

In 1978 Walter Fiers in Ghent, Sherman Weissman at Yale University, and colleagues, using the elegant DNA sequencing techniques of Maxam and Gilbert, worked out the entire sequence of 5243 DNA base pairs constituting the five genes of SV40, the first animal virus for which this was done.

When YOSIF ALONI and Khoury looked at the structure of late messenger RNA, they found that viral mRNA molecules were not colinear with the DNA from which they had been copied, but rather corresponded to two separate DNA regions. This phenomenon of RNA splicing was first seen in adenovirus transcripts by Philip Sharp and his colleagues at MIT and by Broker and Chou at Cold Spring Harbor. Now many groups have shown that first an RNA molecule colinear with DNA is formed in the cell nucleus. Subsequently parts of this transcript are excised and noncontiguous portions are linked. The spliced RNA is then transported to the cytoplasm, where it directs the synthesis of viral proteins. Such splicing of mRNA is also observed in uninfected cells.

It is of great interest to know how genes are transcribed, but the process that determines *which ones* will be transcribed is perhaps a more profound mystery. How does a cell with many thousands of genes dictate which subset will be used at a particular time in its life cycle? Similar mechanisms for gene selection operate during a cycle of virus growth. Even for a simple virus like SV40, mRNA molecules are specified by two genes early in infection and by the other three genes later.

EDWARD BIRKENMEIER, MOSHE SHANI, and Salzman tested a model of regulation of transcription proposed by French investigators. The different forms of viral DNA found early and late in the infectious cycle were postulated to be responsible for the different transcripts generated at these times. Presumably, input viral DNA could serve as the template for early transcription, and later, when DNA synthesis had started, replicating DNA molecules would code for late transcription. However, late transcription complexes were characterized in which the DNA template still held growing RNA strands. The template was found to be the same as the input viral DNA (SV40 Form I), indicating that the proposed model was invalid. Gariglio and Chambon subsequently confirmed these results and demonstrated that SV40 DNA (Form I) was present as a nucleoprotein complex.

Two major questions relating to both cell and virus transcription remain unanswered: What are the mechanisms of RNA splicing? How is the selective expression of genes regulated?

SV40 DNA Replication

Virus growth within a cell is totally dependent on enzymes synthesized by the cell. Hence we can use a virus to probe the nature of the cell that supports its growth. As we explore the steps in viral DNA synthesis, we define the biosynthetic specificities of the enzymes that the uninfected cell contains. Cellular DNA replication cannot be studied in the same way as viral DNA replication, since cellular DNA (a million times larger) is far more complex. Viral DNA synthesis now becomes a model of the way cellular DNA synthesis is likely to occur.

In 1967 Bernard Hirt in Lausanne described a simple but important observation. Since SV40 DNA has a lower molecular weight than cellular DNA, the two can be separated effectively by virtue of the insolubility of the heavier DNA in 1M NaCl. GEORGE FAREED, THOMAS KELLY, EDWARD SEBRING, and Salzman used this procedure in studying how a small number of covalently closed DNA molecules can generate thousands of faithful copies during a lytic cycle of growth. They found that viral DNA synthesis starts at a specific site on the circular molecule, that chain growth is bidirectional, and that it terminates 180° from the initiation site. Danna and Nathans studied the incorporation of radioisotopes into DNA fragments generated by restriction enzymes and reached the same conclusion with this completely different approach.

Fareed and Salzman reported that the process of chain growth was discontinuous. Subsequently, Peter Reichard in Uppsala and Melvin DePamphilis at Harvard Medical School showed by in vitro studies that DNA fragments initiate synthesis with short RNA primers. MICHAEL CHEN, Sebring, Birkenmeier, and Salzman found that the two parental DNA strands continuously unwind as replication proceeds, and that completion of DNA chain growth occurs after the two daughter strands have separated. Ching-Juh Lai and Nathans at Johns Hopkins showed that specific signals are not required for termination of DNA replication and the generation of daughter molecules—that termination occurs at any sequence 180° from the origin.

Studies of DNA replication and transcription revealed that the initiation sites of both these vital functions in SV40 are in a clustered control region. There is no apparent reason why initiation sites for early and late transcription and for DNA replication occur together in the SV40 molecule, but knowledge of this juxtaposition has been of enormous value.

Since 1978 DNA recombinant techniques have proved to be the molecular biologist's most effective tools. Vectors containing genes from prokaryotic (nonnucleated) or eukaryotic (nucleated) cells ligated to the unique SV40 control region have allowed these genes to be cloned in animal cells and the proteins they specify to be produced. These techniques were pioneered by Paul Berg at Stanford. DEAN HAMER and PHILIP LEDER at NIH have used them to clone and express the globin gene in animal cells.

The special character of this SV40 region is also illustrated in more recent experiments by MAXINE SINGER at NCI. Monkey cells are the normal hosts for SV40. Singer searched a monkey DNA genomic library, using the SV40 origin region as a probe, and detected 80 to 100 copies in which partial homology with this region was shared. When inserted into recombinant plasmids, these regions of the monkey genome are seen to have an important regulatory function in transcription.

SV40 Recombines with High Frequency and
Generates a Variety of Recombinant Molecules

Huebner, Rowe, and JANET HARTLEY adapted adenovirus to grow in monkey cells. At that time it was not known that the cells were contaminated with SV40. This infection of monkey cells with unrealized mixed viruses resulted in the generation of hybrid virus in which the entire SV40 or a part of it became covalently linked to part of the adenovirus DNA. GREGORY O'CONOR and ALAN RABSON in NCI, who were studying SV40 and adenoviruses and trying mixed infections with the two, showed that human adenoviruses could only grow in monkey cells when they were coinfected with SV40. Subsequent studies by ANDREW LEWIS and ARTHUR LEVINE offer a precise description of these adeno-SV40 hybrids, and Kelly and JAMES ROSE in NIAID have provided a direct visualization of DNA sequences inserted into recombinant genomes.

For numerous viruses, many defective particles are obtained after several cycles of replication when high levels of virus have been used repeatedly to infect cells. These particles show extensive rearrangements in the viral genome or contain viral and cellular DNAs that are joined together prior to packaging in virus particles. The phenomenon was first observed in SV40, by Konito Yoshiike in Tokyo, Japan, and Ernest Winicour in Rehovot, Israel. Fareed and Malcolm Martin characterized such defective particles and found that the region where Fareed, CLAUDE GARON, and Salzman had mapped the initiation site of DNA replication was always preserved, and that a single molecule might contain multiple repeats of the region. Singer showed that as few as 80 base pairs in the origin region were sufficient to allow replication of the defective particles.

Described above are adeno-SV40 recombinants and defective viral particles, formed after several cycles of lytic infection, in which SV40 DNA had recombined with cellular or SV40 sequences. The most remarkable and biologically interesting category of recombinants is generated when viral DNA, covalently integrated into cellular DNA, results in the virus transformation of cells. For each of these cases, the same questions have been asked regarding the mechanism of generation: Are there specific DNA sites where recombination occurs? Do DNAs that recombine share common sequences in order to allow homologous recombination?

To answer these questions, investigators have determined the sequence of the nucleotides in the DNAs where new connections have been made between cellular and viral sequences, or at newly formed virus-virus junctions. Summarizing the results, it would be fair to say that no clear mechanism can be seen to explain how recombinants arise or why they are formed with high frequency. Current studies on DNA transfection, however, indicate that DNA insertions and rearrangements occur at a much higher rate than was previously imagined and that DNAs not likely to share homology with the host can be covalently linked at multiple sites. Current findings on DNA rearrangements and on chromosomal translocations may be of major importance in understanding how malignancies are induced.

SV40-Like Viruses in Humans

The BK virus, which is similar to SV40, was isolated by Sylvia Gardner from the urine of a patient who had received a renal transplant. Another isolate, the JC virus, was obtained by Padget and Walker from the brain of a patient with progressive multifocal leucoencephalopathy. KENNETH TAKEMOTO in NIAID showed that antibodies to these viruses were present in many adults as a result of inapparent exposure during childhood. PETER HOWLEY compared the BK and JC viruses with SV40 on the basis of serologic crossreactivity and nucleic acid homology, and RAVI DHAR, ISABELLE SEIF, and Khoury based such comparisons on the nucleotide composition. In all these cases, the human virus isolates were found to share many properties with the simian virus. There is little evidence, however, that any of these viruses have a causal role in human cancer.

How Do Viruses Transform Cells?

Molecular studies on the role of viruses in malignant transformation grew out of a number of biologic studies initiated at NIH. Stewart and Eddy's demonstration that polyoma virus grown in cell cultures could cause a variety of tumors at many sites in rodents was a major impetus to oncologic research. Habel's detection of viral-specified antigens in tumor cells was another major finding (1961). PAUL GERBER in the Division of Biologics Standards observed that when rodent cells transformed by SV40 were grown together with untransformed monkey cells able to support growth of the virus, the two cell types fused and released infectious SV40.

Two early findings that helped to define the mechanism of transformation were Thomas Benjamin's observation that RNA of cells transformed by SV40 had hybridized with the viral DNA, and Joseph Sambrook and Heiner Westphal's observation that the viral DNA was integrated with the cell genome. A way to quantitate the number of viral DNA molecules in these transformed cells was described by LAWRENCE GELB, BILL HOYER, and Malcolm Martin. The test is precise, sensitive, and widely used.

Genetic analyses of point and deletion mutations and DNA sequencing studies have shown that two proteins for SV40 and three for polyoma virus are specified by the early transforming region. Mutations in these early proteins yielded viruses that were temperature sensitive. Such "ts" viruses only transformed cells at a permissive temperature, and in some cases cells that had apparently transformed would revert to normal at another temperature.

It has been demonstrated, using restriction enzymes, that the piece of DNA that codes for the early transcripts is sufficient to transform cells. From the large number of specific mutations of polyoma and SV40, it appears at present that the large T (tumor) antigens of SV40 and the middle T antigens of polyoma have a primary role in transformation. Efforts in this remarkably focused field have involved dozens of investigators for the past 10 years. NIH workers include Robert Martin, MARK ISRAEL, Malcolm Martin, and PETER MORA. There are a number of solid leads on how SV40 and polyoma transform cells, but no definite mechanism has been revealed.

Looking Back

Looking back over the last 20 years, one would certainly say that the efforts of the many scientists working with SV40 have produced a high yield. DNA recombinant techniques have emerged from basic studies of SV40 replication and have revolutionized the way almost all investigators do research. We understand a great deal about the formation and structure of virus macromolecules. Mysteries remain concerning the regulation of viral biosynthetic processes and the mechanism of transformation.

Much of the current interest in viral transformation has shifted from DNA- to RNA-containing oncogenic viruses. One might have predicted a different direction of research these past years on the basis of the initial primary interest in SV40 as an oncogenic virus. As is often the case in science, detours and side roads may pass through areas more rewarding than those along the highway.

Introduction

STUDIES ON SLOW VIRUS DISEASES

From earliest times diseases have been arranged in categories by the writers of medical texts, drawing upon the science of disease classification, nosology. Characteristically, whenever a new class is discovered, numerous examples are soon found that were previously undetected or misclassified.

Today we group the bacterial infections, such as typhoid fever, pneumococcal pneumonia, and meningococcal meningitis. We distinguish protozoal infections, such as amebiasis and malaria. There are the viral infections, such as influenza and hepatitis. And there are the nutritional deficiencies, such as scurvy, beriberi, and pellagra. The latest class of diseases to be discovered are the "slow virus diseases"— chronic progressive disorders with long incubation periods, caused by either conventional viruses, like that of measles, or by a newly defined group of "unconventional viruses," which cause scrapie in sheep and kuru in man. So far, there are a very limited number of known slow virus diseases, but we may forecast with confidence that other examples will be revealed.

The slow viral infections have certain puzzling characteristics. In none has a viral particle been visualized. The diseases show a remarkable absence of inflammatory reaction or immunologic response. There is no doubt that they are transmissible from host to host, but the nature of the transmitting agent is still cryptic. It appears to contain little or no nucleic acid, elicits no immune response, and resists the killing action of many common antibacterial and antiviral drugs.

D. CARLETON GAJDUSEK, Nobel laureate and discoverer of the pathogenesis of kuru, postulates that other degenerative diseases of the central nervous system now classified as of unknown etiology may turn out to be slow virus diseases. The reader will wish to be informed of current thinking on the causation of such important health problems as multiple sclerosis, amyotrophic lateral sclerosis, Parkinson's disease, and Alzheimer's disease.

D. S.

395

20

STUDIES ON SLOW VIRUS DISEASES

D. Carleton Gajdusek
Clarence J. Gibbs, Jr.

The NIH Laboratory of Slow, Latent and Temperate Virus
Infections was the first such laboratory in the world, and its
work in the 1960s phrased the problem of slow virus infections. In 1963 the National Institute of Neurological Diseases
and Blindness (now Neurological and Communicative Disorders
and Stroke) sponsored the first meeting on slow virus infections. Two years later a monograph entitled "Slow, Latent
and Temperate Virus Infections" was published. These events
and the subsequent transmission of kuru and Creutzfeldt-
Jakob disease (CJD) from man to primates, demonstrating the
viral etiology of both diseases, launched worldwide awareness
of slow virus infections in man.

Our work and that of JOHN SEVER's laboratory, also in
NINDB, was largely responsible for the demonstration of slow
and delayed measles infection as the cause of Dawson's type-A
inclusion encephalopathy, which the Institute renamed subacute
sclerosing panencephalitis (SSPE) during the first international meeting on this disease, held at NIH in 1967. It
was the demonstration that chronic noninflammatory human
disease was caused by long-term incubating viruses that led
to the demonstration of a papovavirus etiology for progressive
multifocal leukoencephalopathy and a measles etiology for
SSPE, and to tick-borne (Russian spring-summer) encephalitis
virus in Soviet Siberia and Europe as a cause of chronic
infection in man and primates. Subsequently SSPE-like syndromes caused by the rubella virus were established, and
other chronic and persistent central nervous system virus
infections caused by adenoviruses, echoviruses, and herpes-
viruses were identified.

*D. CARLETON GAJDUSEK, M.D., Chief, and CLARENCE J. GIBBS, Jr.,
Ph.D., Deputy Chief, Laboratory of Central Nervous System
Studies, National Institute of Neurological and Communicative
Disorders and Stroke.*

Thus, investigation of the transmissibility and virus etiology of kuru and a presenile dementia of the Creutzfeldt-Jakob type (discussed in detail in GAJDUSEK's Nobel lecture) has permitted these unconventional viruses to be identified as a new group of microbes. Their very atypical physical, chemical, and biological properties have stimulated a world-wide effort to elucidate their structure and to resolve the enormous clinical and epidemiological problems they pose. The demonstration of slow infections by unconventional viruses and of the agents' peculiar properties has challenged the basic tenets of modern molecular biology and led to a series of discoveries with wide implications for neurological diseases of man. These discoveries may be summarized as follows:

The first recognized group of microbes revealing no immune response or nonhost antigen. "Unconventional" viruses are the unique example in microbiology of infectious agents that lack antigenicity. ⊤n spite of the fact that these viruses first invade the cells of the reticuloendothelial system, particularly low-density lymphocytes, they fail to induce an antiviral antibody response or any immune response directed against nonhost viral components. Sera from infected hosts are not capable of neutralizing virus infectivity. Moreover, high titers of infectious materials have failed to elicit an immunologic response against nonhost components, even when adjuvants are used and the response is measured by sensitive hybridoma technology. Thus, these highly pathogenic viruses, the first group of microbes in which such immunologic inertness has been demonstrated, evoke the speculation that they replicate without production of virus-specified nonhost proteins or antigenic substances.

Further, they are transmissible through implanted surgical electrodes, contaminated surgical instruments, and corneal transplantation. This necessitated changes in autopsy and operating room techniques throughout the world and development of precautions in handling older and demented patients. Gentle organic disinfectants, detergents, the quaternary ammonium salts often used for disinfection, and even hydrogen peroxide, ether, chloroform, iodine, and acetone have been found inadequate for inactivation of these viruses. The same is true of the ethylene oxide sterilizer. These findings demand revision of standard procedures for decontamination and disinfection.

Demonstration of single Mendelian autosomal dominant gene patterns; determination of familial CJD. Creutzfeldt-Jakob disease became the first human infection in which a single gene was demonstrated to control susceptibility and occurrence. The autosomal dominant pattern of CJD in families, including its appearance in 50 percent of siblings who survive to the age at which it usually appears, has led to an intensive worldwide study of familial dementias. The presence of CJD in families in which the familial form of Alzheimer's disease has occurred, and the familial occurrence of the transmissible spinocerebellar ataxic form of Creutzfeldt-Jakob disease, called by us the Gerstmann-Straussler syndrome, have led to renewed interest in familial dementias of all types.

Autoimmune antibody to a 10-nm neurofilament appearing in SSVE subjects.

SOTELO and others demonstrated that a very specific autoimmune antibody was directed against 10-nm neurofilaments but no other component of the central nervous system in over 60 percent of patients with kuru and CJD, a phenomenon appearing late, not early, in the disease. This was the first immune phenomenon observed in the subacute spongiform virus encephalopathies (SSVE). It opened an exciting new approach for the study of transmissible dementias.

These autoimmune antibodies, like many other rheumatoid factors, the anti-DNA antibody in lupus, and the antithyroglobulin antibody in Hashimoto's thyroiditis, are typical in prevalence and behavior in that they are occasionally present in normal subjects but occur more often in close relatives of patients with degenerative brain diseases. While found in more than half of patients with transmissible virus dementia, they do not appear in 40 percent of patients with classical CJD. The antibody develops in various gray matter diseases, including Alzheimer's and Parkinson's, but at lower incidence than in CJD or in control subjects without chronic neurological disorders. Furthermore, it is not present in patients with other immune diseases, such as disseminated lupus erythematosus and chronic rheumatoid arthritis. BAHMANYAR and colleagues have demonstrated that this autoimmune response is directed specifically against the 200,000-dalton protein component of the 10-nm neurofilament triad.

Absence of demonstrable virus in other neurological diseases.

Demonstration of the transmissibility of kuru, a heredofamilial disease, and Creutzfeld-Jakob disease, a fatal dementia that occurs sporadically and in familial forms, awakened the suspicion that many other chronic diseases may be virus-induced slow infections. Indeed, data from laboratory studies and epidemiological investigations have suggested that multiple sclerosis and Parkinson's disease, disseminated lupus erythematosus, juvenile diabetes, polymyositis, some forms of chronic arthritis, and acquired immune deficiency syndrome

(AIDS) may be slow infections with a masked and possibly defective virus as their cause.

Attempts, however, to establish a viral etiology for Alzheimer's disease, Parkinson's disease, multiple sclerosis, schizophrenia, autism in childhood, amyotrophic lateral sclerosis, and a wide variety of other chronic degenerative diseases have failed except in the group we classify as the subacute spongiform encephalopathies. But our long-standing negative data have become increasingly important as research on these diseases, even including the hereditary Huntington's disease, has gravitated toward the slow virus hypothesis for their etiology and pathogenesis. In addition to long-term observations of inoculated nonhuman primates and laboratory rodents, we have been using in vitro tissue culture techniques to detect viruses that may reside in brain. Inoculated cultures are screened for cytopathic changes and the presence of viral antigens and are examined by electron microscopy for viruslike particles. In addition, evidence of virus is sought by means of the extremely sensitive technique of in situ hybridization, with nucleic acid probes made to the nucleic acids of known viruses.

Thus the current, much-investigated concept of slow virus infections had its roots at the National Institutes of Health. It was from research on the exotic disease called kuru in an endocannibal stone-age culture in the interior highlands of eastern New Guinea that a virus was first shown to cause chronic, progressive, degenerative, even noninflammatory and heredofamilial disease of man. Such infections are now recognized as possible causes of chronic, progressive human diseases with incubation periods of months, years, or even decades between initial infection and clinical manifestation. Of all studies at NIH, the slow-virus project probably has the widest international collaboration.

Origins of the Study of Slow Virus Infections in Man

Slow-virus investigation at NIH evolved in an unforeseeable and circuitous manner. The project was created by a United States citizen (Gajdusek), who had returned from New Guinea in 1958 to become an NIH Visiting Scientist. It was established on our campus as part of the Neurological Institute's study "Child Growth and Development and Disease Patterns in Primitive Cultures" under Gajdusek's direction. For a time the project was sequestered in the Rare and Diminishing

Species Program of the Department of Interior's Fish and Wildlife Service on 40,000 acres of restricted lakes, marshes, and
woodland at the Patuxent Wildlife Research Center, Laurel,
Maryland. Gajdusek was initially assigned to the Office of
the Director, NINDB, and later to the Institute's Collaborative and Field Research Program. Thus a "clandestine" international endeavor found its way into the NIH structure. During
its first few years, it moved successively from the Office of
the Director, NINDB, to four off-campus buildings in Bethesda
and Silver Spring. Eventually it so parasitized and infil-
trated NIH, even to the point of using NCI space and NICHD
positions, that it had to be administratively accounted for
in some way. It finally came officially into the Intramural
Program.

Gajdusek was recruited to NIH by JOSEPH E. SMADEL, then
Deputy Director of NIH for Research. Papers written with VIN-
CENT ZIGAS described the discovery and characteristics of kuru
in the Territory of Papua New Guinea. These had phrased the
important implications that an elucidation of the etiology
of kuru would have for the whole problem of idiopathic degenerative disease of the central nervous system, even problems
of aging and heredofamilial disorders. Smadel sought to accommodate Gajdusek's wide-ranging interests, having known him
well from Walter Reed Army Medical Service Graduate School
days in which he had done his compulsory military service.
Gajdusek took charge of a program ranging in content from
music, dance, language, cognitive styles, and diverse forms
of symbolic thought, to endocrinology, virology, immunology,
biochemistry, population genetics, neurology, and research
cinema technology, to diverse patterns of sexual behavior,
reproduction, growth, puberty, and aging.

In 1961 Gajdusek and J. ANTHONY MORRIS obtained permission
from Carleton Hermann and his superior at the Patuxent Wildlife Research Center to hold large animals in isolation, including many species of monkeys, gibbon apes, and chimpanzees.
It was yet a year before an NIH contract financing the operation caught up with the fait accompli. To head this off-campus
operation in virology and infectious disease, Gajdusek chose
CLARENCE J. GIBBS, Jr., as his co-worker in the long-term
search for human diseases with slow-virus etiology, particularly kuru—which few thought promising.

In 1963 Gajdusek and Gibbs called the first meeting on
slow virus infections. Two years later the proceedings were
published as the first monograph in the field. The team was
joined by close collaborators from Papua New Guinea (Zigas,
MICHAEL ALPERS, Frank Schofield), England (Elisabeth Beck),
France (FRANÇOISE CATHALA), and others from many countries.
Several young career investigators, particularly PAUL BROWN

and DAVID ASHER, participated. This eclectic team soon established slow virus infections as a cause of chronic disease in
man through demonstration of the transmissibility of kuru to
chimpanzees. Later the disease was extended to New World monkeys. Gajdusek and Gibbs initiated and inspired investigations of many other chronic degenerative diseases of the central nervous system as possible slow virus infections.

Early in the studies on kuru, WILLIAM J. HADLOW, working
with W. S. Gordon on scrapie disease of sheep and goats at the
Agricultural Research Council's laboratory in Compton, England, pointed out similarities between this strange disease
in animals and kuru in man. Gajdusek visited the Compton
group, and also Scottish workers under J. T. Stamp in Edin-
burgh and Pall Palsson and his veterinary virologists in the
laboratory of Bjorn Sigurdsson in Iceland, where slow virus
infections of animals were first defined in the 1950s. This
led to the establishment of a similar program at NINDB to investigate kuru and a wide range of chronic diseases of the
brain that were of unknown etiology, including Dawson's subacute type-A inclusion-body encephalitis, multiple sclerosis,
amyotrophic lateral sclerosis, Parkinson's disease, progressive supranuclear palsy, progressive multifocal leukoencepha-
litis, Alzheimer's, Pick's, and Creutzfeldt-Jakob diseases,
muscular dystrophy, the dementias of Guamanian amyotrophic
lateral sclerosis and Parkinsonism, and even schizophrenia.
The success of the kuru studies attracted widespread interest,
and the pursuit of slow virus infections in man was on!

In 1967 Sever, Wolfgang Zeman, Gajdusek, and Gibbs called
an international meeting on "Delayed and Slow Measles Encephalopathy." Their purpose was to embrace new data from many laboratories, including their own, Arthur O'Connell's in Belfast,
and Edwin Lennette's in San Francisco, indicating that Dawson's subacute inclusion-body encephalopathy of children represents a hyperimmune response to measles. Measles antigen
was demonstrated in the patients' brains, piquing intense
national and international interest in this fatal disease of
infants, children, and young adults. For purposes of the
meeting, the four conveners compromised on a new name for
the disease, then designated in the English-speaking world
as Dawson's type-A subacute inclusion encephalitis, in the
French-speaking world as Van Bogart's subacute sclerosing
leukoencephalopathy, and in the German-speaking world as
Pette-Doring panencephalopathy. They settled on subacute
sclerosing panencephalitis (SSPE), which the disease is now
officially called.

Although investigators at the University of Wisconsin,
University of Pennsylvania, The Johns Hopkins University, and
many other institutions have contributed importantly to the

understanding of slow virus infections, NIH has always played a major international role in their study.

Characteristics of Slow Virus Infections

Kuru was the first chronic subacute degenerative disease of man shown to be a virus-induced slow infection characterized by an incubation period measured in years and progressive cumulative pathology always leading to death. Thus, slow virus infections, first observed in sheep and goats, became recognized as a problem in human medicine. Kuru has led, however, to a more exciting frontier in microbiology than the demonstration of a new mechanism of pathogenesis of infectious disease. It has revealed a new group of viruses with "unconventional" physical and chemical properties and with biological behavior far different from that of any other known group of microorganisms. Conversely, these agents are sufficiently classical in behavior and function, including their need for a metabolizing cell to replicate, to be called viruses.

The unconventional viruses are known to cause six natural diseases: two of man, kuru and CJD; and four of animals, scrapie in sheep and goats, transmissible mink encephalopathy, and the chronic wasting diseases of captive mule deer and captive elk. For a decade, only primate hosts were available as indicators for the viruses causing human disease; but more recently, the CJD virus has been adapted to cats, guinea pigs, mice, goats, and sheep, and kuru to mink. It has been impossible to characterize these agents well. Knowledge of the properties of unconventional viruses is based mostly on investigation of the scrapie virus adapted to mice and hamsters and, more recently, of the CJD virus in mice.

The unusual resistance of the viruses to various chemical and physical agents separates them from all other microorganisms. In fact, their resistance to ultraviolet and ionizing radiation, their atypical ultraviolet action spectrum for inactivation, and their lack of any demonstrable nonhost protein make these infectious particles unique in the biology of replicating infectious agents. Indeed, we must turn for analogy to the newly described viroids causing natural diseases in plants.

In plant virology we have been forced to modify our concept of a virus to include subviral pathogens, such as those causing potato spindle tuber disease, chrysanthemum stunt disease, citrus exocortis disease, Cadang–Cadang disease of coconut palms, cherry chloratic mottle, cucumber pale fruit disease, hop-stunt disease, avocado sunblotch disease, tomato bunchy top disease, tomato *planta macho* disease, and burdock

stunt disease.   There are also virusoids that cause velvet
tobacco mottle disease, solanum nodiflorum mottle disease,
lucerne transient streak disease, and subterranean clover mottle disease.   All are small circular RNAs without structural
protein or membrane, which have been sequenced and their
fine structures determined.   They have partial base pairing
and contain only 246 to 574 ribonucleotides.   They replicate
by a "rolling circle" copying of their RNA-sequences in sequential rotations and produce an oligomeric copy, which is
cut into monomers or dimers.   Protein is not synthesized from
their genetic information; only the replication machinery of
the cell is used.   These subviral pathogens have stimulated
much thought on possible similarities to the unconventional
viruses.   While we have shown that the unconventional viruses
differ from the plant viroids on many counts, these subviral
pathogens of plants have served to alert us to the possibility
of extreme departure from conventional virus structures.

The delta antigen of infectious hepatitis, a defective
particle with only 1,700 bases on its genome (68,000 daltons)
and requiring the infectious hepatitis B virus for its replication, offers further intriguing analogies to the unconventional viruses.

These atypical infections differ from other diseases of
the human brain subsequently demonstrated to be slow virus infections—i.e., they do not evoke a virus-associated inflammatory response in the brain, usually show no pleocytosis, and
are not accompanied by a marked rise in protein in the cerebrospinal fluid throughout the course of infection.   Furthermore, they evidence no immune response to the causative virus
or recognizable virus particles in brain sections examined by
electron microscopy.

The more conventional viruses that cause slow infections
of the central nervous system include measles virus, papovaviruses (JC and SV40), rubella virus, cytomegalovirus, herpes-
virus, adenovirus types 7 and 32, and Russian spring-summer
encephalitis (RSSE) virus.   Unlike these, however, the unconventional viruses of the spongiform encephalopathies are unusually resistant to ultraviolet and ionizing radiation, ultra-
sonication, heat, proteases, nucleases, and many potent organic substances such as formaldehyde, beta-propiolactone,
ethylenediaminetetraacetic acid (EDTA), and sodium deoxycho-
late. They are moderately sensitive to most membrane-disrupt-
ing agents such as phenol, chloroform, ether, urea (6M),
periodate (0.01M), 2-chloroethanol, alcoholic iodine, acetone, chloroform-butanol, sodium hypochlorite (0.5 to 5.0
percent), and 0.1 to 1.0N sodium hydroxide.   Chaotropic ions
(thiocyanate and guanidinum trichloroacetate), proteinase-K,
and trypsin inactivate partially purified virus.

The fact that virions (whole virus particles) are not recognized on electron microscopic study has led to the speculation that the infectious agents lack a nucleic acid and constitute a self-replicating protein (and derepressor of cellular DNA) or a self-replicating membrane fragment that serves as a template for laying down abnormal plasma membrane, including itself. A major effort in our laboratory is directed toward elucidation of the nature and structure of these atypical viruses.

The scrapie virus has been partially purified by density-gradient sedimentation in the presence of specific detergents. ROBERT ROHWER succeeded in purifying scrapie virus relative to other quantifiable proteins in brain and showed the virus to be susceptible to proteinase-K and trypsin but not to nucleases. Paul Brown, using cesium chloride, sucrose, and metrizamide gradients, banded the virus into two peaks of high infectivity with densities of 1.14 to 1.23 g/cm^3 and 1.26 to 1.28 g/cm^3. On electron microscopic examination, highly infective fractions revealed only smooth vesicular membranes with mitochondrial and ribosomal debris and no structures resembling recognizable virions.

The resistance of scrapie virus to ultraviolet inactivation should not be taken as proof that it lacks genetic information coded in the nucleic acid molecules, since work with the smallest RNA viroids indicates a similar resistance thought to depend on the small RNA size. On the other hand, the unconventional viruses resemble classical viruses in numerous properties, some of which suggest far more complex genetic interaction between virus and host than one might expect for genomes with a molecular weight of only 10^5. They are susceptible to inactivation and are not so dangerous that we cannot work with them. Despite unusual resistance to heat, they are rapidly inactivated by temperatures above 85°C. Autoclaving (120°C at 15 lb/in^2 for 60 minutes) completely inactivated scrapie virus in suspensions of mouse brain.

Conventional Viruses Causing Chronic Disease

The other chronic diseases of man that have been shown to be slow virus infections are caused by conventional viruses that in no way tax our imagination. Here we find diverse mechanisms of viral replication, various modes of pathogenesis, and different kinds of involvement of the immune system.

In subacute sclerosing panencephalitis, the offending measles virus is apparently not present as a fully infectious virion. Only a portion of the virus genome is expressed, and replication is defective. In the case of progressive multi-focal leukoencephalopathy (PML), on the other hand, fully assembled and infectious virus particles are produced. Electron microscopy examination of this papovavirus showed that fewer defective particles were produced than in any known in vitro system for cultivating papovaviruses. Thus, these ordinary viruses cause slow infections by very different mechanisms.

Some diseases caused by conventional viruses have been associated with immune defects. PML, for example, may follow immunosuppression, either from natural primary disease (leukemia, lymphoma, sarcoid disease) or an induced suppression (as in renal transplantation or cancer chemotherapy).

The RSSE virus causing Kozhevnikov's epilepsy (epilepsia partialis continua) in the Soviet Union, Japan, and India, and the rubella virus in adolescents with recrudescence of a congenital rubella infection, show defective replication; whereas wholly infectious virus is demonstrable in chronic recurrent echovirus infection of the central nervous system in children with genetic immune defects, and in subacute brain infection with adenovirus type 7 or 32.

In recent years many chronic diseases in animals have been used as models for human diseases. Various mechanisms of whole or partial virus replication are involved. The host's genetic composition and age at the time of infection are often crucial to the type of pathogenesis that occurs. The immune system may be involved in different ways. Immune complex formation is important in some cases and not in others.

Slow Virus Infections in Man

Kuru. It was from the investigation of the exotic disease called kuru in a cannibal tribal culture in the interior highlands of eastern New Guinea that a virus was first implicated in chronic, progressive, degenerative, noninflammatory, and heredofamilial disease of man. Characterized by cerebellar ataxia and a shivering-like tremor, kuru progresses to complete motor incapacity and death in less than one year from onset of symptoms (see Figure 1).

Kuru means shivering or trembling in the Fore language. The disease is confined to a number of adjacent valleys in the mountainous interior of New Guinea and occurs in 160 villages with a total population just over 35,000. More than 80 percent of the cases occur in the Fore cultural and linguistic group, which formerly experienced a yearly incidence rate of about 1 percent. In the early years of investigation, the disease was found to affect all ages beyond infants and tod-

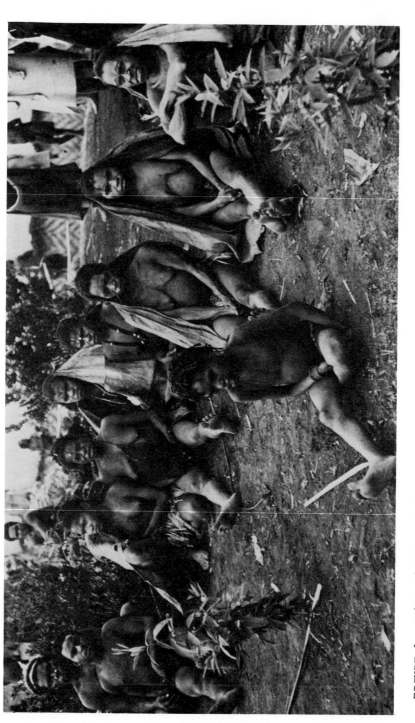

FIGURE 1. Nine victims of kuru from several villages of the South Fore region of New Guinea. All died of the disease within one year of this 1957 photograph.

dlers. It was common in male and female children and adult
females, but rare in adult males. This marked excess of adult
female over male deaths led to a male-to-female population
ratio of more than 3:1 in some villages and of 2:1 for the
whole South Fore group (Figure 2).

Kuru has been disappearing gradually since the early 1960s
and is no longer seen in children, adolescents, or young
adults under 25 years of age. This appears to result from
cessation of ritual cannibalism by women and small children
as a rite of mourning and respect for dead kinsmen, with its
resulting conjunctival, nasal, skin, mucosal, and gastrointestinal contamination. Our most significant new contributions have been the documentation of incubation periods of
30 years and more in human kuru and the identification of the
contaminating episode for several dozen patients occurring in
recent years. Over 90 percent of the infants and children of
women who participated in cannibalism have come down with
kuru.

Continued epidemiological surveillance (1956–1963) has
revealed no alteration in the pattern of kuru as a disappearing manmade epidemic. Kuru virus clearly has no reservoir in
nature and no intermediate natural biological cycle for its
preservation except in humans, nor is there transplacental or

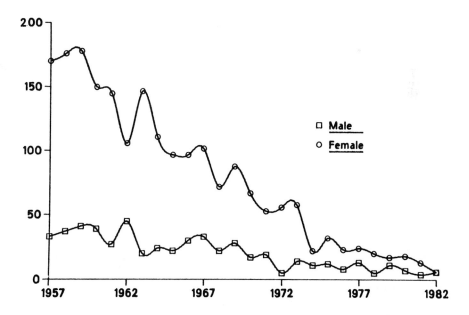

FIGURE 2. Number of kuru deaths in males and females from 1957
to 1982. Deaths have declined since the cessation of cannibalism between 1957 and 1962.

neonatal transmission, even as an integrated genome or as a
milk factor from a mother who has kuru or is incubating the
causal agent.

The clinical course of kuru is remarkably uniform. It is
conveniently divided into three stages: ambulant, sedentary,
and terminal. After a variable latent period, the cerebellar
symptomatology starts insidiously without antecedent acute
illness and progresses to total incapacitation and death usually within three to nine months.

For several years all work on the kuru virus was done
with chimpanzees, the first species to which the disease was
transmitted. Eventually other species of nonhuman primates
were infected. We recently infected mink, ferrets, and domestic goats. The disease in goats resembles scrapie. In contrast, nonprimate and avian hosts of dozens of other species
have been inoculated without evidence of the disease after
many years of observation.

The virus has been regularly isolated from the brain tissue of kuru patients. It attains high titers of more than
10^8 infectious doses per gram. In peripheral tissue, namely
liver and spleen, it has been found only rarely on autopsy and
in much lower titers. Blood, urine, leukocytes, cerebrospinal
fluid, placenta, and embryonal membranes of patients have not
yielded the virus.

Transmissible Virus Dementias (Creutzfeld–Jakob Disease).

CJD is a rare, usually sporadic, presenile dementia found
worldwide. In about 10 percent of cases, it has a familial
inheritance pattern usually suggestive of autosomal dominance.
The typical clinical picture includes myoclonus, paroxysmal
bursts of high-voltage slow waves on electroencephalography
(EEG), and evidence of widespread cerebral dysfunction. The
disease is regularly transmissible to chimpanzees, to New
and Old World monkeys, and on some occasions to domestic
cats and laboratory mice and guinea pigs. At the cellular
level, pathology in the animal is indistinguishable from
that seen in the natural disease or experimental kuru. Highly
diluted human brain tissue inoculated into goats produces a
disease indistinguishable from scrapie, but does not do so
in sheep. Since the host range and incubation periods of
different isolates of the CJD virus vary greatly, many different strains are now available in the laboratory. These
differing biological properties may help identify common
source infections.

A wide range of clinical syndromes involving dementia in
middle and late life are suspected to result from such slow
virus infections associated with neuronal vacuolation or
status spongiosus of gray matter and a reactive astrogliosis.

These even include cases that, at some time in their clinical course, have been correctly diagnosed as brain tumors (glioblastoma, meningioma), brain abscess, Alzheimer's disease, progressive supranuclear palsy, senile dementia, stroke, or Köhlmeier-Degos' disease. Hence, the urgent practical problem is to delineate the spectrum of subacute and chronic neurological illnesses that are caused by or associated with slow virus infection. Some 14 percent of the cases show amyloid plaques akin to those found in kuru, and many show changes similar to those of Alzheimer's disease, in addition to the status spongiosus and astrogliosis of CJD. Other cases involve both CJD and another neurological disease. Thus, we have started to refer to the transmissible disorder as transmissible virus dementia (TVD).

Since our first transmission of CJD, we have obtained brain biopsy or early postmortem brain tissue from more than 500 pathologically confirmed cases. Virus has been isolated in 226 of these. The prevalence of CJD has varied markedly in time and place throughout the United States and Europe. We have been aware of occasional clustering in small population centers and the unexplained absence of cases over periods of years in some large population centers where cases were more frequent at an earlier date. However, this geographic and temporal clustering does not apply to a majority of cases and is not explained by those that are familial. W. B. Matthews has recently noted two clusters in England, and there are two reports of conjugal disease: husband and wife dying of CJD within a few years of each other.

We have noted a trend toward more frequent diagnosis of CJD in many neurological clinics, probably a result of the attention drawn to the syndrome by its transmission to primates. For many large population centers of the United States, South America, Europe, Australia, and Asia, we have found a prevalence approaching 1 per million, with an annual incidence and a mortality of about the same magnitude, since the average duration of the disease is 8 to 12 months. Matthews found in one of his clusters an annual incidence of 1.3 per million, which was more than 10 times the overall annual incidence for England and Wales over the previous decade. Kahana and colleagues reported the annual incidence of CJD as ranging from 0.4 to 1.9 per million in various ethnic groups in Israel. In recent years an annual incidence of at least 1 per million has been reported for Sweden and Finland. We have demonstrated a single autosomal-dominant gene pattern of occurrence in familial cases in spite of the fact that the disease is caused by a virus. This is the first example in man of an autosomal-dominant single-gene inheritance controlling the appearance of an infectious disease.

Transmission of CJD has been observed in a recipient of a corneal graft from a donor diagnosed retrospectively as having had the disease. The onset was 18 months after the transplant, corresponding to the average for chimpanzees inoculated with human CJD brain tissue. From suspension of brain from the corneal graft recipient, we succeeded in transmitting CJD to a chimpanzee though the brain had been at room temperature in 10 percent formol-saline for seven months. More recently we learned that two of our patients with confirmed TVD had been professional blood donors until shortly before the onset of symptoms. To date, CJD has not been transmitted from the blood of human patients. Finally, the recognition of TVD in a neurosurgeon and two physicians has raised the question of occupational infection, particularly in those exposed to infected tissue during surgery or autopsy.

An unexpectedly high incidence of CJD in cases of earlier craniotomy, noted first by Nevin and others, then by Matthews and us, suggests that brain surgery may afford a mode of entry for the agent or precipitate the disease in patients carrying a latent infection. There is support for the former possibility in the transmission of CJD to two young epileptics in whom silver electrodes sterilized with 70 percent ethanol and formaldehyde vapor had been implanted after use in a CJD patient. Subsequently, after sterilization and storage in formaldehyde vapor for an additional two years, these same electrodes induced disease in a chimpanzee.

The resistance to inactivation of the unconventional virus has altered decontamination and sterilization procedures in all autopsy rooms, surgical theaters, and clinics in the world. Continued study of the inactivation and physical properties of these agents is mandatory to the establishment of standards for prevention of iatrogenic transmission.

The problem of resistance to inactivation is pertinent to the hepatitis-B vaccine prepared from hepatitis antigen in sera of human volunteers. Some donors may be incubating the Creutzfeldt-Jakob dementia syndrome. No known assay is sufficiently sensitive to prove the vaccine safe. Even a chimpanzee assay would require decades, and still the results would be uncertain.

In primates the peripheral routes of inoculation give irregular "takes" and exceedingly long incubation periods. For example, a formalinized louping-ill vaccine contaminated with scrapie virus resulted in tens of thousands of cases of fatal scrapie in British sheep previously free of the disease. The moral, ethical, and legal implications of continuing to use the hepatitis-B vaccine once this problem has been appreciated are enormous. A clonal hepatitis-B vaccine should be sought.

Some Slow Virus Infections in Animals

Scrapie. A natural disease of sheep and occasionally of goats, scrapie is distributed widely in Europe, America, and Asia. Affected animals show progressive ataxia, wasting, and frequently severe pruritis. The close resemblance of scrapie to kuru clinically and histopathologically suggested to Hadlow that the two diseases might have similar etiologies.

As early as 1936 Cuillé and Chelle transmitted scrapie in sheep. Its filterable nature and viruslike properties had been known for more than three decades. Much more virological information is available about the mouse- and hamster-adapted strains of scrapie than about those that cause human disease. It has been transmitted in our laboratory to five species of nonhuman primates. Sheep, goat, mice, and squirrel monkeys have been experimentally infected by the oral route.

Although scrapie has been studied longer and more intensively than the other diseases, the mechanism of its spread remains uncertain. The infection appears to pass from ewes to lambs, even without suckling; the placenta itself is infectious. Transplacental versus oral, nasal, optic, or cutaneous infection in the perinatal period are unresolved possibilities. Older sheep are infected only after long contact with diseased animals, though lateral transmission has not been proved. However, susceptible sheep have developed the disease in pastures previously occupied by scrapie sheep.

Field studies and experimental work with sheep suggest genetic control. In mice, there is evidence of genetic control over the length of incubation and anatomic distribution of lesions, with variation according to the strain of agent used.

Transmissible Mink Encephalopathy. TME is very similar to scrapie both in clinical picture and in pathological lesions. The disease occurred where the carcasses of scrapie-infected sheep had been fed to mink, and presumably the disease is scrapie. TME is indistinguishable from disease induced in mink by inoculation with scrapie from sheep or mouse and, like scrapie, has been transmitted by the oral route. Transplacental or perinatal transmission from the mother has not been demonstrated. Physicochemical study has revealed no differences between TME and scrapie virus.

The disease has been transmitted to the squirrel, rhesus, and stump-tailed monkey and to many nonprimate hosts, including the sheep, goat, and ferret. It has not been transmitted to mice. In monkeys the illness is indistinguishable from experimental CJD in these species.

Transmissible Spongiform Encephalopathy of Mule Deer and Elk. In 1978 a chronic wasting disease was noted in the mule deer herd at Fort Collins, Colorado. Clinically and neuro-pathologically it closely resembled scrapie in sheep or goats. The disease is experimentally transmissible to other mule deer, and Bahmanyar has demonstrated amyloid plaques in brain tissue from affected animals. A similar chronic wasting disease with a subacute spongiform encephalopathy has recently occurred in an adjacent herd of captive elk.

Conjectural Natural History of Kuru, CJD, and Slow Virus Infections of Animals

Unanswered crucial questions posed by all of these agents are related to their biological origin and mode of survival in nature. They cause naturally occurring diseases, not artificial phenomena produced by researchers tampering with cellular macromolecular structures, as some would have it. Mystery surrounds their mode of dissemination and long-term persistence. For kuru we have a full explanation of the unique epidemiological findings and their change over the past two decades: the viral contamination of close kinsmen at the opening of a kuru victim's skull at the rite of cannibalism, in which all females and prepubertal males participated. But this does not provide us with a satisfactory explanation for the origin.

Was kuru the unlikely event of a sporadic case of world-wide CJD that produced in the unusual cultural setting of New Guinea a unique epidemic? We now have a report of spontaneous CJD in a 26-year-old Chimbu New Guinean from the central highlands, whose clinical diagnosis was confirmed by light- and electron-microscope examination of a brain biopsy specimen. Serial passage of brain-infected virus in successive cannibalistic rituals may have resulted in modification of virulence and a change in the clinical picture.

Speculatively, serial brain passage of a ubiquitous virus may have yielded a new strain that has been modified into a defective, incomplete, or highly integrated or repressed neurotropic agent in vivo in the course of its long-masked state. Such a new breed of virus might no longer be recognizable either antigenically or structurally because of failure of full synthesis of viral subunits or of their assembly into a known virion.

The possibility is easily entertained that the viruses of all six of the spongiform encephalopathies are not just closely related agents but different strains of a single virus modified in different hosts. Figure 3 presents a conjectural schematic history of the origin of CJD, kuru, and TME from

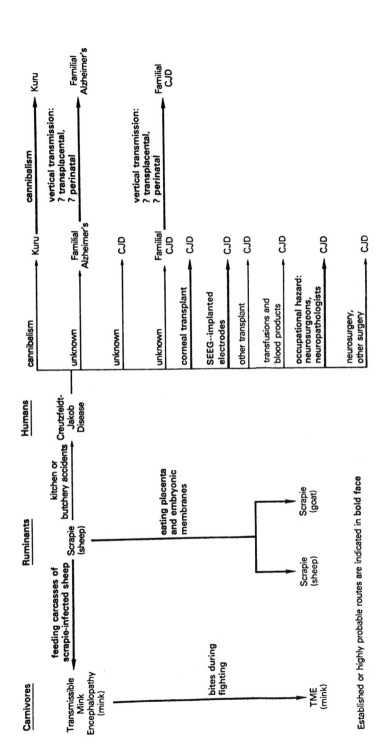

FIGURE 3. Conjectural origin of transmissible mink encephalopathy, Creutzfeldt–Jakob disease, kuru, and familial Alzheimer's disease from natural scrapie in sheep.

natural scrapie of sheep. Such speculations, however, provide schemata that cannot be tested.

Scrapie has caused disease in Old and New World nonhuman primates that is indistinguishable from experimental CJD. In some instances passage of the virus through primates alters its host range so that it no longer causes disease in sheep or goats. The same alteration occurs when the virus has been passed through mink or ferrets.

Strains of CJD and kuru viruses also vary, as do their host responses. In squirrel monkeys, CJD or kuru may produce an acute central nervous system disease with death in a few days, following an asymptomatic incubation period of two years or more. In contrast, these same strains produce a slowly progressive, chronic clinical disease in spider monkeys. In addition, the strain of virus and the species of host influence type and severity of pathological lesions in the brain: A strain of kuru or CJD may induce severe status spongiosis in the cerebral cortex of chimpanzees and spider monkeys, with little or no pathology in the brain stem or spinal cord, whereas the same strain in squirrel monkeys causes extensive brain stem and cord lesions. Thus it is clear that data on incubation periods, host range, and the distribution and severity of neuropathological lesions will not alone unravel the relationships of the unconventional viruses causing subacute spongiform encephalopathies, nor can we expect to arrive at answers in the absence of proven antigenicity or identifiable infectious nucleic acid.

Prospect

Elucidation of the etiology and epidemiology of a rare, exotic disease restricted to a small population isolate—kuru in New Guinea—has brought us to worldwide considerations with importance for all of medicine and microbiology. For neurology, specifically, we have new insights into the whole range of presenile dementias and particularly the large problems of Alzheimer's disease and the senile dementias. The implications of vertical transmissions and host genetic control of the pathological expression of these slow infections, as well as the possible relationship of their causal viruses to neoplasia, are obvious.

Still, the etiology of major degenerative diseases— multiple sclerosis, Alzheimer's disease, amyotrophic lateral sclerosis, parkinsonism, schizophrenia, and autism—remains unresolved despite tantalizing laboratory and epidemiological data pointing to the possible role of viruslike agents. Perhaps the masked and defective slow infections with conventional viruses, seen in PML and SSPE, may provide the best leads.

Association of the high incidence of two diseases, parkinsonism dementia and amyotrophic lateral sclerosis, among the Chamorro people on Guam and the Japanese of the Kii Peninsula remains a continuing challenge. Our discovery of a small but intense focus of motor neuron disease associated with a high incidence of parkinsonism, parkinsonism dementia, and other bradykinetic and myoclonic dementia syndromes among the Auyu and Jaqai people in western New Guinea suggests some common environmental etiological factor underlying these syndromes that occur strangely in subpopulations but not in surrounding general populations.

The models of lysogenicity and subviral, genetically active macromolecular structures from the study of bacterial viruses, bacterial genetics, and the viroid and virusoid subviral pathogens of plants supply ample imaginative framework for ideas of possible mechanisms of infectious pathogenesis in man. Molecular biology is challenged to relate the characteristics of unconventional viruses to those of bacterial and plant viruses, in view of strongly suggested parallels.

That a now-disappearing disease in a small primitive culture has brought us this far is ample reason to address intensively the questions and opportunities posed by the still unexplained high incidence and peculiar profusion of neurological syndromes, pathologically distinct yet apparently somehow related, that have been discovered in several isolated population enclaves.

ENDOCRINOLOGY

It is now generally believed that a chemical messenger is involved whenever information is transmitted from one tissue to another. The mechanisms of hormonal and neural transmission are essentially the same, but with a distinctive difference in the distance usually traversed. Neurotransmitters cross a minute gap between nerve cells and receptors, whereas classical hormones travel great distances via the bloodstream from the endocrine glands to the effector organs.

The subject matter of endocrinology deals largely with the individual hormones: their chemical structures, the nature of their cells of origin and chemical precursors, the mode of their discharge into the blood and their capture by effector cells, and the way in which they create their effect. The endocrinologist is also concerned with disturbances of these processes. Considered together, such disturbances are the endocrinopathies—the diseases of the endocrine system. We now clearly recognize diseases that are due to abnormalities in the production, delivery, or reception of the chemical messenger.

Probably soon after the development of the earliest multicellular organisms—certainly very early in our phylogeny—the need arose for one cell type to communicate with another. Both neural and humoral channels are found in very primitive animals. Complex organisms are highly dependent on the integrity of these information delivery systems. In view of the disruptions that we encounter daily in communication between persons, it is not surprising that disorders of an individual's neural and humoral systems also occur.

Neuropathies and endocrinopathies constitute a substantial part of medical practice. In the following chapter, we learn that problems of endocrinology have concerned almost all the Institutes at one time or another. The reader will find an account of some of our more important adventures in this interesting field of biology and medicine.

D. S.

21

ENDOCRINOLOGY

Jacob Robbins

Mortimer B. Lipsett

The Early Years

Probably the first endocrinologist at NIH was ROY HERTZ, who in 1941 joined HENRY SEBRELL's laboratory in what would soon become the Experimental Biology and Medicine Institute (EBMI). While working on biotin (a B-complex vitamin) and avidin (antibiotin), Hertz also found time to follow his interest in the endocrinology of reproduction. He transferred to the National Cancer Institute (NCI) in 1945 and there continued his experiments on folic acid, a nutritional factor that greatly enhanced the response of the chick oviduct and the rat and monkey uterus to estrogen. Folic acid antagonists were later applied effectively in treating choriocarcinoma, a uterine cancer in women. In 1949 Hertz opened the first NIH clinical endocrinology unit at George Washington University. The unit studied the interrelation of cancer and the endocrine system, including tumors that produced, responded to, or were induced by hormones.

The second endocrinologist to mount an NIH research program with preclinical and clinical aspects was FREDERIC BARTTER, who had entered the Public Health Service the same year as Hertz. In 1946, after a tour at the Sheepshead Bay PHS Hospital in Brooklyn, he was assigned to work under the great endocrinologist Fuller Albright at the Massachusetts General Hospital. There, for the next five years, he conducted studies on subjects that characterized his later career: calcium metabolism, antidiuretic hormone, and the adrenal

JACOB ROBBINS, M.D., Chief, Clinical Endocrinology Branch, National Institute of Arthritis, Diabetes, and Digestive and Kidney Diseases. MORTIMER B. LIPSETT, M.D., Director, National Institute of Child Health and Human Development.

gland. In 1951 he established an NIH endocrine unit in LUTHER TERRY's department at the Baltimore PHS Hospital.

In 1947 the first NIH laboratory devoted to basic endo-crinology was developed in the newly established EBMI. EVELYN ANDERSON, who had discovered anti-TSH* and the principle of antihormones in Herbert Evans' laboratory at Berkeley, headed an Endocrine Section in EBMI's new Laboratory of Nutrition and Endocrinology under FLOYD DAFT (later DOFT). There she con-tinued studies on the pituitary gland and pursued a new inter-erest in the hypothalamus. Early members of her laboratory were KATHRYN KNOWLTON, HILDEGARD WILSON, and ROBERT SCOW. In 1949 BERNARDO HOUSSAY, the Argentine Nobel laureate and expert in the pathophysiology of diabetes, worked with the section for about four months.

Several other endocrinologists entered NIH laboratories during the late 1940s and early 1950s. In 1948 SEYMOUR WOLL-MAN, a biophysicist, joined EGON LORENZ's biophysics labora-tory in NCI and pursued an interest in thyroid physiology, us-ing iodine radioisotopes. Collaborating with Scow, he worked on the iodide-trapping phenomenon, and with HAROLD MORRIS on transplantable thyroid tumors in mice. He also collaborated with MONTE GREER in studying neuroendocrine control of the thyroid gland.

In 1951 G. DONALD WHEDON, while still at Cornell-New York Hospital, was appointed to organize the Metabolic Diseases Branch of the National Institute of Arthritis and Metabolic Diseases (NIAMD). He brought to the NIH campus the following year a strong background in the effects of immobilization on bone metabolism.

Many of these early endocrinologists remained at NIH throughout most of their careers. Hertz retired in 1966 as Scientific Director of the National Institute of Child Health and Human Development (NICHD); Bartter in 1979 as Chief of the Hypertension-Endocrine Branch of the National Heart, Lung, and Blood Institute (NHLBI); and Whedon in 1981 as Director of NIAMD. Scow and Wollman are still active NIH scientists.

Expansion and Changing Patterns

With the opening of the Clinical Center in 1953, endo-crinology at NIH began a progressive expansion in avenues of inquiry. Endocrinology laboratories of three Institutes moved into the new quarters, and Roy Hertz admitted the first pa-tient, a man with prostatic cancer, for a study of estrogen

_____
*A substance capable of counteracting TSH, pituitary thyroid-stimulating hormone.

turnover. In NCI the Endocrinology Branch, headed by Hertz, included WILLIAM TULLNER working on reproductive physiology of monkeys, MIN CHIU LI on choriocarcinoma, and Greer on goitrogens in food and on the hypothalamic control of thyrotropin secretion. Later DELBERT BERGENSTAL, MORTIMER LIPSETT, and GRIFF ROSS joined the group, expanding the work on cancer and on reproductive biology.

Early members of Bartter's group, in the National Heart Institute (NHI), included GRANT LIDDLE, EDWARD BIGLIERI, PHILIP CHEN, IVOR MILLS, and DONALD GANN. The group later became the Clinical Endocrinology Branch.

Three laboratories of NIAMD conducting endocrinology research were transferred to the Clinical Center:

Anderson's section, in addition to Knowlton and Wilson, included GORDON FARRELL, ROBERT BATES, and later PETER CONDLIFFE. Bates and Condliffe's hormone chemistry studies led to the isolation of human TSH and the subsequent development of a radioimmunoassay.

Donald Whedon headed the Metabolic Diseases Branch, with HOWARD HIATT, PAUL MARKS, and DAVID THOMPSON as his first fellows. ROBERT HEANEY began his work on radioactive calcium kinetics. A metabolic chamber, built in the early 1950s, was staffed by RON THOMPSON and ELSWORTH BUSKIRK. GERALD AURBACH, who had begun his NIH career in Hertz's laboratory, succeeded Whedon as branch chief in 1964.

The new adrenal steroid drugs used in treating rheumatoid arthritis and related diseases were studied in the Arthritis and Rheumatism Branch, directed by JOSEPH BUNIM. RALPH PETERSON investigated the kinetics of corticosteroid and aldosterone metabolism. Simultaneously, NORMAN BOAS pursued his studies on tissue glycoproteins and mucopolysaccharides.

In 1955 J. EDWARD RALL organized a new Clinical Endocrinology Branch in NIAMD, with emphasis on basic and clinical thyroid studies. It included JACOB ROBBINS, who had arrived in 1954 and later succeeded Rall as branch chief, and JAN WOLFF, HANS CAHNMANN, HAROLD EDELHOCH, and CHARLES LEWALLEN. Later, CEB expanded into pituitary and metabolic studies with JAMES FIELD and STANTON SEGAL. JESSE ROTH and IRA PASTAN, other early members, conducted studies on polypeptide hormone receptors.

In 1966 Hertz established an intramural research program within the newly organized NICHD. Lipsett and Ross moved their laboratory from NCI to NICHD in 1971, adopting the name Reproduction Research Branch, with Lipsett as head. Lipsett left NIH in 1975 and Ross became chief. In 1977 Lipsett returned as Director of the Clinical Center, Ross became Deputy Director, and KEVIN CATT succeeded him as branch chief. Lipsett was appointed Director of NICHD in 1982.

It is evident that the NIH community of endocrinologists proliferated after 1953. RUSSELL WILDER, Director of NIAMD from 1951 to 1953, had been a senior endocrinologist at the Mayo Clinic. He played a key role in launching endocrine studies in Bethesda. The various endocrine groups, organized within disease-oriented Institutes, naturally followed different lines of study. Interests overlapped, however, leading to a great deal of interaction. This took the form of joint seminars, discussion groups, and collaborative research projects. In time the remarkably broad resources of this community were tapped in the first inter-Institute training program at NIH for fellows, clinical associates, and eventually medical students. BRUCE WEINTRAUB became the first director of this popular program in 1972. Although clinical endocrinology was its primary focus, the training program drew much of its strength from the basic endocrine research groups dotting the NIH campus.

In a discipline such as endocrinology, which impinges on every organ system of the body and on virtually every disease entity, the great size and diversity of NIH provided a unique opportunity. A structure of unparalleled breadth and distinction developed. This was the inevitable outcome of a system that attracted and nurtured excellent scientists and encouraged their exploration of promising avenues of research. No other institution can boast an endocrine "department" of such scope. Each of the Institutes promoted endocrine research in relation to its own mission; but just as the body's hormones arise in one locus and affect another, endocrinologists at NIH have exerted an influence beyond their organizational boundaries. Furthermore, the central role of endocrinology in biology and biochemistry assured that it would assert itself in many different forms and places. An important and felicitous trait of NIH is that these manifestations of creative science were not forced into specific molds.

A few examples will illustrate these points. The interest of Hertz and his group in hormones and cancer led to the formation of a team of scientists investigating gonadal steroids as they impinged on the pathophysiology and therapy of various tumors, such as those of the prostate and breast, and on gonadotropins (hormones affecting the gonads) as related to the placental cancer choriocarcinoma. To advance these interests, the group worked on the bioassay, chemical assay, and immunoassay of these hormones and on their role in normal development and sexual function. When the time came to staff for reproduction research in the new NICHD, it became apparent that no finer group than that in NCI could be found for this work. The result was a transfer of the NCI laboratory, but with little change in its general objectives. These were approached through studies on pituitary gonadotropins, sex steroids, the menstrual cycle, fertility, and diseases of sexual development. At the same time, NIAMD's Clinical Endocrinology and Metabolic Diseases Branches and several NHLBI laboratories supported research programs in hormone production by malignant tumors and in cancers of various endocrine glands. Thus work on hormones and cancer continued at a high level despite NCI's loss of its major endocrinology laboratory.

On the other hand, an NIAMD scientist, Pastan, was invited to establish a Laboratory of Molecular Biology in NCI. He had begun at NIH as a Clinical Associate with an interest in thyroid hormones, TSH, and the mechanism of hormone action. Gradually he extended his work to the control of protein synthesis in bacteria and to cell control and transformation in higher forms. Again, as cancer "recepterology" became important, MARC LIPPMAN directed a section in NCI concentrating on steroid receptors and breast cancer metabolism.

In contrast to these self-directed shifts in emphasis, other endocrine groups arose according to the missions of their disease-oriented Institutes. Thus Roth, beginning as a Clinical Associate with an interest in acromegaly, the immunoassay of pituitary growth hormone, and later the cell surface receptor for TSH, became head of a new Diabetes Section in NIAMD. He soon launched an extensive study of insulin receptors. In a similar way Bartter's group in the Heart Institute became deeply involved in the endocrine aspects of hypertensive disease, with studies on aldosterone, renin, and electrolyte metabolism; while other groups in NHI concentrated on hormones of the adrenal medulla, the catecholamines. NICHD, to advance its mission in the study of human development, established a new pediatric endocrinology unit under JAMES SIDBURY and MARVIN CORNBLATH. In addition, the endocrine group under ROBERT GREGERMAN in Baltimore had been active since 1967 in the Gerontology Branch, later the National Institute on Aging.

Another aspect of the growth and development of endocrinology at NIH was the response to service needs of the Clinical Center. The various endocrinology groups, as they grew in expertise, provided increasingly broad consultative service to other clinical investigators. Simultaneously, the various clinical research and service departments made significant contributions to endocrinology. Outstanding in this respect have been endocrine surgery under MURRAY BRENNAN in the NCI Surgery Branch and arteriography and venous catheterization under JOHN DOPPMAN in Diagnostic Radiology. In this way, many departments have been deeply involved in furthering endocrine investigation.

NIH has had a major impact on endocrine science, not only

through the accomplishments recounted in the remainder of this chapter but also by its development of well-trained and highly motivated investigators. We will not attempt to list those who only stayed a few years at NIH before moving on to active careers in endocrinology, many achieving distinction in the United States and abroad.

The Endocrine Systems

We begin this account with the major endocrine systems, most of which were early foci of study. Interest in the gastrointestinal hormones came later as the field evolved. Some systems, such as adrenal aldosterone and the placental hormones, are discussed in later sections on cardiovascular disease and cancer. Collaboration among laboratories and constructive overlap of subject matter have greatly contributed to the achievements discussed below.

The Anterior Pituitary and the Hypothalamus

The advent of radioimmunoassay made it possible for members of the NCI Endocrinology Branch to examine a variety of regulatory mechanisms. BILL ODELL and BOB UTIGER developed an assay for TSH, using materials supplied by Bates and Condliffe of NIAMD; and Ross, working with them, developed and adapted assays for hCG, FSH, and LH.* With Lipsett, Ross produced the first comprehensive description of the menstrual cycle, described the short luteal phase, and predicted the interactions between the ovary and pituitary. Simultaneously, Lipsett with MARVIN KIRSCHNER developed a method for plasma testosterone assay and demonstrated the negative feedback aspects of the testis-pituitary axis.

It was during this period that Odell first used radiation inactivation to estimate the molecular weights of the pituitary hormones. PETER KOHLER measured the metabolic clearances of FSH and LH, thus providing the first estimates of their secretion rates. ABBA KASTIN, working with Ross, studied the regulation of MSH** in the frog. He continued these studies with Schally in New Orleans, where he has contributed extensively to our knowledge of the behavioral effects of central nervous system peptides.

---

*Human chorionic gonadotropin; follicle-stimulating hormone; luteinizing hormone.
**Melanocyte-stimulating hormone.

The group of scientists working with Ross concentrated on the structure and function of hCG. With JUDITH VAITUKAITIS and E. V. Van Hall, Ross showed that sialylation of hCG* was responsible for its long plasma half-life and thereby explained the discrepancies among different bioassays. He and Chen were the first to demonstrate the presence of hCG in normal subjects, thereby supporting the hypothesis of "leaky genes."

Vaitukaitis joined the group in the late 1960s and, after developing assays for the hCG subunits, showed how they could be used to mark tumors and to distinguish recurrent choriocarcinoma from pregnancy. These assays have been applied extensively in NCI. BRUCE NISULA proved that the thyroid-stimulating activity of hCG, noted during therapeutic trials of women with choriocarcinoma, was intrinsic to the hormone and not due to a contaminant of either subunit. The properties of the hCG subunits were intensively explored by many researchers in the Branch.

At about this time, SAUL ROSEN in NIAMD described the first case of anaplastic carcinoma of the lung associated with high levels of hCG. He broadened these studies and, with Weintraub, greatly enhanced appreciation of the unbalanced synthesis of gonadotropin subunits in tumorous tissues. These investigators are now engaged in defining the translational changes involving glycosylation** of the gonadotropins in tumorous tissues.

NICHD's DAVID RODBARD, physician and mathematician, aided all of these studies immeasurably. He devised new ways of observing ligand-receptor interactions, both in radioimmunoassays and in hormone-receptor binding, and his computer programs to analyze these events are in worldwide use. Other important contributions to this area resulted from ANDREAS CHRAMBACH's efforts. A physical chemist in NICHD, Chrambach placed polyacrylamide gel electrophoresis and isoelectric focusing on firm ground, making possible the characterization and separation of small amounts of protein hormones.

LYNN LORIAUX's Developmental Endocrinology Branch, NICHD, has moved one step further in the study of regulatory mechanisms, working with analogs of LHRH, CRF, and GRF.*** With FLORENCE COMITE, Loriaux has shown the dramatic effects of long-acting agonists (stimulators) of LHRH in reversing pre-

---

*Combination with sialic acid, a common component of tissues.

**Combination with glycosyl groups, derivatives of carbohydrate.

***Luteinizing hormone releasing hormone; corticotropin releasing factor; growth hormone releasing factor.

cocious puberty. This builds on the demonstration by Catt and others of the loss of LH receptors following constant stimulation by LHRH. Loriaux and GORDON CUTLER carried out extensive studies on the adrenarche,* exploring factors concerned with the secretion of dehydroepiandrosterone and its sulfate, and have obtained further evidence of the role of a still-unidentified pituitary factor critical to this process.

Roth's previous work on growth hormone with Solomon Berson and Rosalyn Yalow, in New York, led him to continue this interest at NIH. He and PHILLIP GORDEN systematically studied the natural history of acromegaly, correlating growth hormone levels with response to therapy. In so doing, they challenged current thoughts about the efficacy of X-ray in the treatment of underlying pituitary tumor, showing that radiation was as effective as attempts to remove the tumor surgically.

Adrenals, Gonads, and Steroid Hormones

The interests in endocrine-related cancers and reproductive endocrinology remained intertwined for two decades. Definition of the hormonal milieu that favored the growth of breast, uterine, or prostate cancer required development of successively more sophisticated types of analysis. Thus Lipsett, first using colorimetric measurement of urinary steroids, progressed from paper chromatography to fluorimetry to vapor phase chromatography. He developed, with Kirschner, vapor phase chromatography for such measurement. Subsequently, ligand-binding assays, first using natural constituents of plasma such as CBG and TeBG** with high binding affinities for steroid hormones and later antibodies against such hormones, were developed and incorporated into the Branch's technology.

Lipsett and his co-workers STAN KORENMAN, LARRY FISHMAN, WAYNE BARDIN, WYLIE HEMBREE, Loriaux, TERUYA YOSHIMI, EBERHART NIESCHLAG, and YUKITAKI MIYACHI carried out basic studies on metabolism and interconversion of the steroid hormones and their metabolites. They studied and delineated androgen excess in adrenal and ovarian disorders and analyzed problems of the estrogen system, including the role of plasma estrone sulfate. They demonstrated the temporal relationships of ovary and placenta in progesterone synthesis and found that 17α-hydroxyprogesterone was a prominent steroid secretory

---

*A physiologic change usually occurring at age 8 or 9, involving augmented adrenal cortex secretion.

**Corticosteroid-binding globulin and testosterone-binding globulin.

product of the Leydig cells and corpus luteum. Later, Lipsett with GEORGE MERRIAM, SHINZO KONO, and Loriaux placed the study of catechol estrogens on firm ground by developing a reliable immunoassay and establishing that these compounds had high clearance rates. These findings refuted claims of a physiologic role for the catechol estrogens in peripheral blood.

DICK SHERINS and Loriaux devoted considerable effort to dissecting the hormonal regulation of the gonadotropins in normal men and proved that both androgens and estrogens exert regulatory effects. Sherins established a male fertility clinic that continues to yield new data about male hypogonadism. He showed that only small amounts of FSH* were necessary to initiate spermatogenesis, characterized the spectrum of hypogonadotropic hypogonadism, demonstrated that only a few million normal spermatozoa were necessary for impregnation, and established the importance of testicular estrogen in spermatogenesis.

As the work on steroids progressed, Ross and his collaborators made strides in understanding ovarian function. They demonstrated the necessary role of estrogen in follicular growth and the sensitivity of pituitary gonadotropins to low doses of estrogens. They showed that androgen synthesized in the ovary caused follicular atresia** and studied the process morphologically and biochemically. With JIM SCHREIBER, Ross characterized a follicular androgen receptor. In studies of the human menstrual cycle, they demonstrated the relationship of the ovarian follicle to FSH levels, defined the diagnostic maneuvers necessary to characterize primary and secondary amenorrhea, and characterized the responses of various types of ovarian follicles to gonadotropin stimulation.

GARY HODGEN, who had worked with Ross, became Chief of the Pregnancy Research Branch. He conducted basic studies on the physiologic control of ovarian function in the pregnant rhesus monkey and extended observations bearing on the regulation of folliculogenesis, the selection of dominant follicle, the resumption of follicular growth during the puerperium, and a series of intraovarian events.

The Thyroid Gland and Iodine Metabolism

Jacob Robbins was one of the Clinical Associates who served as junior "house officers" in lieu of military service, gaining an opportunity to continue their research careers.

---

*Follicle-stimulating hormone.
**Degeneration of the ovarian follicle before maturity.

After a year he joined the new CEB, then headed by Rall, with whom he had worked at the Memorial-Sloan Kettering Cancer Center in New York. Rall soon succeeded in creating a thyroid research group strong in basic science as well as clinical investigation.

The group included Jan Wolff, who graduated from medical school in 1953 and came immediately after his internship. He had received his Ph.D. at Berkeley in 1949 under I. Chaikoff. In that laboratory, noted as a center of thyroid research, he had described the phenomenon known as the Wolff-Chaikoff effect: inhibition of thyroid hormone synthesis by a high concentration of iodide ion. At NIH he launched a far-reaching study of the mechanism of iodide transport into the thyroid cell, the first step in thyroid hormone production.

Harold Edelhoch, a physical chemist with extensive experience in protein research at Princeton, Harvard, Wisconsin, and Kansas, joined the group at an invitation to pursue his own interests. Surrounded by thyroidologists, he quickly recognized the importance of thyroglobulin, the little-studied protein of the thyroid follicles. His systematic investigation of this essential vehicle for thyroid hormone set a new standard.

Hans Cahnmann, an organic chemist trained in Munich under Heinrich Wieland, had moved one step ahead of the Nazis to Jean Roche's laboratory in Paris and then Marseilles. Presently, escaping to New York, he entered industrial chemistry and patented the synthesis of vitamin A. At NIH he first worked on chemical carcinogens under ROBERT J. HUEBNER, then moved to CEB and began a distinguished career in thyroid hormone chemistry and synthesis. In 1976, at age 70, he became Scientist Emeritus and, after his "retirement," solved the structure requirements for synthesis of thyroxine, the thyroid gland hormone that exerts the main influence on metabolic rate.

Another member of the group was Charles Lewallen. As a physician at the Brookhaven National Laboratory, he had assisted Rall and Rulon Rawson in their studies on the treatment of thyroid cancer with radioactive iodine. He came to CEB to continue this work and pursue an interest in the kinetics of iodine metabolism. Robbins and Rall extended two lines of inquiry begun under Rawson in New York: the transport of thyroid hormones by plasma proteins and the function of differentiated thyroid cancer.*

This heterogeneous team of independent but interacting scientists created one of the world centers for thyroid re-

---

*A differentiated cancer is one comprising mature type cells that resemble those of the tissue of origin.

search. A succession of fellows came from many countries for training and inspiration. The group has been remarkable for the stability of its senior staff. Rall became Scientific Director of NIAMD but continued to supervise his laboratory, working toward a molecular definition of the mechanism of thyroid hormone action in liver cell (hepatocyte) nuclei. In 1983 he became Deputy Director for Intramural Research, NIH.

A description of two research directions can illuminate the way in which the thyroid group has functioned for 25 years. The thyroid cell, like all cells, is surrounded by a plasma membrane. The thyroid cell membrane is endowed with specialized functions. One is to serve a key peculiarity of this cell: its ability to recognize the element iodine, a minor component of the environment, and to incorporate it in the production of thyroxine, an iodinated amino acid.

In the 1940s Chaikoff's laboratory at the University of California (Berkeley) was one of the few centers to explore the functions of the thyroid cell in biochemical terms. Wolff, growing up in this environment from laboratory assistant to graduate student, became a biochemically oriented cell biologist. When he joined CEB, he decided to study the iodide-trapping mechanism, which he assumed to be a function of the plasma membrane. He was able to define the cell's iodide transport properties, including its energy requirements and its relation to membrane components. PETER SCHNEIDER, REED LARSEN, and DONALD ALEXANDER participated in some of this work.

At about the same time, Robbins and Monte Greer, who were attending the thyroid clinic that Greer had organized at D.C. General Hospital, encountered a newborn girl with an unusual congenital goiter. She was included in a case study of congenital cretinism published in 1958 by DANIEL FEDERMAN, a Clinical Associate working with Rall and Robbins. This was actually the first reported case of congenital absence of the iodide transport mechanism. Wolff and Robbins published a detailed study of the patient, showing that iodide ion transport was lacking at certain body sites and that the patient's hypothyroidism could be reversed with iodide alone. Twelve years later Wolff and MARVIN GERSHENGORN systematically investigated the relation between iodide supply and hormone synthesis in this patient, who had been kept under observation in the CEB clinic.

Wolff meanwhile had redirected his major interest to other functions of the thyroid plasma membrane—those involved in hormone secretion. This led him into work with JOHN WILLIAMS and others on mechanisms of basic cellular functions: adenylate cyclase response to TSH, the formation of colloid droplets in the thyroid gland, the involvement of microtubules and calmodulin.* His interest was not confined to thyroid cells but extended to steroid-secreting endocrine glands and even to bacteria. Wolff's and ERIC HEWLETT's work on the release of adenylate cyclase from certain pathogenic bacteria is of great potential interest for disease mechanisms and can provide information about how hormones act.

The freedom of a scientist to follow wide-ranging interests is important, not only for personal satisfaction but for the advancement of science in unexpected directions. On a practical level, Wolff's expertise in thyroidology was tapped repeatedly for information about radiation damage to the thyroid gland. Together with Rall and Robbins, he served as consultant to the Brookhaven Laboratory in followup studies of the Marshall Islanders after their exposure to radioactive fallout. He also served on the National Council for Radiation Protection's expert committee that defined the use of high doses of iodine to block the thyroid gland's uptake of radio-iodine. Like many NIH scientists with training in medicine, he could devote himself to basic research while contributing importantly to clinical science.

Another episode reflects the fertile soil of NIH for such scientists. In 1969 STEPHEN BERENS, a young Associate in the Laboratory of Clinical Science at the National Institute of Mental Health, asked Robbins for suggestions about the effects of lithium on the thyroid gland. In a study of lithium therapy for cyclic depression, Berens had learned that the treatment frequently causes a goiter. He was invited to do some animal experiments in CEB. These revealed clearly that lithium's major effect on the thyroid gland is to slow hormone secretion. This of course raised the question whether lithium might have a role in treating hyperthyroidism.

A study was launched by Wolff, Robbins, and two Clinical Associates, ROBERT TEMPLE and HAROLD CARLSON. Patients with Graves' disease (a form of hyperthyroidism) were admitted to the Clinical Center, and MONES BERMAN of NCI's Laboratory of Mathematical Biology helped design a study of iodine kinetics. It demonstrated that lithium is a unique therapeutic agent with possible importance for treating severe thyrotoxicosis, so-called thyroid storm. Berens and Wolff carried out an impressive series of laboratory experiments to elucidate the mechanism of the lithium effect. Robbins later investigated the potential use of lithium to slow the release of radio-activity in the treatment of thyroid cancer with radioiodine.

Thyroglobulin, the major protein of the thyroid gland involved in hormone synthesis, was a focus of attention in CEB

---

*Calmodulin: a protein that binds calcium ions; a metabolic regulator.

for several years. Robbins and Rall, in their studies on thyroid cancer begun in New York, were interested in whether tumors were abnormal in their ability to make this protein. As it turned out, thyroid tumors produce normal thyroglobulin, but aberrations in protein iodination explain the occurrence of unusual iodoproteins both in cancer and in other thyroid diseases.

A part of these studies employed a unique resource at NIH: strains of rats bearing transplantable thyroid tumors, developed in Wollman's laboratory in NCI. These tumors proved to be a source of some remarkable abnormalities. One, studied by Wolff, Robbins, and Rall, revealed preservation of the iodide-trapping mechanism but no organification—that is, linking of iodine with carbon compounds to form thyroxine. Another abnormality, later described by Robbins, Cahnmann, and MOTOMORI IZUMI, was an inability to make normal thyroglobulin. Yet another was studied by two visiting fellows from MARIO ANDREOLI's laboratory in Rome. GIOVANNI SALABE demonstrated a defect in the release of thyroglobulin from intracellular particles in tumor cells, and FABRIZIO MONACO later ascribed this to lack of sialic acid addition, thus revealing a key factor in the secretion of thyroglobulin and its subsequent iodination.

These and other studies on thyroglobulin abnormalities— for example, the congenital goiter in Afrikander cattle brought to CEB from South Africa by ANDREIS VAN ZYL—complemented fundamental discoveries about the chemistry of this protein. Harold Edelhoch's group defined its molecular properties and the special role of its iodine-containing constituents. Edelhoch played a particular part in the training of many thyroid scientists. The knowledge of physical chemistry gained in his laboratory strongly enhanced their work, which varied as widely as immunochemistry (HENRY METZGER), molecular biology (BENOIT deCROMBRUGGHE), cellular growth factors (PETER NISSLEY), thyroglobulin biosynthesis (ARTHUR SCHNEIDER), and thyroid cell membranes (SALVATORE ALOJ, now in the active NIADDK thyroid laboratory of LEONARD KOHN).

Collaboration with Italian scientists has been an interesting aspect of the NIH work on thyroglobulin. Andreoli came to CEB to study thyroxine transport proteins in the blood. In the same period, GAETANO SALVATORE arrived with similar interests but, stimulated by the new environment, turned his attention in unexpected directions. He and his wife, MARISA, working with Cahnmann and Robbins, applied powerful new separation techniques (gel filtration and density gradient ultracentrifugation) to the preparation and characterization of natural thyroglobulin polymers. This began a long, productive collaboration between CEB and the major thyroid laboratory that Salvatore established after returning to Naples. Salvatore is a frequent working visitor to Bethesda, most recently as a Fogarty Scholar. There were also notable contributions from Japanese scientists, among them, TERUO MATSUURA and TETSUO SHIBA (with Hans Cahnmann) and YOICHI KONDO (with Robbins and Rall).

This account has slighted many ventures in thyroid research that took place in CEB and other thyroid laboratories at NIH, such as the work on electron microscopy and structure-function relationships by Seymour Wollman and on functions of the thyroid plasma membrane by Leonard Kohn. Studies on the pituitary and TSH were conducted by Jim Field, an early member of the staff, by Ira Pastan, who did the first experiments identifying a receptor for this hormone on the surface membrane of the thyroid cell, and most recently by Bruce Weintraub, the latest addition to the CEB senior staff, now doing advanced work on the role of glycosylation in TSH biosynthesis. Clinical investigations proceeded side by side with laboratory research: early work on genetic alterations in thyroxine-binding proteins, recent work on the syndromes of thyroid hormone resistance, studies in the diagnosis and treatment of thyroid tumors. This interpolation of clinical and laboratory research, and exposure to such distinguished Visiting Scientists as ROSALIND PITT-RIVERS and JAMSHED TATA from London, RAYMOND MICHEL and JACQUES NUNEZ from Paris, and NOBUO UI from Japan, have provided a fertile milieu for many trainees in endocrinology.

The Parathyroids, Calcium Metabolism, and Gastrointestinal Hormones

Two laboratories in the new Clinical Center set out to study the endocrinology of bone diseases. At that time the primary tool in calcium studies was metabolic balance analysis, and the Heart and Arthritis Institutes established and shared a special diet kitchen for this work. Both Fred Bartter and Don Whedon, heading these laboratories, attempted to solve the enigma of osteoporosis, a condition of bone depletion or atrophy associated with aging. Despite significant findings, the essential mechanism of osteoporosis remains elusive.

Beginning in 1963, with the coming of the Space Age, Whedon led the development of calcium balance techniques to monitor the effects of weightlessness in space flight. He was a key member of the Space Metabolism Advisory Group of the National Aeronautics and Space Administration, contributing to the first balance study in Gemini 7 and the first comprehensive experiment in Skylab, 1973-1974. This was a direct continuation of his earlier work on immobilization in paralyzed patients. Immobilization in bed and weightlessness in space can both result in pronounced negative calcium balance, demonstrating that mechanical stress is required to maintain a normal calcium content in bone.

A frequent problem in patients with high blood calcium is the occurrence of kidney stones. CHARLES PAK, working with Bartter on the factors leading to stone formation, discovered that cellulose phosphate was an effective preventive.

A new era of research in metabolic bone disease began in 1959 when Gerald Aurbach came to NIH as a Research Associate. At an Associates' seminar, he presented some of his earlier findings under Edwin Astwood at Tufts on the parathyroid hormone (PTH). BOB CANFIELD heard the report and described it to JOHN POTTS, a colleague in CHRIS ANFINSEN's laboratory in the Heart Institute. Potts suggested to Aurbach that they work together on the purification and structure of PTH. After finishing their tours as Associates, Aurbach was appointed to Evelyn Anderson's laboratory in NIAMD and Potts stayed on as a permanent member of NHI under DONALD FREDRICKSON. Aurbach and Potts isolated PTH from 330 kg of bovine parathyroid glands with the assistance of JOHN KERESZTESY's facility in NIAMD for large-scale preparations.

The Aurbach-Potts collaboration continued after the two moved, Aurbach in 1965 to the Metabolic Diseases Branch, then under BOB GORDON, and Potts in 1969 to Massachusetts General Hospital. In January 1970 they reported the sequence of 34 amino acids in bovine PTH and then synthesized a portion of the molecule, showing it to be biologically active. Meanwhile, Clinical Associate BRYAN BREWER undertook to solve the complete sequence of 84 amino acids. He published in December 1970, one month before Aurbach and Potts also reported the complete sequence. Both laboratories continued the race to solve the structure of human PTH, and in 1974 both were successful at about the same time.

The large-scale purification of PTH was not only the key to the structure of the hormone but also to developing a radioimmunoassay. LOU SHERWOOD applied the new assay in studying PTH secretion in cows, setting the stage for its important introduction into clinical medicine.

A fortuitous encounter occurred in 1966 when Potts and Aurbach, together with Ira Pastan and Peter Condliffe, were conducting a seminar course for Research and Clinical Associates on the mechanism of hormone action. Earl Sutherland of Vanderbilt University was a guest speaker. He discussed cyclic adenosine monophosphate (cAMP), a key metabolite that mediates the action of numerous hormones, and described finding it in bacteria and in urine. The seminar had far-reaching consequences. Pastan began work on the role of cAMP in bacterial metabolism, and MARTIN RODBELL in fat and liver cells. Aurbach was stimulated to investigate the possible influence of PTH on urinary excretion of the metabolite. An indication that PTH might have such an influence was its known effect on calcium ion flux in the kidney. Aurbach and Clinical Associate LEW CHASE soon demonstrated in rats and then in man that the major factor regulating the urinary excretion of cAMP was indeed PTH.

The possibility that this information as well as the new radioimmunoassay for the hormone might be used in the diagnosis of parathyroid disease inspired Aurbach to begin a major study of hyperparathyroidism. This ultimately led to the development of methods for the diagnosis and treatment of patients who had failed parathyroid surgery. John Doppman, chief of the Radiology Department in the Clinical Center, developed venous catheterization for sampling PTH and radiological techniques for visualization of parathyroid tumor.

In the context of this group effort, Murray Brennan of NCI's surgery department became one of the nation's outstanding parathyroid surgeons. Another NCI surgeon, SAM WELLS, developed methods for cryopreservation of parathyroid tissue. If surgical removal of tissue for parathyroid hyperplasia proves excessive, the frozen tissue can be reimplanted, as demonstrated on NIH patients. The studies on hyperparathyroidism also led STEVE MARX, a young colleague in Aurbach's group, to discover the syndrome of familial hypocalciuric hypercalcemia (FHH), which resembles hyperparathyroidism in presenting elevated blood calcium. It must be distinguished from hyperparathyroidism for proper treatment, since parathyroidectomy is contraindicated.

Aurbach's developing interest in cAMP and the parathyroid glands had other ramifications. Drawing on basic findings by Rodbell and LUTZ BIRNBAUMER, Aurbach and AL SPIEGEL showed that a guanine nucleotide regulatory protein (G-unit) is responsible for the failure of patients with pseudohypoparathyroidism to respond to PTH and for the simultaneous failure of other glands such as the thyroid.

Related work on turkey red blood cells, in which the adenylate cyclase system is under the control of catecholamines such as epinephrine, led to a number of other important developments in Aurbach's laboratory. This work attracted JERRY GARDNER, a Clinical Associate in the Metabolic Diseases Branch with an interest in the membrane transport of sodium and potassium ions. Gardner undertook to study the role of adenylate cyclase in the action of gastrointestinal hormones and, after becoming head of his own laboratory, continued these studies in depth. Gardner and BOB JENSEN showed in 1975 that the gastrointestinal hormones secretin and vasoactive intestinal peptide (VIP) acted by stimulating cAMP production in the intestinal mucosa, whereas gastrin and cholecystekinin mobilized intracellular calcium ion. In 1976 they demonstrated the binding of VIP to pancreatic acinar cells and extended this work to receptors for other gastrointestinal hormones.

The Endocrine Pancreas and Diabetes

When the Clinical Center opened, there were no members of the staff with an interest in clinical diabetes mellitus, though basic research in many related areas was under way. Field, after working on carbohydrate metabolism as a Research Associate in HANS STETTEN's lab, joined CEB and undertook to study the effects of pituitary hormones on intermediate carbohydrate metabolism in the target endocrine organs. He also carried out clinical studies on syndromes of insulin resistance, such as those induced by high alcohol intake. When Field left NIH in 1963, his colleague GLENN MORTIMORE continued to study the mechanism of insulin action in the perfused rat liver.

About 1965 the Congress began to urge a greater research effort in diabetes at NIH. Grant support of diabetes research was increased, but little happened intramurally despite Stetten's superb lecture series on frontiers of diabetes research for the NIAMD staff. To meet the challenge, a Diabetes Section was established in CEB under Stanton Segal, who had been working on galactosemia and cystinuria. Segal left, however, before he could launch a research program. Jesse Roth succeeded him as section chief in 1967.

Roth had completed his clinical associateship with Robbins and had moved quickly into the status of independent investigator. His early work in CEB included the application of a growth hormone immunoassay in acromegaly, an outcome of his aforementioned association with Berson and Yalow, and the development of other immunoassays useful in endocrine research. The systems covered in the latter study included ACTH (adrenocorticotropic hormone) and, with GARY ROBERTSON, the posterior pituitary hormone. Under Roth the Diabetes Section soon began a study of the forms of insulin in blood. With a flair for catching the eye of the scientific public, Roth and Phil Gorden reported their finding of "big insulin." This large molecular form was present in blood in various clinical situations. When Donald Steiner presented his discovery of the insulin precursor molecule, proinsulin, it became evident that these two substances were identical.

In close proximity in the Clinical Center, Condliffe, Pastan, and Roth had many discussions on the mechanisms of hormone action. Pastan and Roth demonstrated that there are receptors for TSH on the surface of the thyroid cell. This discovery led Roth to undertake similar research with insulin. Finding evidence for insulin receptors on the surface of the liver cell, Roth, Gorden, and a succession of colleagues demonstrated that interaction of insulin and its receptor was the first step in the hormone's action. Insulin receptors were found on many types of cells, and were shown to decrease when exposed to insulin, a phenomenon called "down regulation." They were also affected by overnutrition and other influences. These findings led to an explanation of the insulin resistance sometimes seen in obesity. Later, Roth with JEFFREY FLIER and RONALD KAHN, studying certain nonobese patients, discovered insulin receptor antibodies that could effectively block insulin action in certain autoimmune states. Though diabetic, these patients did not respond to insulin in enormous doses.

The expanding research on diabetes and insulin led to the establishment of a Diabetes Branch under Roth's leadership in 1975. Many scientists—PIERRE DeMEYTS, PIERRE FREYCHET, DAVID RABIN, ROBERT LEFKOWITZ, and a number of others—worked and trained in this active laboratory.

Almost simultaneously with the burgeoning of diabetes research in NIAMD, REUBIN ANDRES, Clinical Director of the National Institute on Aging, was examining carbohydrate metabolism in the elderly. In order to study insulin secretion in vivo, he devised, with Berman's help, the now widely used glucose clamp technique. This permits the assessment of insulin secretion at varying blood sugar levels achieved by continuous infusion of glucose.

Endocrinology and Cardiovascular Disease

Fred Bartter was frequently asked by the leaders of the Heart Institute to justify their support of a laboratory whose major interest was endocrinology and metabolism. He would remind them that ATP* was responsible for every beat of the heart. This holistic view of research created an atmosphere in which important interactions between endocrinology and the cardiovascular system were investigated. In Bartter's own research, this relationship surely buttressed his work on aldosterone, an adrenocortical hormone with a major role in

---

*Adenoside triphosphate, hydrolysis of which releases energy for muscular and other types of cellular activity.

sodium and potassium metabolism. A major result was the discovery of Bartter's syndrome, a disease characterized by kidney cell hyperplasia and associated metabolic aberrations causing mental retardation and short stature.

Hypertension, one of the commoner and more dangerous cardiovascular ailments, has a multitude of causes. One heterogeneous subset may be called endocrine hypertension, two forms of which were a focus of attention in the Heart Institute over many years. During early studies in the Clinical Center, ALFRED CASPER, a superb animal surgeon, adrenalectomized several dogs every day to supply assay subjects for Liddle and Bartter's studies on hypercortisolism.* This diplomatic supervisor of the animal laboratory also supplied adrenalectomized dogs to Bartter's "competitor" JAMES DAVIS, who used them to assay for aldosterone. In these laboratories, with Casper as a link, the interrelations of aldosterone and other factors—renal excretion of sodium and potassium, changes in blood volume and pressure, and the renin-angiotensin system (see below)—were explored.

The complex interplay of these factors generated vigorous controversies in the search for the point of endocrine control. About 1960 several NIH scientists—Gordon Farrell, Ivor Mills, Ed Biglieri, and CATHERINE DELEA, as well as those just mentioned—building on the syndromes of primary aldosteronism (excessive aldosterone secretion) caused by adrenal tumors and hyperplasia, began to clarify secondary aldosteronism and its role in hypertension and edema. The central influence of the kidney, both as a site of renin production by the juxtaglomerular cells and through its conservation or excretion of sodium and potassium ions, became evident. This led Bartter and JOHN GILL to recognize the syndrome of juxtaglomerular hypertrophy and oversecretion. Cells lining small renal arteries, sensitive to volume and pressure changes, secrete renin, which in turn initiates a protein breakdown leading to the production of angiotensin. This stimulates aldosterone secretion and also affects the blood pressure. Increasing knowledge of the mechanism has led to a better understanding of the causes and control of hypertension.

Later, in NICHD, interest in glucocorticoid receptors led GEORGE CHROUSOS, Loriaux, and Lipsett to delineate a rare, treatable form of hypertension due to a defective glucocorticoid receptor. They also described an animal model of the disease. This is another example of the advancement of endocrinology through new insights developing from unexpected quarters.

---

*Excessive secretion of cortisol (hydrocortisone), a major hormone of the adrenal cortex.

In still another area of interplay between endocrinology (in the broad sense) and the circulatory system, EUGENE BRAUNWALD, chief of the Cardiology Branch, explored the controlling effects of the sympathetic nervous system on the heart. The neurohormones epinephrine and norepinephrine are produced not only at sympathetic nerve endings but also in the adrenal medulla, the core of the adrenal gland. Tumors of this organ, the pheochromocytomas, were investigated by ALBERT SJOERDSMA, chief of the Experimental Therapeutics Branch. This led to his discovery of methyldopa, a drug affecting the sympathetic nervous system and ultimately resulting in a reduction of blood pressure. Methyldopa remains a major therapeutic agent.

In a turnabout role, Braunwald and his young colleague TOM GAFFNEY investigated the possible use of catecholamine inhibitors for treating the cardiovascular manifestations of hyperthyroidism. They showed that reserpine and guanethidine were effective therapeutic agents but were fraught with side effects. Others later developed a less troublesome inhibitor, propranolol. GERALD LEVEY, first with NIAMD and then NHLBI, played a major role in this development.

Earlier, Sjoerdsma and his colleagues in NHLBI delineated the clinical and biochemical features of the carcinoid syndrome, a symptom complex associated with serotonin-secreting tumors of the gastrointestinal tract. Their investigations of serotonin metabolism and the development of the pellagra-like syndrome remain landmarks in the study of this disease. HARRY KEISER, now Clinical Director of NHLBI, continued studies of pheochromocytomas and carcinoids and investigated the roles of the kallikreins and prostaglandins in these syndromes and in hypertension.

An early and central department of the Heart Institute was the Laboratory of Kidney and Electrolyte Metabolism, organized by JAMES SHANNON about 1950. ROBERT BERLINER, JACK ORLOFF, and MAURICE BURG included in their spectrum of interest the antidiuretic hormones of the posterior pituitary gland and their role in the kidney's handling of water and electrolytes. Fred Bartter, sharing this interest, defined the water intoxication syndrome known as SIADH—the syndrome of inappropriate secretion of antidiuretic hormone. This hormone, also called vasopressin, is the major force that allows the kidney to excrete urine hypertonic with respect to blood plasma. Viewed otherwise, vasopressin prevents the kidneys from drawing water out of the blood. Bartter and William Schwartz showed that an excess of the hormone could cause dilution of the blood, as in hemorrhage and trauma, neurological diseases, endocrine diseases, vasopressin-secreting tumors, cardiac failure, and cirrhosis of the liver. Many drugs can also produce the syn-

drome. In such conditions water restriction and slow restoration of sodium can be life-saving.

Beginning in 1976 HAROLD GAINER in NICHD and MICHAEL
BROWNSTEIN in NIMH began a series of experiments on the biosynthesis of vasopressin and of oxytocin, the second hormone
of the posterior pituitary gland. Built on information contributed by many others, their work culminated in the demonstration of precursor polypeptides synthesized in the hypothalamus. Vasopressin and oxytocin, parts of these precursors, are released from storage in the posterior pituitary
gland by proteases (proteolytic enzymes, or "protein split-
ters"). The carrier proteins linked to the hormones are
called neurophysins, and such a carrier system is known to
occur with many protein secretions.

Neurobiologists, working intensively in the field of
neuropeptides, made a contribution to more classical endocrinology. These vignettes dramatize once again the interpolation
of endocrinology into distantly related medical disciplines
and its broad involvement in the history of NIH.

Endocrinology and Cancer

In 1955 Min Chiu Li came from Olof Pearson's laboratory in
the Sloan-Kettering Institute to NCI as a Clinical Associate.
There he initiated a most important chapter in chemotherapy.
While at Sloan-Kettering he had participated in the study of a
patient with malignant melanoma who had a positive pregnancy
test, presumably a result of hCG production by the tumor.
During treatment with aminopterin, a folic acid antagonist,
the test became negative. This experience suggested to Li
that folic acid antagonists might be effective in choriocarcinoma, a cancer characterized by copious hCG secretion.
Li proposed such studies on arriving at NCI and, despite initial opposition, eventually received approval to try methotrexate for the treatment of women with metastatic choriocarcinoma, using his own scheme of intensive short courses.
In 1956 the first paper showing that this cancer, even when
metastatic, could be cured by chemotherapy appeared in the
*Proceedings of the Society of Experimental Biology and Medi-
cine*. Over the next 15 years, Hertz and his group, including
Bergenstal, Lipsett, Ross, and many Clinical Associates, expanded their studies and showed that other chemical agents
were also effective. In treating women with hydatidiform mole
who were at high risk for choriocarcinoma, they developed the
first chemoprophylaxis against cancer.

The use of specific inhibitors of steroid synthesis had

its roots in this Branch. William Tullner noted that amphe-none, an antiadrenocortical drug, caused enlargement of the adrenal glands in rats. He showed subsequently that it blocked conversion of cholesterol to steroids. It was in-effective, however, in the treatment of adrenal cancer. Bergenstal, Lipsett, and Hertz then investigated the use of op'DDD, a compound that caused necrosis of the adrenal cortex in dogs, and demonstrated that it could induce regression of metastatic adrenal cancer in about 25 percent of those af-fected. In the course of these studies, the group examined many aspects of the hormonal function of adrenal cancers. Hildegard Wilson joined Lipsett for this work, and they showed that Cushing's syndrome due to adrenal cancer was character-ized by a high excretion of tetrahydro substances. The bio-synthetic patterns in adrenal cancer were explored.

A major interest in functional tumors of the endocrine glands continues throughout NIH. Robbins is still exploring diagnosis and therapy of functional thyroid tumors; Lipsett and his co-workers studied many functional tumors of testis and ovary; Roth, Gorden, Kahn, and Gardner have made major discoveries in diagnosis and therapy of pancreatic and gastro-intestinal tumors; Rosen and Weintraub are dissecting the biosynthesis of glycoprotein hormones by nonendocrine cancers; and Loriaux and his colleagues are studying the natural his-tory of prolactinomas.

Hormone Transport and Metabolism

The central fact about a hormone is that it leaves its cell of origin to exert an action on more or less distant target cells. To do so, in the classical sense of an endo-crine substance, it must traverse the blood, the extravascu-lar spaces, and the target-cell membrane. As a consequence, endocrinologists must concern themselves with the nature and kinetics of this transport phenomenon and with the metabolic transformations that the hormone may undergo. Furthermore, measurements of hormone levels in blood (since blood is a convenient fluid to sample) are used extensively in clinical medicine to assess the functional status of the secreting endocrine glands. NIH scientists have made major contribu-tions to the understanding of these phenomena, especially as they pertain to the thyroid and steroid hormones.

Robbins and Rall were among the first to recognize the existence of specific proteins for the transportation of thy-roid hormones in blood plasma. As information developed about changes in these proteins influenced by inheritance, pregnancy, steroid hormones, and a host of diseases and drugs, it became clear that the concentration of free hormone in blood, in contrast to hormone bound to protein, was the key factor in hormone action. This led to an understanding of the relationship between thyroid hormone levels and thyroid state and eventually to the measurement of free hormone in the clinical evaluation of thyroid disease. Robbins and Rall enunciated the "free hormone hypothesis" at the Laurentian Hormone Conference in 1956 and in *Physiological Reviews* in 1960. These articles and their mathematical formalization of the equilibrium interaction between hormone and protein had a major impact on acceptance of the concept, now a basic tenet of thyroidology.

An effort to understand the chemical and other properties of the transport proteins paralleled attention to the free hormone question. The technique of affinity chromatography, developed by PEDRO CUATRECASAS, Anfinsen, and MEIR WILCHEK, enabled a group at Case Western Reserve University to purify the elusive thyroxine-binding alpha globulin (TBG).* Subsequently Cahnmann, Robbins, Edelhoch, and a succession of fellows including Marvin Gershengorn and SHEUE-YANN CHENG showed TBG to be a single polypeptide chain with unusual, irreversible instability.

Returning to an earlier period, another story about thyroxine transport proteins illuminates the way in which collaboration between NIH scientists and colleagues in widely dispersed institutions can extend frontiers of knowledge. BARUCH BLUMBERG (later to win the Nobel Prize for establishing the relation of Australia antigen to infectious hepatitis) joined NIAMD in 1957. He was interested in applying the new techniques of starch gel electrophoresis to investigate genetic polymorphism (concomitant existence of types) in proteins. In the course of these studies, Blumberg and Robbins discovered that thyroxine-binding prealbumin (TBPA)** was polymorphic in the rhesus monkey. Then basic work of various contributors enabled Robbins, Cahnmann, Edelhoch, Cheng, and others to clarify the molecular and thyroxine-binding properties of prealbumin in monkeys and humans. (This coincided with developments in the United States and Sweden showing that TBPA also functions in vitamin A transport.) In England X-ray diffraction studies on prealbumin crystals were pursued. These efforts led to the first, nearly complete characterization of a hormone-binding protein. It is

---

*A plasma protein with a strong binding affinity for thyroxine.

**A plasma protein with a binding affinity for thyroxine which is somewhat less than that of TBG.

now possible to define in molecular terms the alternate binding of thyroxine at two otherwise identical sites, discovered
by Robbins, Edelhoch, and their colleagues. Knowing how a
hormone can interact with a protein is basic to understanding
how hormones work.

Since a hormone spends part of its life in the blood, one
can learn a great deal about the dynamics of its production
and metabolism by taking samples over time. The thyroid hormone lends itself well to such kinetic studies because it can
be tagged with radioactive iodine. The isotope can also be
measured in the thyroid gland and in excreta as well as in the
blood and other tissues. Rall persuaded Mones Berman, who had
become interested in this system, to join the newly organized
Mathematics Research Branch of NIAMD. Berman developed a powerful computer program—the SAAM (System Analysis and Modeling)—that could be adapted to the study of many problems in
biological kinetics.

Gradually Berman incorporated new bits of information into
his calculations: the identification of triiodothyronine as a
hormone separate from thyroxine, the discovery that most of it
was derived from thyroxine in tissues outside the thyroid
gland, the movement of iodide through organs other than the
thyroid, etc. This mathematical approach enabled Berman to
explore unexpected metabolic pathways. An example was his
collaboration with Wolff, Robbins, Robert Temple, and Harold
Carlson to study how lithium affects iodine metabolism. Surprisingly, kinetic analysis revealed a slowing of peripheral
thyroxine metabolism.

Ralph Peterson and JAMES WYNGAARDEN (now Director of NIH)
conducted early studies on steroid hormone metabolism in the
Arthritis and Rheumatism Branch of NIAMD. A major interest of
the branch was to explore the use of cortisone in the treatment of arthritis and related diseases, following dramatic
applications of this adrenal hormone at the Mayo Clinic in
1948 (Hench, Kendall, and others). The group was encouraged
to pursue investigations on the metabolism of labeled corticosteroids (steroid hormones of the adrenal cortex).

Aldosterone, the newly recognized corticosteroid, was difficult to measure because of its low concentration and metabolic transformation. Peterson devised a novel method known
as double-isotope derivative dilution for measuring hormones
in body fluids. Based on the interrelation of a labeled hormone and a chemically formed derivative tagged with a different isotope, the method permits the metabolic turnover of
an injected hormone to be accurately determined from fluid
samples. Peterson not only measured the production rates of
the corticosteroids, but offered a new way to study many hard-
to-measure compounds.

The Mechanism of Hormone Action

The manner in which hormones exert their myriad effects in the body comes down to the central question of the biochemical mechanisms of their interaction with cells. Endocrinologists have gradually extended the frontiers of this problem, and NIH scientists have significantly contributed. We have previously referred to several contributions; here we note other examples.

In the 1960s Sutherland at Vanderbilt University, studying the action of glucagon on liver metabolism, detected an unknown compound that eluded identification. Simultaneously, David Lipkin at Washington University found that ATP and barium hydroxide in vitro gave rise to an unknown product. Both of these men sought the help of LEON HEPPEL, the NIAMD expert in nucleotide chemistry. Leon recognized that they were studying the same compound, which he identified as 3',5'-cyclic adenosine monophosphate. Now called cyclic AMP, the well-known "second messenger" results from the interaction of many hormones with the target cell's surface membrane. This discovery had enormous impact on the study of hormone action. Many other contributions in this area were made by scientists throughout NIH, including Aurbach, Rodbell, Pastan, and Gardner, as mentioned earlier.

GORDON TOMKINS, NIAMD, pioneered and initiated several fields of steroid research. He delineated the rate-limiting step in cortisol metabolism and explained the effects of thyroid hormone on this reaction. These findings stimulated Bartter and his colleagues to describe the different disposal rates of cortisol in hyperthyroidism and myxedema. Tomkins initiated studies in the molecular biology of glucocorticoid hormones, using hepatic cells in culture. Glucocorticoid induction of the enzyme tyrosine aminotransferase still serves as a model system for those interested in hormone action, and BRAD THOMPSON in NCI, who started with Tomkins, continues along these lines.

An interesting chapter in molecular biology began in the Endocrinology Branch of NCI. In the 1940s Hertz had shown that progesterone specifically increases the amount of egg white factor, avidin, in the chick oviduct. Stan Korenman, after working with Mort Lipsett for three years, spent a year with Chris Anfinsen and then returned to the Branch to study the effects of hormone action. Mort pointed out the advantages of working with the chick oviduct, and Stan, using this system, developed an assay for avidin. That year, BERT O'MALLEY, who had started his research with Lipsett, joined Korenman. When Stan left the following year for California, Bert, still a first-year Clinical Associate, took over the project. This was the beginning of Bert's use of the chick oviduct system to delineate the molecular events of steroid hormone action that led, in succeeding years at Vanderbilt and Baylor, to his remarkably productive work on the molecular biology of the progesterone receptor gene in eukaryotes.

It was in this milieu that BILL McGUIRE began his studies on estrogen receptors and the mechanism of estrogen action in breast cancer. This work was the basis of his major research effort in breast cancer after moving to San Antonio.

Another current of research took form when a husband-wife team, Kevin Catt and MARIA DUFAU, joined the Branch in 1970. Their work over the next decade focused on mechanisms of peptide hormone action, particularly the gonadotropins, gonadotropin-releasing hormone (GnRH), and angiotensin. They were gifted in developing analytic techniques: the Dufau bioassay for LH, using the dispersed Leydig cell system, remains the standard of reference. They contributed to the understanding of gonadotropin binding, initiation of adenylate cyclase activity, GnRH activation of gonadotropin release, and angiotensin action at the receptor level. They developed the concept of spare receptors and demonstrated that receptors could be transferred from testis to ovary and remain active.

In his NIADDK laboratory, Ed Rall formed a new group, with VERA NIKODEM and MARK MAGNUSON working on the mechanism of action of thyroid hormone. In the initial phase, they succeeded in cloning the gene for malic enzyme, a liver protease responsive to thyroid hormone.

Epilogue

The fabric of endocrinology at NIH that we have described is interwoven with contributions from most of the Institutes. Given the number and preparation of NIH intramural trainees and their worldwide dissemination, the product is indeed far greater than the sum of its parts. We have attempted to show how the wise selection of scientists with an inclination to study various aspects of the discipline has created a dynamic core from which important scientific accomplishments have issued. Individuals and groups are free to pursue their own special interests, even if these seem to overlap. Actually, there has been little true redundancy, reflecting the innate tendency of good scientists to avoid repetition and explore new ground. Emphasis on quality of the people and evaluation of their work ensure that endocrinology at NIH will continue to be an invaluable national resource.

Introduction

SPECTROSCOPY AND CHEMICAL PHYSICS

Almost all portions of the electromagnetic spectrum serve the biologist, the biochemist, the biophysicist, or the physician at one time or another. This brings into play a wide diversity of instruments and of persons skilled in their use. The mission of NIH is predominantly to explore the biological world, so the development of new optical and other instruments is essential. If our investment in this effort is small compared, for instance, with that of the National Bureau of Standards, we have nonetheless a distinguished record of accomplishments in such areas as X-ray crystallography, electron microscopy, nuclear magnetic resonance (NMR) spectroscopy, and tomographic scanning, as in positron emission tomography (PET).

Over the past few years, it has been particularly interesting to observe the movement of some of this sophisticated technology from the laboratory to the clinic. It appears at this time that future diagnostic procedures will draw heavily on laboratory developments, especially in the field of PET scanning and NMR. At such points in the history of science, the advantages of NIH, with its relatively close wedding between the basic research laboratory and the clinic, become most obvious.

The succeeding pages recount a number of NIH developments in the general area of spectroscopy. Besides the instruments and the results they have produced, I find some of the associated individuals to be of particular interest. One of the most colorful is FREDERICK BRACKETT, who was the first to photograph the solar spectrum in the infrared region of 900 to 960 nm, at Mount Wilson Observatory. He then went on to discover in 1921, while still quite young, a series of lines in the spectrum of hydrogen atoms that is known throughout the world as the Brackett series.

Brackett's discoveries must have created a stir in the world of astronomy, but as far as I am aware these were his last ventures in that field. He carried out innovative laboratory research in spectroscopy and then turned his attention to matters of photobiology, such as the absorption of light by chloroplasts, the chlorophyll-containing particles in green leaves.

Then, a few years ago, we succeeded in sending cameras to the moon and, for the first time, were able to map its entire surface. By tradition, craters on the moon are named after dead astronomers, but the craters proved to be very numerous while dead astronomers are relatively scarce. Finally someone recalled the name of Brackett, who had not published in astronomy for 50 years and was therefore presumed dead. A handsome crater was named for all time Brackett Crater. This is the only crater on the moon named for a nonastronomer or a living scientist. We at NIH take some satisfaction from this high honor.

D. S.

22

SPECTROSCOPY AND CHEMICAL PHYSICS

Edwin D. Becker

Norman E. Sharpless

In this chapter we examine the role of some aspects of physics and physical chemistry in the development of the NIH intramural program. NIH is renowned primarily for its work in biology and medicine. In the purely physical sciences, it may never achieve the prominence of such institutions as the National Bureau of Standards or Bell Laboratories. But its scientists have made, and continue to make, significant advances in chemical physics. More important, however, has been the development of new physical techniques at NIH and the introduction of the physical scientist's rigorous thinking into the milieu of biological applications.

Two recent examples illustrate the importance of the physicochemical approach to biological problems. Since the 1950s sickle cell disease has been recognized as resulting from the substitution of a single amino acid in hemoglobin, the oxygen-bearing protein of blood. This fact has provided guidance for hundreds of investigations into the mechanism by which the aberrant erythrocytes (red blood cells) assume their characteristic crescent shape. During the last few years, WILLIAM EATON, JAMES HOFRICHTER, and PHILIP ROSS have made an important advance in understanding the disease and perhaps in treating it.

They observed a substantial delay time between the deoxygenation of sickle cell hemoglobin (Hb-S) and the onset of a rapid polymerization of this protein. Careful study of the kinetics of the polymerization process revealed that the delay time is critically dependent on hemoglobin concentra-

EDWIN D. BECKER, Ph.D., Associate Director for Research Services, National Institutes of Health, and Chief, Nuclear Magnetic Resonance Section, Laboratory of Chemical Physics, National Institute of Arthritis, Diabetes, and Digestive and Kidney Diseases. NORMAN E. SHARPLESS, Ph.D., Research Physical Chemist, Laboratory of Chemical Physics, NIADDK.

tion, temperature, and pH. If the delay could be lengthened somewhat—say, by appropriate drug therapy—there would be a greater likelihood that erythrocytes could pass through small capillaries without sickling, hence without initiating a "sickle cell crisis." Such a result would not actually cure the disease, but might prevent its serious consequences. The physicochemical contributions here lie both in the formulation of the kinetic hypothesis and in the development of methods for in vitro testing of possible therapeutic agents by comparing the changes they induce in delay time. [See Section V of chapter entitled "Genetic Diseases."]

This work on sickle cell disease was not the first time that physical methods had been applied to the problem at NIH. In the 1960s MAKIO MURAYAMA and collaborators made detailed studies of the effects of pressure and magnetic field on the polymerization process and used optical spectroscopy to investigate the organization of the polymer.

A recent advance has been made by DENNIS TORCHIA, ALAN SCHECHTER, and their collaborators, applying nuclear magnetic resonance (NMR) to assess the amount of Hb-S that has polymerized within the erythrocyte. This NMR work draws on the most advanced technology developed for the study of solids.

A second example stems from the work of WILLIAM HAGINS and his collaborators, who are engaged in an elucidation of the molecular and ionic processes in vision. These investigators made crucial deductions on the photochemical quantum yield of the visual process by careful analysis of the noise accompanying electrical signals in retinal rods when absorbing electromagnetic radiation. This information, together with quantitative measurements of electrical currents from the retinal cell membranes in the dark and in light, has led to our present understanding of the critical role of cytoplasmic calcium ions as the sensory transmitters.

Origins

How did the disciplines of physical science make their way into what was once an entirely classical biological and medical research laboratory?

Physics and physical chemistry have a long history at NIH, as it was recognized very early that biology was directly associated with chemistry and physics and that indeed many biological problems were essentially chemical. In the early 1920s the Division of Chemistry of the Hygienic Laboratory, forerunner of NIH, conducted a series of studies on electrode potentials in oxidation-reduction systems, following earlier published observations in bacteria. [See reference to WILLIAM MANSFIELD CLARK on first page of Witkop chapter.]

In the 1930s the Division of Industrial Hygiene (DIH) established laboratories at NIH to investigate health hazards in industry. The causes of many industrial sicknesses are subtle, and new and sophisticated techniques were required. The problems were met by a fortunate meld of medicine, engineering, and chemistry. For example, detection of small amounts of lead, arsenic, and other heavy metals required emission spectroscopy; determination of ultraviolet hazards utilized sensitive radiation detectors; and demonstration of free silica (the cause of silicosis) in rocks and dusts employed X-ray diffraction.

The director of DIH, ROYD R. SAYERS, had long recognized that only basic research could answer many of the questions raised by the industrial hygienist. To provide a nucleus for the necessary work in basic biophysics, he offered laboratory space to the Washington Biophysical Institute. WBI eagerly accepted the offer, and most of its personnel were later incorporated into the Civil Service. Among these was WBI's director, FREDERICK S. BRACKETT.

Brackett was one of the first to use the newer available techniques and instruments, many of which he designed himself. A well-known physicist when he came to NIH, notably for his discovery of the Brackett series in the spectrum of hydrogen (1921), he expanded and developed techniques in ultraviolet and infrared spectroscopy and furthered the design of spectroscopic instrumentation.

Brackett worked on the recording and evaluation of ultraviolet levels in sunlight, creating, in collaboration with the Westinghouse Laboratories, an integrating cell that was unusually accurate and stable. He achieved prominence also through the development of double-beam infrared spectrometers. Modern spectrometers use double-beam optics exclusively. Brackett was also interested in photochemistry and photobiology. In conjunction with PETER COLE, he investigated the conversion of ergosterol to calciferol (vitamin D) as a function of the wavelength of the exciting light. This required design and construction of a double monochromator, containing the world's largest natural quartz prisms, for the excitation and analysis of samples by photographic absorption spectrophotometry.

There were fruitful offshoots of these programs. RODNEY OLSON investigated photosynthesis. ALEXANDER HOLLAENDER studied the wavelength dependence of radiation in biology (using microorganisms), and Peter Cole developed its logical sequel, ultraviolet microscopy. Using quartz optics microscopes with light at various wavelengths, Cole obtained photomicrographs that gave clues, through differential absorption, to the chemical composition of various regions in unicellular organisms.

In the early 1940s, politics intervened. DIH was split over results of an investigation into the hazards of lead arsenate in the apple industry in Washington State. The purely industrial hygiene functions, with medical and engineering personnel (field investigations, plant surveys, etc.), were transferred to Cincinnati, and the laboratory research functions stayed at NIH as the Industrial Hygiene Research Laboratory. The director, PAUL A. NEAL, who had headed laboratory research in DIH, planned to lead the new laboratory into high-quality basic research by building on existing expertise.

During World War II the many war-related interests of NIH included the toxicity and pharmacology of DDT. X-ray powder diffraction was used to identify the first known metabolite of DDT in warm-blooded animals, bis(p-chlorophenyl) acetic acid.

The advent of the atomic bomb, the availability of radioactive tracers, and the increased use of X-rays necessitated investigation of both the biophysical aspects and the health hazards of ionizing radiation. This line of research, which began in the late 1940s, was organized and led by HOWARD L. ANDREWS. It included studies of dosimetry and basic radiation physics, as well as the beginnings of radiochemistry as applied to amino acids, proteins, and living organisms.

These studies were organized on the basis of increasing complexity of the substrate. CHARLES MAXWELL and NORMAN SHARPLESS investigated amino acids, and WILLIAM CARROLL investigated proteins and thymus gland extracts. GILBERT ASHWELL studied the effects of radiation on mouse spleens, specifically phosphorylation ratios. This led to the discovery of ribose phosphate, an intermediate in carbohydrate metabolism. [See Horecker section in chapter entitled "Development of Enzymology."]

Brackett's genius in instrumental design was tapped by the Army Air Corps during World War II, when he was asked to design a simulated bombsight to train student bombardiers. Working with LAWRENCE CRISP in what is now the Biomedical Engineering and Instrumentation Branch, Division of Research Services, Brackett designed a suitable instrument, only to have the drawings confiscated by the FBI. They said he had discovered the principle of the Norden bombsight, one of America's top-secret weapons during the war. Undaunted, Brackett and Crisp made new drawings and constructed the simulator. Brackett recalls that working bombardiers praised it, reporting that it gave them the "feel" of a real bombing run, but some high-ranking officers found it too difficult to use. Brackett responded by making two models, one for the students and a simpler one for the generals.

RALPH W. G. WYCKOFF was already well known as a crystal

chemist when he came to NIH in 1945, and his book *The Structure of Crystals* was a classic. Although he continued his
research in X-ray diffraction here, he worked primarily on
electron microscopy. He was among the first to define the
structure of viruses and to visualize them within diseased
tissues. Much of his work in electron microscopy was done in
collaboration with DAVID SCOTT, later to be Director of the
National Institute of Dental Research.

Before the establishment of the National Science Foundation in 1950, the support of basic science depended largely
on mission-oriented Federal agencies. Perhaps the area of
research at NIH that was least relevant to health, yet of
substantial scientific interest, was the study of cosmic rays.
HERMAN YAGODA, who had worked at NIH as an analytical chemist
in toxicologic research, became interested immediately after
World War II in the measurement of radioactive particles in
photographic emulsions. With the advent of NIH investigation
into the health effects of high-energy radiation, Yagoda became an international authority on the detection of high-
energy particles. During the 1950s he sent specially designed
photographic plates on some of the early high-altitude balloon
and rocket flights and analyzed the nuclear reactions induced
by cosmic rays, at that time the only source of sufficient
energy to initiate such "events."

A Period of Rapid Expansion

Through expansion of the field, the terms *spectroscopy* and
spectrometry now cover a broad range of techniques, having in
common the identification and measurement of substances by
examining their characteristic spectra of absorbed or emitted
energy. In the decade from the mid 1950s to the mid 1960s, a
period of rapid growth for NIH coincided with this expansion
of interest in spectroscopy of various types.

Brackett's continuing influence was strong in attracting
both senior scientists and young investigators who were destined to play leading roles in later NIH research. In 1955
URNER LIDDEL joined Brackett's Section. He had pioneered in
infrared spectroscopic investigations of hydrogen bonding,
then had turned to the administration of nuclear physics programs in the Office of Naval Research. At NIH, again investigating hydrogen bonding by infrared spectroscopy, he perceived the advantages of using the emerging technique of
nuclear magnetic resonance (see below).

In 1955-1956 two young infrared spectroscopists, EDWIN D.
BECKER and ELLIOT CHARNEY, joined the group. Both contributed
to the advance of vibrational spectroscopy, especially in

clarifying anomalies in the spectrum and structure of *p*-benzo-quinone and related molecules.

A few years later IRA W. LEVIN joined the Section and made substantial advances in the understanding of vibrational spectra and force fields in small molecules. Some years later, taking advantage of progress in infrared and Raman spectroscopy, Levin applied knowledge gleaned from the study of such small molecules to phospholipid bilayers and biological membranes. The infrared and Raman spectra provide sensitive probes of bilayer reorganizations and conformational changes in lipid chains.

With the formation of NIAMD's Laboratory of Molecular Biology in 1962, H. TODD MILES began a long, comprehensive, and productive spectroscopic investigation of synthetic and natural polynucleotides. In order to use infrared spectroscopy, Miles developed elegant methods for studying samples in aqueous solutions (principally D_2O), despite the prevailing opinion that infrared spectra could not be obtained in aqueous solvents.

Other early physicochemical studies at NIH focused on the analysis of electronic spectra, both absorption and emission (fluorescence). [The role of fluorescence spectroscopy in biochemistry is mentioned in the Witkop chapter.] Absorption spectra in the visible and ultraviolet regions are widely used for analytic purposes, but the work of DAN F. BRADLEY in the 1950s illustrates the use of the methods in a more fundamental way to characterize molecular structure and interactions. Bradley and his co-workers explained how certain dyes intercalate into nucleic acids. Bradley and HOWARD DeVOE were the first at NIH to use quantum mechanical methods in a sophisticated and systematic way to relate molecular structure and spectra to electronic properties of molecules. Electronic spectroscopy continues to be a key method at NIH for the study of molecular structure, with much of the work depending on modern high-technology methods of the sort seldom found in other biomedical research laboratories. RUTH McDIARMID is using a molecular beam apparatus with laser-induced multiphoton detection to study electronic spectra of molecules that are isolated from one another and cooled to only a few degrees Kelvin. Meanwhile, Hofrichter and Eaton have developed a novel pulsed laser spectrometer to study spectra and kinetics in the nanosecond range.

The Study of Chiroptical* Phenomena

As molecular structures were probed ever deeper, the factor of molecular dissymmetry was recognized as biologically important. At NIH, optical activity measurements probably started with CLAUDE HUDSON, working in what is now the Laboratory of Chemistry, NIADDK [see Witkop]. "Hudson's Rules," formulated in 1909, showed that the rotatory contribution of the asymmetric carbon-1 in sugars is unaffected by structural changes in the rest of the molecule unless they are on contiguous atoms.

Rotations were usually measured at the sodium D line, a convenient wavelength, since it could be generated easily by placing a crystal of salt on the grid of a Meeker burner. This spectral line, however, is in a region in which most organic compounds are quite transparent, and thus its usefulness to many molecular symmetry problems is limited. Another limitation of the single line is that one cannot make use of information from the rotatory dispersion—i.e., the wavelength dependence of the rotation.

Optical rotation in a molecule arises from the difference in refractive index of the substance between right and left circularly polarized light. Since refractive index is a function of wavelength, the rotation is also. The resulting plot of rotation vs. wavelength is the rotatory dispersion curve. The analogous effect wherein a difference occurs in the absorption of left and right circularly polarized light (circular dichroism) also yields data that can be used to elucidate the structure of biologically active molecules with the proper dissymmetry.

The basic theory of optical rotatory dispersion as applied to biological systems was originally set forth by William Moffitt and Albert Moskowitz. In collaboration with Moskowitz, ULRICH WEISS, HERMAN ZIFFER, and Elliot Charney at NIH extended the theory to conjugated systems. They also demonstrated its applicability to real systems, especially to the optical rotatory dispersion of dienes (unsaturated hydrocarbons containing two double bonds). One initial delay in the application of theory to experiment was the lack of suitable instrumentation. The initial work in the Laboratory of Physical Biology utilized an accessory specially made by the Perkin-Elmer Corp. to be grafted onto a Cary spectrometer. Meanwhile, the Rudolph Instrument Engineering Co. designed and built for H. K. MILLER, in the Laboratory of Chemistry, the

---

*From Greek *cheir*, hand + optical: optical rotation: right or left rotation of polarized light in passing through optically active substances.

first recording spectropolarimeter. This was the forerunner of many commercial instruments.

Optical rotatory dispersion has been particularly fruitful when applied to nucleic acids and proteins and to the binding of dyes to such macromolecules. Charney and K. YAMAOKA investigated the electric dichroism of dyes bound to various macromolecules in solution, giving insights into drug action.

Nuclear Magnetic Resonance

An excellent example of the interplay at NIH of physical methods and biomedical problems is seen in the development of nuclear magnetic resonance. First discovered in 1946, NMR became of interest to chemists in 1951 with the discovery of the chemical shift. By 1956 Brackett and others at NIH were at work on an incipient instrumental development in NMR, and Liddel had published an article pointing out the potentialities of NMR in the study of hydrogen bonding. Becker was dispatched to California to visit the sole manufacturer of NMR apparatus and assess its utility for NIH's needs. His glowing reports, supported by data (obtained in two days of work) for a paper on hydrogen bonding of ethanol, convinced DeWITT STETTEN, then Scientific Director of NIAMD, that the Institute should invest in this new tool. At $30,000 in 1956 dollars, the 40 MHz NMR spectrometer was the most expensive instrument the Institute had ever purchased.

Becker, as NIH's "expert" (after a week's experience with NMR), was assigned responsibility for NMR development, along with his infrared spectroscopic studies. In a series of collaborations with organic chemists, he assisted in the elucidation of several molecular structures and developed new insights into the correlations of NMR spectra and molecular configuration. He and his colleagues reported the first NMR spectra of porphyrins and were among the first to study ^{15}N NMR by double resonance methods.

In the late 1960s, NMR underwent a major advance. The introduction of Fourier transform methods* greatly increased the versatility and rapidity with which NMR data could be obtained. Becker began a close collaboration with Thomas C. Farrar at the National Bureau of Standards (NBS). Farrar had developed instrumentation for high-power pulse NMR, a key ingredient in the development of a Fourier transform spectrometer. They concentrated on the study of ^{13}C NMR with several

---

*Computerized application of Fourier series—infinite series of sine and cosine functions used to fit a given set of known constants.

collaborators, including REGITZE R. SHOUP, a postdoctoral
fellow; STEPHEN DRUCK, a graduate student doing his Ph.D.
dissertation with Becker; and JAMES A. FERRETTI of the Division of Computer Research and Technology (DCRT).

The potential for organic structural studies was enormous, but the low NMR sensitivity of ^{13}C, along with its relative scarcity in nature (1.1 percent natural abundance), presented formidable obstacles. The initial experiments were primitive and tedious: Data were recorded on a time-averaging device at NBS, transferred to paper tape, and analyzed in a DCRT computer. Nevertheless, these experiments demonstrated the feasibility of the approach, and their fundamental data on relaxation mechanisms for ^{13}C contributed to the rapid advance of studies in the field. Farrar and Becker's introductory book *Pulse and Fourier Transform NMR* provided a primer on the new technology for a generation of graduate students and post-doctorals in magnetic resonance and chemistry.

With the commercial development of Fourier transform instruments and the rapid improvement in magnets, solid state electronics, and dedicated minicomputers, NMR has become in the last decade an essential tool in biochemical studies. From one 40 MHz spectrometer in 1957, NIH's complement of NMR instruments has grown to more than 20 in 1983, ranging up to 500 MHz. Incidentally, the magnet purchased in 1957 as part of the first instrument is still in use. Current applications range from elucidation of organic and inorganic structures to studies of conformation in enzymes and nucleic acids to investigations of metabolic processes in living cells and organs. Since 1974 Dennis Torchia has been among the pioneers in applying to biopolymers many of the sophisticated new NMR methods for the study of solids.

Finally, an exciting development of the last decade is the use of NMR to obtain two- or three-dimensional images of human and animal subjects. This method is already rivaling or surpassing X-ray CT (computerized tomography) scanning. DAVID I. HOULT, who came from Oxford University to the Division of Research Services in 1979, developed much of the fundamental physics in the field and built an imaging device for small animals (see figure). A commercial NMR imaging device is now part of the Diagnostic Radiology Department in the Clinical Center. As NMR imaging and related methods for studying metabolic processes in human subjects are widely implemented at NIH, the whole array of NMR methods previously used only in the laboratory is becoming of direct clinical relevance.

Electron paramagnetic resonance (EPR) is closely related to NMR phenomenologically, but applications of EPR range widely, from the study of paramagnetic ions and unstable free

radical intermediates to that of molecular mobility by means
of stable free radical "spin labels." Although EPR studies at
NIH were begun by Becker in 1958 as an adjunct to the NMR program, the development of the technique here has largely been
in the hands of HIDEO KON, who came to NIH in 1963. He has
contributed principally to the understanding of heme proteins
through studies of ^{57}Fe-substituted hemes, nitrosyl-liganded
iron (II) porphyrin complexes, and iron (III) in cytochrome
P-450. Kon used spin label studies to investigate the defor-
mation of red blood cells, while COLIN CHIGNELL and others
have applied such studies to elucidate membrane structure and
function. PETER RIESZ and his collaborators have used EPR in
extensive studies of free radicals arising from the action
of high-energy radiation.

Laboratory Computers

Almost all instruments for measurement of spectra and
other physical properties now incorporate sophisticated computers. The computer has affected all research at NIH in major
ways, and our scientists have contributed to the revolution.
A scant 20 years ago computers were still large, complex, and
located usually in a central facility. In the late 1950s
Frederick Brackett foresaw the impact that computers would
soon have on the processing of data from spectrometers and
other laboratory apparatus. At a time when data were being
recorded in digital form on cumbersome and unreliable paper
tape, Brackett pioneered in the development of methods to
digitize data on magnetic tape in a format that could be interpreted by the central computer (then a Honeywell 800).
The techniques had an impact on commercial computer interfaces
for spectrometers. Subsequent developments at NIH, particularly by the Computer Systems Laboratory of DCRT, provided
improved networks for acquiring and processing data in a computer hierarchy. [See Pratt, "Computers in Biomedical Research."]

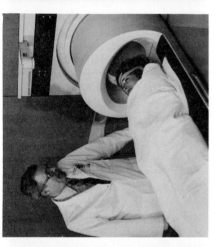

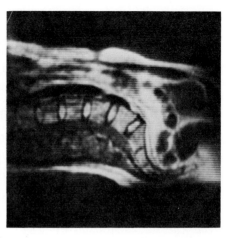

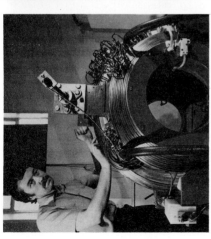

NUCLEAR MAGNETIC RESONANCE serves as an aid to diagnosis of structural and functional abnormalities. NMR permits effects of a magnetic field on atomic nuclei of tissue components to be analyzed and imaged by means of a computer. It does not depend on density, can penetrate all tissues, and is believed to be harmless. Left: DAVID I. HOULT, physicist in the Division of Research Services, adjusts NMR apparatus of his own design. Center: JOHN L. DOPPMAN, Chief of the Clinical Center's Diagnostic Radiology Department, prepares a patient for NMR examination. Right: computer images of 10-mm sagittal sections of (1) head, showing cerebral cortex, brain stem, cerebellum, spinal cord, etc.; and (2) spine, showing vertebral bodies, disks, cross-sections of muscles, etc. With such instruments, it is also possible to study metabolic processes in the heart, liver, and other organs.

COMPUTERS IN BIOMEDICAL RESEARCH

The management of data and other information has passed through many epochs, each of which is associated with a particular type of device. Commencing in the fifteenth century with the introduction of movable type and the printing press, there followed the typewriter, disk and tape recorders, automatic copying devices, calculators, and finally the modern computer with its capacity to process both words and numbers with extreme rapidity. Meanwhile, biomedical science developed from a descriptive science to a quantitative one, and with increased automation the bulk of data that can be collected in a short time has grown enormously.

Early in the development of the computer, JAMES A. SHANNON, then Director of NIH, clearly recognized that computer technology and the biomedical sciences would inevitably come together. In order to further this major development, the Division of Computer Research and Technology (DCRT) was established in April 1964. ARNOLD (Scotty) PRATT has been its only Director. Here he summarizes highlights of its history.

An important byproduct of this revolutionary technology has been the field of computer graphics: the generation of a picture on an oscilloscope screen by means of an appropriate computer. Applying methods developed at DCRT, RICHARD FELDMANN and associates have depicted startlingly realistic models of protein and other molecules wherein each atom is represented by a distinctively colored ball. A selection of such photographs depicting biological macromolecules discussed in this volume may be seen in the frontispiece. It should be understood that these are not photographs of solid molecular models, but rather of fluorescent images generated by feeding physicochemical measurements into a computer. Such pictures are particularly instructive to scientists working at the molecular level.

D. S.

23

COMPUTERS IN BIOMEDICAL RESEARCH

Arnold W. Pratt

The Beginnings of Computer Science

During the past four decades, man's intellectual curiosity has increasingly focused on information—both its nature and its utilization. "Information theory" was a topic of lively discussion and debate immediately after World War II. One recalls that the physicists and mathematicians were the more active participants in these exchanges. But they were by no means alone in expressing this early interest. Attendance at the First International Conference on Information Theory held in London in 1950 was drawn broadly from across science. Included were physiologists, geneticists, mathematicians, physicists, engineers, linguists, anthropologists, and others. The consensus was that important aspects of each discipline were fundamentally dependent on the processing of information.

The advent of the digital computer introduced a most powerful means of contemplating the general concept and specific subject matter of information and information theory. The digital computer is an information machine. This well-known class of machines includes switching circuits, telephone exchanges, missile guidance systems, and so forth. Most of these are special-purpose in the nature of their functions—that is, limited to specific calculations; but the digital computer is capable of a wide variety of calculations and thus may be called a general-purpose machine. Information machines have played an important role in nearly all aspects of human life. As a consequence, there has always been a strong motivation to explore their theoretical and pragmatic bases. Computer science is derivative of these interdisciplinary studies.

The science is not alone in its dependence on a particular instrument or device. Astronomy comes to mind, as do radiology and crystallography among others. And just as astronomers may pursue theoretical studies that do not require a telescope,

ARNOLD W. PRATT, M.D., Director, Division of Computer Research and Technology.

NIH: AN ACCOUNT OF RESEARCH
IN ITS LABORATORIES AND CLINICS

ISBN 0-12-667980-0

the computer scientist can readily engage in research efforts that do not require a computer directly. Whether present-day theoretical research, however, could in any final sense be fully described by the computer scientist (or the astronomer) without access to a digital computer may be left an open question.

Computer science has evolved from three disciplines: engineering, mathematics, and formal linguistics. There is general agreement that

- Turing's work in mathematical logic in the early 1930s led to the discovery of fundamental limitations on mechanical computation and thus provided the mathematical beginnings of computer science.

- The engineering component of computer science emerged with Claude Shannon's demonstration in 1938 that the functions of relay switching networks could be represented in the symbolic notation of Boolean algebra.

- The linguistic contribution to computer science came from Chomsky's specification of formal grammars and language in the 1950s, which in turn provided computer scientists with the basis for developing artificial (programming) languages.

There is now an extensive computer science literature, rich in subject matter, that is both instructive and challenging to students and scientists alike.

As in the case of any science, computer science looks to underlying principles and basic knowledge. The major subdisciplines may be specified and defined as follows:

- Numerical mathematics: study and development of digital machine techniques for evaluating mathematical problems.

- Computer programming languages: generation of formal, artificial languages suitable and sufficient for human beings to communicate with digital computers. Well-known examples are FORTRAN, COBOL, PL1, etc.

- Information storage and retrieval: development of efficient methods for the capture, storage, retrieval, and reporting of alphanumeric (alphabetical and numerical) data and of images.

- Automata theory: abstract study and explication of the

capabilities of computers, typically studies in attempting to define machinery by designating input signals and in turn calculating the probabilities of obtaining desired output signals, given some specified but usually abstract machine.

- Logical design: investigation of methods and strategies for converting original conceptions of machines such as cars, boats, rockets, and computers into objects, as well as their actual design.

- Programming systems and systems architecture: development and description of systems programs that make possible man-machine and machine-machine communications.

Some writers on computer science enjoy pointing out (tongue-in-cheek, one suspects) that the abacus was the first digital computing instrument. Recall that the abacus was invented in the Orient at some early time and introduced into Europe in the Middle Ages. The notion that the abacus is an early relative of the digital computer is generally assessed as superficial and false. Behind this is the concept that some degree of automatism is fundamental to digital computers. The abacus has no potential for automation short of a drastic redesign with resulting loss of most of its basic characteristics.

Pascal, the distinguished French mathematician, is said to have invented the first digital computer in 1642. He built a mechanical calculating device that did addition and subtraction. In the latter part of the seventeenth century, Leibniz extended Pascal's invention to do multiplication and division. The work of Pascal and Leibniz demonstrated the first important principle of automatic digital computation: that the operations of arithmetic could be mechanized.

Further development of the emerging computer languished until an English mathematician, Charles Babbage, built a "Difference Engine" in 1822. This machine was devised for the purpose of computing mathematical tables—for example, tables of logarithms, which in those days were done by hand and riddled with error. It is not clear that Babbage ever produced a routinely functioning Difference Engine, but the evidence strongly suggests that there was a working model and that some tables were calculated by machine.

Roughly a decade later, Babbage introduced the revolutionary notion of an "Analytical Engine." He made complete drawings and even built some parts. The machine was never finished because the technology of the times could not produce the needed assembly of intricate gears, levers, sensors, etc. The drawings, however, clearly established the revolutionary nature of the concept involved. The machine was conceived as a general purpose calculator, a "programmable" instrument that could perform strings of arithmetic and decision operations without manual intervention. Babbage's proposal was to feed instructions and data to the machine in the form of a punched card, which was widely used to control looms. Clearly, Babbage was a man of extraordinary vision who appeared well before his time.

Between Babbage and the third generation of electronic digital computers, which appeared in 1963-1964, were two landmark innovations. In 1937 Howard Aiken of Harvard University proposed the development of an automatic general-purpose digital computer. Mark I, an automatic sequence-controlled calculator developed by IBM, was completed in 1944. It was the largest electromechanical computer ever built. The first digital electronic computer, ENIAC (Electronic Numerical Integrator and Calculator), was completed in 1946 by J. Presper Eckert and John W. Mauchly at the University of Pennsylvania. It used 18,000 vacuum tubes and required rewiring to change programs, a first-generation machine. It was developed for the Army's Ballistic Research Laboratories at Aberdeen, Maryland.

NIH Enters the Field

The National Institutes of Health came latterly to the new world of machine-based data processing. A central data-processing facility was established in 1954. It comprised solely electrical accounting machinery (EAM), traditionally referred to as "punch card equipment." The machines and 22 employees were established in approximately 5000 square feet of space in Building 12. Dedication of such a large area to a nonresearch enterprise drew grumbles from senior NIH staff, but the fact is that the space was unsatisfactory for human occupancy and remained essentially so for the better part of two decades. The building was located near the balky NIH incinerator and directly on the downwind side of some inlet pipes for large gasoline storage tanks, and our building's ventilation system drew efficiently on both these sources of environmental pollution. Lighting a match at one's desk on gasoline delivery day, with our exchange system frequently belching finely charred particulate matter, challenged even the most intrepid souls. Besides, data processing and computation were conducted immediately below the monkey quarters and mouse production areas, and animal odors often permeated the building. On any given Monday morning, it was often necessary for the staff to make a new commitment to self and country. Attainment of standards for human occupancy had to await the tenure of Secretary Elliott Richardson (1970-1973), who reacted vigorously after a public confrontation with a frustrated, exasperated employee who feared for her life and that of her fellow workers.

The EAM was placed initially under HAROLD DORN, who welded his small group of biometricians and the production staff into a cohesive, efficient group. Card processing was done well at NIH; epidemiologists and administrators prospered. Dorn's original and important studies on the association between lung cancer and cigarette smoking were EAM products. But the facility expanded rapidly as more card-processing tasks materialized, to the point where the capability was inundated and had to be augmented by a true digital computer.

In 1958 NIH acquired an IBM 650. The machine, to be sure, was less than state-of-the-art, but it had proved itself. It was a reliable computer and relatively easy to understand. As a "decimal" machine, it retained, as one wag put it, a proper respect for the human being's comprehension of the base-10 number system. It was not one of those newer, ugly machines that performed arithmetic and other symbol-processing tasks in the binary (base 2), octal (base 8), or hexadecimal (base 16) system.

The initial NIH venture into digital computing was tentative and exploratory. Many senior scientists openly questioned the value of computing in their programs. These attitudes were heard and only partially discounted by the NIH leadership, and the provision of resources to the new trans-NIH scientific enterprise was marginal at best. It is not surprising that in the years immediately after 1958, NIH digital computing was turbulent if not chaotic. The central facility was chronically short of materiel and personnel to meet the burgeoning workload. As a consequence, the users were frequently dissatisfied and discouraged with the services. But somehow the turbulence of those early days was resolved, correctly or otherwise. A major factor was the intense effort of individuals across the NIH community to develop competence in the use of the facilities. This phase may have been disorganized and very much "by-one's-bootstraps," but it was typical NIH—and effective.

By late 1959 the machine's impending saturation was obvious and all too soon became distressingly real. New capacity was needed. A Honeywell H-800 computer with substantially greater capacity than the IBM 650 was installed in 1961. Within 4 months the new computer was in operation 20 hours a day 5 days a week and some 20 to 28 hours each weekend. The capacity shortage continued, and in early 1963 a second large

Honeywell H-800 machine/system was installed. But again work-load saturation could be readily foreseen. NIH leaders con-tracted with the National Bureau of Standards for a task force to conduct a study with a view to recommending an equipment configuration that could meet the burgeoning NIH demand. While the NBS task force failed to produce useful equipment specifi-cations, it did perform an important service. In the course of their study, the members interviewed most of the NIH sci-entists and administrators who were getting involved in com-putation and data processing. Thus there emerged a most con-vincing testimony in support of the need for a computer-based data processing competence at NIH.

The NIH Steering Committee

In May 1962 NIH Director JAMES A. SHANNON appointed a steering committee to examine NIH needs, current and future, for automatic data processing (ADP). This action was supported broadly among NIH leaders. The committee membership included representatives from major program areas. After months of thoughtful discussion, interviews with users, site visits to installations both in and out of government—in short, what amounted to an intensive education of the committee members about ADP and about NIH needs—they reached a large area of agreement and finally a consensus. They had done their work well. A clear position on ADP at NIH had been delineated and choices specified. Special credit for the committee's work must be accorded the chairman, THOMAS J. KENNEDY, Jr. Gregarious by nature, Kennedy could be effectively friendly or threatening to committee members and witnesses alike, and his control of any gathering was excellent. He was intellec-tually perceptive and highly articulate. And he enjoyed the full confidence of the NIH leadership.

The steering committee's basic convictions about a suc-cessful computing enterprise at NIH can be readily recaptured by reproducing parts of their summary report:

> The Committee was deeply impressed by the power of this ADP technology and the promise it holds for con-tribution to a new level of insight into problems in the life sciences. It was equally impressed by the magnitude of the resources, fiscal but especially intellectual, that its large-scale applications de-manded.
>
> Computer technology represents a new and extraordi-narily powerful tool within the universe of science.

Applications in the physical sciences and engineering contrast with those in the life sciences in terms of the nature of the problems, the ease with which they lend themselves to mathematical formulation, the mathematical background of users, the essentiality of the methodology to the work, and the "style" of the applications. Comparatively speaking, biological problems are more difficult to formulate in mathematical terms.

Computer and data processing technology will continue to be highly dynamic and be extended rapidly to many fields of endeavor. Machines will be marketed that will store and manipulate data more efficiently and at lower costs per unit of computation. But the sophistication in software will continue to lag far behind the sophistication in hardware, and significant shortages in expert manpower will also continue.

The committee delineated carefully the complex nature of the "problem-mix" of the NIH workload:

A large number of business or administrative procedures amenable to automation.

The needs of the NIH to automate the processing of information on its extramural awards programs in the interest of efficient paper processing, report generation, etc.; substantive analysis to maintain conceptual control over the scientific content of the total support effort; and identification of trends in program evolution.

The increasing number of large-scale biometric and epidemiological studies.

The growing concern with the problems surrounding the management of scientific and technical information to provide the scientific community with better and more timely information services.

The wide spectrum of applications arising from intramural research programs which include, among others, problems in equation solving, model building, model testing, statistical analysis and computation, pattern recognition, vector analysis, simulation, curve analysis, and many others.

The committee commented:

> In-house competence to deal with technological de-
> velopments in this field would offer this institution
> a tremendous number of opportunities to extend the
> frontline of biomedical investigations. . . . To
> realize the anticipated needs with as little confusion
> as possible will require full-time, expert guidance,
> dynamic policy formulation and execution, flexible
> fiscal support mechanisms, and encouragement from the
> high-level administrative echelon of the NIH.

The committee concluded after intensive study:

> Previously the NIH has limited its commitment in this
> area of technology to providing ADP services. Full
> realization of the potentiality of the new method,
> however, will require a broader horizon. An array of
> scientific talent competent in mathematics, mathemat-
> ical statistics, computer science, programming, com-
> puter systems design and engineering, data systems
> analysis and design, and information sciences will
> have to be embedded in the NIH direct operation if
> progress commensurate with promise is to occur. To
> attract such talent, the organization of a viable re-
> search and development program is essential. This
> leads to the recommendation that a "Division of Com-
> puter and Information Sciences" be activated.
>
> The Division will conduct research, development and
> demonstrations programs in mathematical and computer
> sciences . . . ; will seek to create a climate to
> facilitate the permeation of its expertise into other
> biomedical sciences; will provide the leadership to
> make available resources . . . for a vigorous pro-
> gram; and will ensure access to computation and data
> processing services of high quality.

Other conclusions concerned financing and implementation of
the new programs and recommended that a separate appropriation
be considered.

Shannon accepted the steering committee's report with appreciation and praise but not much initial comment. It turns
out that he pondered at some length the report's main thrust:
the need for a new division of computer science. Shannon's
usual method of assessment was to contact directly any col-

leagues, friends, or strangers who had intelligence on the
subject matter; and he assessed the new proposal in typical
fashion.

Birth of DCRT

The profile and biography of Jim Shannon at NIH will have
to be written by others. Suffice it to say here that he was
a complex mixture of impulse, logic, and emotion. Certainly
he was a good scientist and an extraordinarily effective and
dedicated administrator. We know that he respected the power
and day-by-day realities of the legislative and executive components of the Federal establishment. He thoroughly enjoyed
intimidating any of the intellectually empty bureaucratic enclaves that presumed to interfere with the translation of a
promising scientific idea into action. And he was supported
most ably by STUART SESSOMS, his Deputy Director, and G. BUR-
ROUGHS (Bo) MIDER, Director of Laboratories and Clinics, each
with an uncanny ability to predict Shannon's reaction to scientific proposals.

Shannon embraced fully the steering committee's report,
and the Division of Computer Research and Technology was established by the Secretary on April 16, 1964. It came into
physical being in October 1965 under an acting director, JAMES
A. KING. The formal program was launched in August 1966 with
the appointment of the Division's first Director, ARNOLD W.
PRATT.

Mider's solid support in the early years was a key factor
in DCRT's growth and success. He considered the fledgling
DCRT an intramural activity. This meant that the Division
got the same watchful attention that Bo gave to all parts of
"his" intramural research program. Translated, this meant
that the Director, DCRT, could expect strong program support
liberally spiced with constructive comment and advice from
the "Friendly Front Office."

The organization of DCRT has been relatively stable since
its beginning. The few changes have largely reflected shifts
in emphasis as computation and data processing are applied in
the conduct and management of biomedical research. The organization seems to have accommodated well to the explosion of
knowledge and technology in biomedicine over the last 20 years
as well as to the extraordinary revolution in microelectronics
and computer hardware.

The original organization of DCRT (January 1967) comprised
the Laboratory of Applied Studies, Computer Systems Laboratory, Physical Sciences Laboratory, and Computation and Data
Processing Branch. The Heuristics Laboratory (designating an

area of applied mathematics) was added later that year. It
was subsequently abolished, primarily because of diminishing
financial resources and, secondarily, its inability to compete
for the bioscientists' attention and support. In December 1968
the Computation and Data Processing Branch was divided into a
Computer Center Branch and a Data Management Branch. This
move reflected the rapidly growing competence of the young
scientific and technical staff to master the complexities of
the so-called third-generation computer hardware—IBM 360
technology, in this case—and to confront and solve some of
the inordinately difficult problems involved in the data processing requirements for large, multifaceted data files. In
1974 the Laboratory of Statistical and Mathematical Methodology was formed, with the goal of ensuring that the computer
hardware and software for the evaluation of biomedical data
were mint quality in every dimension.

Challenge and Early Achievements

The urgent task of the new DCRT was to develop and maintain a computing service that could meet NIH's developing
needs for data handling. The beginning was bleak in terms
of the promise. In 1967 the NIH central facility consisted
of two IBM 360/50 computers, machines of very modest capacity.
With this hardware, the central computer facility could accommodate an average of 43 defined jobs per day, submitted
as card decks and run on batch mode. Some of these jobs were
large, by the standard of the times. They arose in the NIH
central administrative area and from epidemiologists in the
Institutes, particularly the National Cancer Institute and
the National Institute of Mental Health. An original Computer Center Branch software facility known as SPOUT permitted
upper- and lower-case printing and easily handled large-volume
punched card chores. SPOUT favored administrative and epidemiological jobs. There were no interactive systems, and almost all peripheral storage of data was on magnetic tape. The
minor exceptions were eight disk drives that provided a small
amount of on-line data storage. There were no formal consulting services for users of the facility, and computer classes were essentially nonexistent.

The Computer Utility Today

In contrast to this 1967 modest capability, today's NIH
central computer facility constitutes a large, efficient,
economical resource. Operated as a utility, it provides a

variety of computational services in support of a diverse, dynamic community of nearly 14,000 persons. These include a broad spectrum of users: research scientists, service administrators, program directors, and their supporting mathematicians, statisticians, programmers, secretaries, and clerks.

The primary component of the NIH computer utility is a uniquely configured multiprocessor computer system designed around five IBM 3081 processors with 160 million bytes* of directly addressable memory. The peripheral complex supporting the system includes 115 tape drives, 344 disk drives, 2 mass storage systems, and 11 high-speed printers, with card reader/punches, microfiche output units, and teleprocessing facilities serving over 1200 communications lines. Operating in a multiprogramming mode, the utility provides time-sharing, text editing, and batch-processing services, as well as microfiche, graphics, plotting, and data management facilities 24 hours per day. The IBM System 370 currently processes over 14,500 batch jobs and 13,500 interactive sessions daily. Over 7.3 million jobs-sessions were processed during the past year (fiscal 1983), and more than 93 percent of these were completed and available to the user in less than two hours.

The other major component of the NIH computer utility, the DECsystem-10 time-sharing facility, is designed around one DK and two KL-10 processors with 5 million bytes of directly addressable memory. This facility provides time-sharing services and data communications support to over 2000 laboratory scientists throughout NIH. Ten tape drives, 31 disk drives, and a variety of teleprocessing equipment make up the peripheral complex. Over 120,000 interactive time-sharing sessions were processed on the DECsystem-10 during the past year.

The DCRT central computer facility has evolved from meager beginnings into a modern-day, state-of-the-art facility. In large part this has occurred through acquisition of up-to-date hardware and, to a lesser but highly significant extent, through research and development achievements in computer science by the DCRT staff. Four of these accomplishments warrant special mention—namely, NIH Shared Spool, NIH WYLBUR, Molecular Graphics, and Modeling Laboratory (MLAB). These four software systems represent landmark contributions to basic computer sciences.

NIH Shared Spool. When digital computers were first introduced commercially, it was generally accepted that user organizations, because of the great expense and limited flex-

---

*A group of bits (adjacent binary digits) processed as a unit and forming a character (digit, letter, or other symbol).

ibility of the machines, would need only one. In actuality,
computational needs would soon exceed the computer's capacity,
and a larger and faster one would be installed. This strategy would work quite well until an organization's needs exceeded the processing capacity of the largest, fastest computer available. The obvious solution then was to acquire
multiple computers. Many organizations made this choice and
thereby addressed the capacity problem effectively. But multiple computers introduced complex, expensive scheduling and
load-balancing problems. Since it was impossible to forecast
accurately the time required to process any particular job,
traditional block-time scheduling was cumbersome and ineffi-
cient and full capacity could not be realized. In an attempt
to minimize the problem, various techniques involving the
categorization of jobs were used; but the more effective this
was at resolving the scheduling difficulties, the more in-
efficient the entire system became.

By mid 1970, with three IBM 360/50 computers operating
round-the-clock seven days a week, NIH (like many other organizations) was experiencing severe difficulty balancing its
workload. A small NIH team of well-qualified systems ana-
lysts investigated the problem. They concluded that the crux
of the problem was the division of work into long, independent
queues for each of the three computers. One possible solution
was to shorten the queues, but this would require more manual
handling of jobs, which was inherently slow and subject to
human error. The study team proposed a unique solution: a
system with only one work queue that could be shared automatically among the multiple computers. Individual jobs would
be routed to a particular computer only when it was actually ready to process them. In this manner the team hoped to
achieve automatic optimum scheduling and load balancing.

The "shared-spool" concept was discussed with representatives from industry and academia in the hope of encouraging
computer manufacturers to provide equipment with such a capability. Although the concept was generally accepted, there
was considerable debate about the overhead expected from the
requirement that the computers must compete for access to the
single spool. Computer manufacturers thought the design would
be so complex that implementation would be impractical and declined to participate in such a development project.

The NIH team decided to undertake the project alone. The
first shared spool became operational at NIH on April 19,
1971. Its effectiveness greatly exceeded the designers'
expectations. Overhead was well within reason, and the dynamic
load-balancing increased the throughput dramatically. Word of
the success of this effort spread rapidly among major computer
users throughout the world. Requests for information about the

system were so prevalent that two 2-day seminars describing the design, installation, and use of the shared spool were conducted at NIH in mid 1973. Representatives from private industry, academia, and governments attended; and the NIH system was widely adopted. Its acceptance and popularity among hundreds of organizations worldwide caused computer manufacturers to reevaluate their decision. In early 1975 IBM announced that a Multi Access Spool facility (that is, a shared spool) would be included in new software to be released by the end of the year.

WYLBUR. The WYLBUR program has been one of the main reasons for the phenomenal growth of the NIH computer utility. It has provided ready access to the computer and the computing tools available. The system can be learned easily and used in most facets of computing and word-processing applications.

WYLBUR functions as an on-line interactive text editor and job-entry facility. Terminals connected by telephone lines to NIH's IBM System 370 allow users to communicate with the WYLBUR system and to apply predefined commands to the available facilities. The editing features of WYLBUR provide an easy-to-use mechanism for creating, changing, searching, and displaying all kinds of text, such as computer programs and data, letters, proposals, reports, manuals, and lists. Data sets can be stored on-line. WYLBUR's job-entry facilities allow the user to submit a computer program to the batch job stream and examine the output at the terminal. The document-formatting facility can justify text lines (make them even in length), divide the text into pages automatically, and generate page numbers, headings, footings, tables of contents, and indices. WYLBUR is programmed to evaluate expressions, execute collections of stored commands, and perform comparisons and logical branching.

The current version of WYLBUR, known as NIH Extended WYLBUR, was completely designed, developed, and implemented at the NIH computer facility in Bethesda. It is a successor to the original WYLBUR, which was developed at the Stanford University Computation Center as a limited logical kernel and modified and extended by DCRT to meet NIH needs.

Molecular Graphics. Over the last 10 years computer programs have been developed for representing and analyzing the structure of proteins and nucleic acids. The outputs from these systems serve investigators in the various NIH Institutes and in academic and industrial research institutions in this country and abroad. The key to the growth of capability lay in the realization that any problem of molecular structure, however trivial it may seem at the beginning, nevertheless contains an element of variety that causes either an increase in our understanding or a demand for change in the substance and performance of a computer program(s).

In the early 1970s, when time-sharing computers were first coming into general use, DCRT developed programs for searching various forms of chemical information. The design became the basis for the NIH/EPA Chemical Information System, which is now in general use via commercial computer networks.

In the mid 1970s crystallographers all over the world began to determine the structures of proteins and nucleic acids. Their published papers contained only a few illustrations, often not in stereo, and scientists found difficulty in understanding particular aspects of the molecules. Then it was realized that a part of the NIH central computer facility, a microfiche output device, could be used to generate stereo images of macromolecules.

Before anything systematic could be done, the data had to be organized; so in the next four years, staff collected and purified all the available proteins and nucleic acid structures. (Many of these data sets were used in forming the data base at the Brookhaven National Laboratory.) An atlas of one protein had been prepared by scientists at Yale and Oxford Universities, but had taken three years of handwork. DCRT, using extensive computerization, composed in four years the Atlas of Macromolecular Structure on Microfiche (AMSOM) of 96 macromolecules. The atlas contains 110,000 pages of text and stereographic information. Scientists all over the world bought microfiche viewers to use the atlas in studying macromolecule structure.

The microfiche atlas was the culmination of the first high-level graphics system at NIH. At the end of its 10-year life span, the worn display was being held together by bits and pieces of wire and was always blowing fuses. A new display system was purchased to create an entirely different form of graphic output. Physical models come in two varieties, the so-called Kendrew models, or stick representations, and the CPK (Corey, Pauling, Koulton) models, which are space-filling. An algorithm developed for generating the surface of spheres could in turn represent the surface of a macromolecule. Utilizing this capability, NIH computers can represent molecules either by lines connecting atom centers or by the atom surfaces. The response of the scientific community to these sphere-based images was spontaneous and gratifying. Since 1976 more than 70,000 macromolecular surface images have been produced, many appearing in major scientific journals and textbooks. The culmination of the surface graphics system was the publication of a package of images, Teaching Aids for Macromolecular Structure (TAMS), to be used in universities and graduate schools. The impact of these images in stereo and color will be far-reaching, for young scientists in the course of training will think of proteins and nucleic acids as real objects in three dimensions.

Molecular graphics at NIH is headed in two directions. We still want to be able to determine the structure of a protein from first principles. To this end the third molecular graphics system at NIH is now in the process of design and implementation. It will contain an array processor that will permit the instantaneous calculation and minimization of macromolecular energy. Crystallography will continue to provide the definitive configurations, but we should attain a new plateau of rapid structure determination. On this plateau we should be able to design proteins. The new display system will also support extensive graphic representations of subcellular and cellular structure. These representations should cause the same sort of revolution in thinking that occurred with the computer-generated images of protein surfaces.

Modeling Laboratory. MLAB is a set of computer programs that were started in 1970 and progressively enhanced and developed to form an interactive system for mathematical modeling. These programs allow the user to fit curves, solve differential equations, and produce high-quality graphic plots. MLAB also incorporates a variety of special mathematical, statistical, and graphics operators, including a large collection for cluster analysis (the C-LAB system). Also included are facilities for fast Fourier transforms, smoothing, definite integrals, three-dimensional surface graphs and contour plots, eigenvalues and eigenvectors, and root-finding.

Curve-fitting is a useful analytical tool in many scientific disciplines. One of MLAB's main uses is to fit models to data. The heart of the system is a curve-fitting program that will adjust the parameters of a model function to minimize the sum of the squared errors. A repertoire of mathematical functions, a collection of routines for plotting, and mechanisms for saving data between sessions provide a powerful and convenient utility for data manipulation, arithmetic calculations, and model building and testing. The MLAB language is defined in the *MLAB Reference Manual*.

The Computer in Scientific Instrumentation

The Computer Systems Laboratory (CSL) was one of the original laboratories in DCRT. It was organized in 1967 to exploit the revolution in computer applications to biomedical instrumentation. The computer revolution has been driven in turn by the astounding progress in microelectronics, principally the steady increase in the number of circuits that can be placed on silicon chips with resulting decreases in the cost of memory and logic. Miniaturization has greatly enhanced speed of computation and remarkably improved circuit reliability.

The advent of the minicomputer brought the computer to the scientific laboratory, where it was used to collect data directly from scientific instruments and to perform some limited data processing. A dedicated computer could control an instrument and perform the data-collection process. The early dedicated computers were usually applied to the more costly instruments—X-ray diffractometers, mass spectrometers, etc.; but the advent and evolution of the microcomputer has made possible the incorporation of inexpensive microprocessors in instruments of every type.

An early effort by CSL staff to provide for acquisition and control of laboratory data was made in collaboration with two basic research Laboratories of NIADDK: Chemical Physics and Molecular Biology, which shared adjoining space and some common instrumentation. These two laboratories have become the experimental workplace for CSL professionals, who are changing computer technology. The 15-year collaboration has been mutually profitable. CSL has had first-hand access to outstanding scientists using state-of-the-art spectroscopy, and the scientists in turn profit from having computer science and technology immediately at hand.

Remote Operator Consoles. Discussions between CSL personnel and laboratory scientists in 1967 led to the proposal to establish a central minicomputer facility to serve multiple laboratory instruments. The plan called for transmission of analog signals to a single multichannel analog-to-digital converter, with subsequent transmission of the conditioned signals to an industrial interface that made them accessible to the computer under program control. This design reduced costs significantly; analog-to-digital converters were expensive in 1967, and the cost of providing individual converters for each lab instrument was unacceptable. It was felt that this approach would result in a reliable, stable system for supporting long-term research projects.

Key to the system were the Remote Operator Consoles (ROC), designed and built by CSL staff for each of the lab instruments involved. Each console served as an interface between the scientist and the instrument—via the computer. Each was sufficiently "smart" that a scientist could tell the computer the preferred sequence of computer programs to be invoked in an experiment, then enter the appropriate parameters to control the instrument's operation, as well as acquire, process, store, and display the experimental data.

This experiment in laboratory automation was highly successful. Within an 18-month period, a Honeywell 516 minicomputer was purchased and put in operation, programmed to serve several individual lab instruments. The programming challenge was to improve the machine's response time so as to accommodate on-line, real-time simultaneous data acquisition. Five instruments attached to the computer proved to be the optimal data-processing workload.

Hierarchical Structure. By 1976, after a decade of reliable service, the system had to be replaced. Among other problems, the computer could not be serviced properly; cannibalized machines became the only source of spare parts. And it was evident that the practical limits for adding software enhancements had been reached or exceeded. The recommended replacement, which included a host computer, was based on a microcomputer system. Analysis had indicated that a three-level hierarchical structure with independent communicating microcomputers would be economical and reliable. Such a processing system would be capable of instrument control, local data acquisition, graphic display of data, and data communication between computers at their respective levels.

As now in place, the first line of the hierarchy comprises the lab instrument and its dedicated microcomputer. This arrangement, using customized data-acquisition software, can make the best use of the lab instrument. The second level is a microcomputer, a communication processor that accepts data from the level-1 machine. These data can be stored or transmitted to the level-3 host minicomputer. This machine is a PDP 11/70, itself capable of teleprocessing linkage to the DCRT computer center. Routine use of the replacement system has sustained the opinion advanced in the earlier analysis of the lab instrument data-processing problem: It has proved to be highly reliable and flexible.

Flow Cytometer/Electronic Cell Sorter Computer Systems. In July 1973 CSL started a collaborative project with the Immunology Branch, National Cancer Institute, to develop a system for the acquisition, storage, and analysis of the enormous volume of data being produced by their newly acquired flow cytometer/electronic cell sorter (FC/ECS). This instrument, built for NCI by Becton-Dickinson Electronics Laboratory, was modeled after a prototype at Stanford University. It provided for analysis and, optionally, separation of viable stained cells in a fluid stream. Analysis was by cell fluorescence and low-angle light scatter.

A computer-based system that would have capability for data acquisition, storage, and processing was recommended, with CSL responsible for interfacing the FC/ECS and for developing software. By August 1975 the system was in routine use. It was subsequently expanded to accommodate a second FC/ECS developed by Los Alamos Scientific Laboratories. The computer used was a Digital Equipment Corporation PDP 11/40. Data could be collected from either or both instruments while previously collected data were being processed. In 1977 the NCI FC/ECS was upgraded. Because the combined sample volume from two fluorescence channels saturated a single system, each instrument now required a dedicated computer.

Computer-generated data presentations strongly assisted researchers in data interpretation. To increase sample volume, the software was improved by sequencing automatically with preselected parameters through data files, reducing the time spent at the computer console.

Research-quality flow devices, available within the past four years, include integral microcomputers for instrument control and data acquisition. These microcomputers offer some data-processing capabilities but are not designed for high-sample volume. CSL is presently developing the interprocessor links that will allow researchers to connect FC/ECS instruments equipped with integral microcomputers directly into a large computer running a multiuser operating system.

Voice–Output Terminal for the Blind. In the late 1970s, CSL contributed to effectiveness and expanded job opportunities for blind computer programmers by developing a voice-output terminal. A microcomputer, combined with a speech synthesizer, is connected between a standard alphanumeric computer terminal and a host computer. Data from the host computer intercepted by the microcomputer are converted to phonetic codes by a software program that applies rules of English pronunciation. The phonetic codes, in turn, are converted to speech by the synthesizer. Data are entered into the computer in the usual way, via the keyboard of the computer terminal. The full-word audible output of the voice terminal frees the blind programmer from laboriously reading text one character at a time with optical-to-tactile converters or braille printers.

Not only is the audible output from the voice terminal faster than tactile devices; it is also more natural and efficient, being the primary means by which the blind communicate with others. Furthermore, the voice terminal permits a kind of interactive dialogue with computers similar to that which sighted programmers find so useful.

The prototype of this voice output terminal was originally

developed in 1978 in collaboration with a blind computer programmer. It was exhibited at the 1979 annual meeting of the President's Committee on Employment of the Handicapped. Subsequently, additional CSL terminals helped four other blind Federal employees improve their productivity. The design of the voice-output terminal has been given to a number of companies in the private sector. Several are now selling similar terminals, at least two based on CSL's work.

Radiation Counter Data Recorder.

Since 1977 much of the tedium of managing data from liquid scintillation counters and gamma counters has been eased through use of the radiation counter data recorder developed by CSL. There are now hundreds of such counters at NIH, many of which produce data that require subsequent processing.

In 1976 DAVID RODBARD, an NICHD scientist with extensive experience in computer processing of radiation counter data, suggested that a better means of recording was needed. He cited the problems of transcribing teletype printouts or reading punched paper tape torn and crumpled from hostile laboratory environs. In response, CSL developed a data logger designed to connect easily to a wide range of radiation counters. Using microprocessor control, the data logger performs simple editing and validation checks on the data and then records them onto digital magnetic cassette tape. At the conclusion of an experiment, the tape may be quickly, quietly, and reliably played back to a computer for analysis, using a commercially available cassette tape data terminal. The format of the recorded data is compatible with the DECsystem 10, the IBM 370, and numerous minicomputers.

CSL initially fabricated a number of radiation counter data recorders in its own laboratory facilities. Demand for the devices, however, led in 1979 to a contract for their commercial manufacture. Since their introduction, more than 100 data recorders have been installed in laboratories throughout NIH.

These examples have been arbitrarily selected to say something about the rapid and diverse evolution of computer applications in scientific instrumentation at NIH. The NIH experience is far from unique. Discussion of computer-dependent, multidimensional instrumentation—CAT scanners, quadrupole mass spectrometers, nuclear medicine scanners, etc.—has been bypassed here, for instrumentation can only be described adequately in the context of specific application. Suffice it to say that the NIH scientific cadre is broadly engaged with the newer instrumentation in both laboratories and clinics.

Computers in Clinical Research

Information, whether in the form of specific data or generalized knowledge summaries, is the currency of medical research, medical care delivery, and medical education. Optimal performance of clinical and laboratory informational tasks has for years tended to exceed the cognitive capability of the human mind because of the volume and sheer complexity of the data describing biological systems. This has been particularly true in clinical science.

Improvement of computer and telecommunications technology in recent years has made possible the development of very potent and versatile tools for the management of clinical information. The NIH Clinical Center utilizes a broad array of computer services that have emerged from the collaborative efforts of Clinical Center staff, DCRT computer scientists and engineers, and dedicated research physicians and their coworkers. The Clinical Center staff is proud of its technological achievements, which provide solid support to the care of patients and the conduct of research.

The earliest Clinical Center computer activities began in the Clinical Pathology Department in the "precomputer era" of the late 1950s. These efforts, using electronic accounting machines, key punches, and plugboard wiring apparatus to tabulate and collate laboratory results in the chemistry service, were labor-intensive, slow, tedious, and rudimentary. Yet they provided some insight into the potential of electronic data manipulation while laying the groundwork for education of senior medical investigators and their technologist colleagues. Card-processing operations and staff were maintained, extensive space and resources allocated, and large collections of paper reports generated for inclusion in the medical record.

By today's standards, the efforts were remarkably primitive. For example, shelves had been installed by 1975 to permit a stack of reports approximately 6 feet high and 25 feet long to be stored along each wall of the secretarial office. Today all of these reports can be stored on a small quantity of microfiche, a direct access file, a mass storage device, or magnetic tape. And not only are cost and ease of access important considerations; a safety factor is also involved. These reports were eventually removed on the basis of a calculation of the likelihood of retrieval versus the risk to the secretarial staff of a stack falling off a shelf!

The punch-card laboratory reporting system was maintained until the mid 1960s, at which time a prototype computer was installed in the laboratory to attempt direct connection of laboratory instruments to the computer so that data might be collected efficiently, rapidly, and "untouched by human hands." As one of the world's first efforts to accomplish this task in a clinical setting, it was successful to the extent of demonstrating feasibility with the instrumentation and engineering knowledge then available. It was also a major contributor to staff education and the testing of state-of-the-art constraints in medical computer science.

As an aside, the contracting process was much simpler in those days. The specifications under which the half-million dollar system was acquired consisted of less than two pages, and the winning proposal was five pages long.

This prototype system for needs in clinical pathology operated from 1967 to 1975, 14 hours a day, 5 days a week, collecting instrument data through special-purpose electronics and primitive computer terminals. The technologists described this as a "one-way" system because they were able to enter data but not retrieve them. System capabilities were limited: test requests were entered in the morning, results obtained in the afternoon, and reports printed at night. Simultaneous functions and software sophistication were also limited. And support was not available to the laboratory during off hours.

When a successor system was considered, the technologists wanted a machine with a "big memory that wasn't one-way." By this they meant one that could retrieve information by patients' names, remember the associated lab results, select results based on reasonable criteria, and store at least several weeks of data on each case. Such a system was installed in 1975 and continues in use today. Its success reflects the advantages of involving NIH staff and computer professionals in the selection and adaptation of advanced technology systems. Furthermore, it is sufficiently flexible to permit the insights of clinical scientists, computer professionals, and system users to be melded for effective system evolution.

Other needs of the clinical investigators and the hospital administration stimulated DCRT and the Clinical Center to develop a prototype on-line admitting, census, and statistics program. The result was an admitting system and a discharge diagnosis system that served in conjunction with the clinical laboratory system to permit physicians to call for logical searches among patients with multiple diagnoses. This three-way information nucleus was considered in its time a major facilitator of certain clinical research activities. Physicians could request computer retrievals using multiple parameters, such as "For all patients two months post mitral valve replacement who are anemic and have elevated reticulocyte counts, print laboratory values, biographic data, and associated diagnoses if any." These and similar retrievals were used in identifying patients for further research or in extracting data for subsequent statistical analysis.

At about the same time, a clinical researcher in the Arthritis Institute began an experiment using WYLBUR to record and follow patients on the 9E nursing unit. He was interested in a variety of clinical parameters, including medications, physical findings, automatic generation of the medical care kardex, and associated medical and nursing management issues. The combination of these efforts led to requests for further access to computer-stored information of the general type: "Now that we have lab results, diagnoses, and biographic information, can you give us medications, X-ray results, anatomic pathologic data, and everything else?"

With these requirements for research support and clinical care in mind, a multidisciplinary group was formed to assess the feasibility of introducing a large-scale computerized patient care and clinical research data system into the Clinical Center. The request initiated an era of extensive learning and exposed Clinical Center and Institute medical staff to the excitement and vagaries of modern computer science. It also brought an endless stream of visitors anxious to participate and to learn from an NIH experiment in the application of computer science to patient care and clinical investigation. Approximately one year (1975-1976) was required to prepare for operation of the system for the first nursing unit. Installation on the last nursing unit was completed in late 1978.

This was a stimulating, though traumatic time in the adaptation of technology to the hospital and the hospital to emerging technology. In 1974 the large-scale hospital-wide Medical Information System (MIS) was successfully interfaced to the clinical laboratory system. This represented the first interface of its type between such highly sophisticated, yet independently designed clinical operations.

Concurrent with the implementation of MIS, a committee was involved in the development of the Clinical Information Utility (CIU), a collaborative DCRT-Clinical Center undertaking. The intent was to extract clinical data from all existing Clinical Center systems, to collate and reorganize the data, and to make them available for clinical investigators in a timely, accurate, cost-effective, and easy-to-use fashion. This effort continues today. It is widely used by clinical investigators at NIH and has become the standard method of extracting pertinent clinical variables from the medical record while avoiding the drudgery of chart reviews and transcriptions for a significant percentage of clinical data. The CIU also permits investigators to develop independent data bases at DCRT to which they need add only their personal experimental data, knowing they can tap the CIU for many parameters of clinical care. In particular, an interactive statistical system, BRIGHT, operating on the DECsystem 10, can access the IBM/370-based CIU conveniently and easily through DCRT-developed resources.

The combination of the CIU, BRIGHT, and many other DCRT services for the scientific analysis of medical data has proved a hypothesis developed in the early 1970s by DCRT and the Clinical Center: High-speed, specialized computer support systems may be tailored to (1) meet direct needs associated with the provision of medical care and, at the same time, (2) allow the extraction and transport of clinical data and observations to the computer center for sophisticated statistical and scientific analyses.

Other specialty computer systems have evolved through collaborative NIH-wide efforts. The Nuclear Medicine Department of the Clinical Center was an early computer user through a highly fruitful collaboration with DCRT. The interfacing of gamma counters to minicomputer systems, the analysis of data on both NMD and DCRT computers, and the development of image-processing algorithms, electronic technology, and physiologic data collection have set a new standard for sophisticated imaging technology in clinical systems. Further collaborative efforts of DCRT, the Clinical Center, and the Institutes involve intensive care units, postsurgical cardiac care units, and ECG data processing.

As we look to the future, we expect computers to play an increasingly prominent role in Clinical Center activities. Continuing improvements are foreseen in the provision of clinical information for physicians, including high-speed terminals, graphic and flow sheet presentation for immediate patient care purposes, access to larger data bases over extended periods as the outpatient activities expand, better integrated departmental and clinical care systems, and continuing evolution in the exciting areas of digital imaging. There are new challenges in nuclear magnetic resonance, computerized tomograpic scanning, positron emission tomography, ultrasound, and the integration of these modalities to yield the maximum amount of diagnostic and clinical followup information.

Looking Ahead

Any retrospective look at computation and data processing at NIH reveals that the recent past has been exciting and productive. The computer facilities at our disposal have served well the biomedical statistician and mathematician and have provided a reliable technology that greatly enhances the scientist's ability to define, conduct, and evaluate experiments. As fruitful as the past has been, the future promises even more as the ideas and aspirations of 20 years of pioneering computer science are realized in the laboratory and the clinic.

Acknowledgment

The author wishes to thank THOMAS LEWIS, DANIEL SYED, PERRY PLEXICO, and ARTHUR SCHULTZ for their contributions to this paper.

Introduction

CARDIAC SURGERY

In 1902 Dr. Luther Leonidas Hill successfully repaired a penetrating stab wound of the left ventricle of the heart, operating, it is said, on a kitchen table. It was the first such procedure to be reported in the United States, and so American heart surgery was born. Luther Hill named his son after his preceptor, Lord Lister; and Lister Hill, as Senator from his native state of Alabama, served for many years as chairman of those Senate committees having most to do with health research. With the collaboration of Congressman John Fogarty, Lister Hill gave strong support to the then burgeoning National Institutes of Health and to its director, JAMES A. SHANNON. Certainly his family background in medicine contributed to a lifelong interest in Federal support of medical research.

LUTHER TERRY served successively as branch chief, clinical director, and assistant director of the National Heart Institute. He subsequently became Surgeon General, PHS. He, too, was associated, in a sense, with Luther Hill, who was a friend of the Terry family and the inspiration for their son's name. By these channels, NIH has close associations with the origins of cardiac surgery in this country.

Since 1950 particularly, the rapid development of cardiac surgery has depended heavily upon concurrent developments in physiology and engineering. The introduction of catheterization procedures and the interpretation of results led to a precise understanding of the flow and pressure relationships of blood in and about the heart. As the surgeons became bolder and more skillful, and especially after the invention of the heart-lung machine, procedures that had previously been impossible were introduced and perfected.

Among the more interesting of these was the replacement of heart valves by various prostheses. In the development of such devices, close cooperation was required between surgeons and engineers. It is precisely in areas requiring multidisciplinary approaches that NIH has provided the most unusual opportunities. In the following chapter the reader will find accounts of some of the surgical advances that have taken *place in the operating rooms and laboratories of the National Heart, Lung, and Blood Institute, where surgeons are restoring function to the deformed or damaged heart by exquisite methods now available.*

D. S.

24

CARDIAC SURGERY

Charles L. McIntosh

I have considered that it is only by means of objective postoperative measurements that we can determine, with certainty, the extent to which a given
procedure has restored normal cardiac function and,
perhaps most important of all, to what extent the
operation has influenced, favorably or unfavorably,
the natural course of the disease in which it was
applied.

Andrew Glenn Morrow
(at dedication of NIH cardiac
operating rooms, 1963)

The Clinic of Surgery of the National Heart Institute was
established in August 1953 under the direction of ANDREW GLENN
MORROW, who served as chief until 1982. Morrow received his
surgical training under Alfred Blalock at Johns Hopkins and
Geoffrey Wooler at the General Infirmary in Leeds, England.
The Clinic of Surgery—Morrow's title for the clinical component of the Surgery Branch—became a training institution for
a number of outstanding senior investigators and 138 clinical
associates. Nine of these trainees now occupy university
chairs of surgery, 20 are chiefs of departments of cardiovascular surgery, and approximately 83 are on the faculties of
outstanding medical schools throughout the world. It is a
little-known fact that the Cardiology Branch was originally
a section under EUGENE BRAUNWALD in the Surgery Branch (until
1960).
The discipline of cardiac surgery was in its infancy in
the mid 1950s, and we have seen that fertile areas of clinical
and experimental research lay ahead. The development of the
field depended on the simultaneous growth of many others,
including cardiology and cardiovascular physiology, pharma-

CHARLES L. McINTOSH, M.D., Ph.D., *Attending Cardiac Surgeon,*
Surgery Branch, National Heart, Lung, and Blood Institute.

NIH: AN ACCOUNT OF RESEARCH
IN ITS LABORATORIES AND CLINICS
ISBN 0-12-667980-0

cology, and technical development, all found within the "cottage industry" NIH. Cardiac operations performed in the mid 1950s before the introduction of the heart-lung machine included closed aortic and mitral commissurotomies, closure of persistent ductus arteriosus, resection of coarctation of the aorta, pericardiectomy, and closure of atrial septal defects by various methods. The goals of this department were to chart the natural history of various types of congenital and acquired heart disease once a cardiac operation was deemed necessary, and to utilize the data obtained from these patients as a rational basis for changing or maintaining various surgical procedures and philosophies.

An important aspect of clinical cardiovascular research at NIH is the facility in which it is conducted: Building 10A, which was designed for heart surgery and neurosurgery. The two cardiac operating rooms were unique in 1963 in that they were dedicated to cardiac surgery and involved special systems for monitoring, lighting, communications, and storage and retrieval of large amounts of research data. They were state-of-the-art at that time and have continued to function well as "operating laboratories." In 1983 these facilities were named the Andrew Glenn Morrow Cardiac Operating Rooms.

The clinical research protocols developed over the past 25 years have been largely a collaborative effort of the Cardiology, Surgery, and Pathology Branches. The topics chosen for discussion here were the major areas of interest historically in which important contributions were made to cardiac surgery.

Diagnostic Techniques

Performing an operation with reasonable safety and maximal benefit to the patient requires precise a priori knowledge of the pathologic anatomy to be corrected or palliated. Prior to the clinical use of the heart-lung machine for correcting intracardiac lesions, numerous diagnostic techniques were developed and perfected by the Surgery and Cardiology Branches. Detection of an abnormal circulatory shunt in patients with congenital heart disease was made possible by use of a radioactive tracer, krypton-85 (1). The patient inhaled the isotope, which would diffuse through the pulmonary capillaries, pass through the left cardiac chambers, and be virtually removed from the circulation by the tissues (see Figure 1). Thus little ^{85}Kr would be returned to the right-side chambers. Ten to thirty seconds after inhalation, samples were withdrawn through catheters placed in the pulmonary artery and a systemic artery. The presence of more than 12 percent ^{85}Kr in

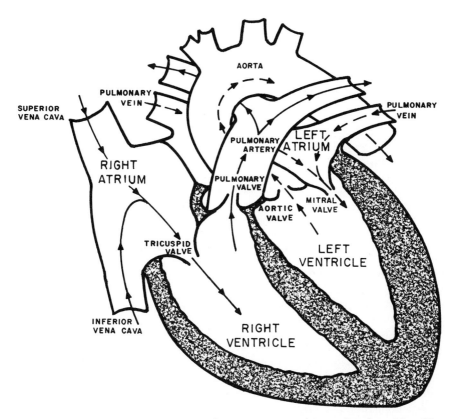

FIGURE 1. *The human heart in cross section, showing the flow of blood. Oxygen-poor blood (solid-line arrows) from the body flows through the right atrium to fill the right ventricle, which pumps it out through the pulmonary artery to the lungs. There the blood gives up carbon dioxide and gains oxygen. Freshly oxygenated blood (broken-line arrows) enters the left atrium via the pulmonary veins and flows into the left ventricle, which pumps it into the aorta, the main artery to the body. (Actually, the same muscular action pumps the blood from the two ventricles simultaneously.) From the aorta the blood enters smaller arteries, then arterioles and capillaries of the body tissues, and finally returns via the veins to complete the cycle.*

the pulmonary artery indicated a significant left-to-right shunt in the heart.

The indicator-dilution technique developed in this clinic makes localization and quantitation of the shunt more practical (2). Green dye is injected into the heart and detected

in blood samples through a densitometer. By timing the appearance of the dye in the various chambers sampled, one can
determine the localization, direction, and magnitude of the
shunt. This technique is in use today for preoperative evaluation and intraoperative confirmation that the shunt has been
completely closed (3).

Techniques developed at NIH to assess left atrial and
ventricular pressures and transvalvular gradients include
the transbronchial method (4), transseptal left heart catheterization (5,6), and direct left ventricular puncture (7).
These techniques, which measure chamber pressures across a
valve, permit intraoperative evaluation of the mitral valve
following closed mitral commissurotomy* (8). Currently the
decision to replace a valve following a reconstructive procedure still depends on data derived from these methods.

Congenital Heart Disease

Congenital heart disease has been a major interest of the
Institute, which is credited with reference observations concerning the operative treatment in congenital aortic stenosis
(9-11), congenital discrete subaortic stenosis (12), and the
incomplete form of persistent atrioventricular canal with
cleft mitral valve (13,14).

Morrow's major interest for 20 years centered on the study
and treatment of a congenital heart disease termed obstructive
hypertrophic cardiomyopathy, or idiopathic hypertrophic subaortic stenosis (IHSS). In the early 1960s it became evident
to cardiologists, clinical physiologists, and surgeons that a
form of left ventricular outflow obstruction had previously
gone unrecognized. The feature that differentiated this obstruction from the familiar valvular, subvalvular, and supra-
valvular forms of aortic stenosis was that the stenotic
orifice was dynamic rather than fixed. Studies in the heart
catheterization laboratory and the operating room eventually
revealed that the obstruction resulted from contact of the
anterior leaflet of the mitral valve against the outflow tract
of the hypertrophied left ventricle and that the severity of
the obstruction depended on the factors governing the contractile state of the remainder of the heart. The obstruction
was made more severe by agents that produced positive inotropism, or a more forceful contraction of muscle. Conversely,
obstruction was lessened by interventions resulting in nega-

---

*Mitral commissurotomy: opening of the fused mitral valve
leaflets by an instrument or finger.

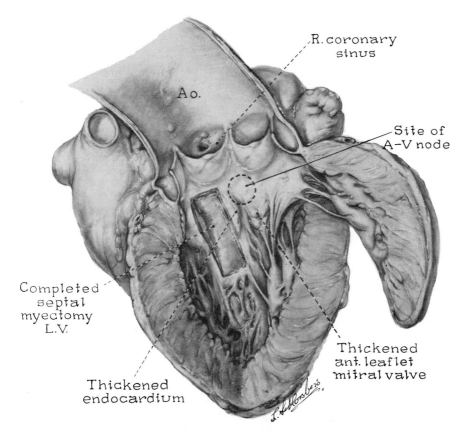

FIGURE 2. Morrow operation (completed) for palliating a congenital heart disease, idiopathic hypertrophic subaortic stenosis. The opened left ventricle and aorta demonstrate the rectangular block excised from the surface of the interventricular septum. This produces a new, adequate outflow tract from the left ventricle, relieving outflow obstruction and symptoms in virtually all patients.

tive inotropism or those causing an increase in the lateral distending pressure of the ventricle (15).

With this understanding of the physiology of the disease, a method for operative treatment could be devised. The operation that has evolved, called the "Morrow operation," is generally accepted throughout the world as the most effective means of relieving IHSS obstruction. In the procedure (see Figure 2) the ascending aorta is opened, and through the opened aortic valve a rectangular block is excised from the surface of the interventricular septum. This produces a new and adequate left ventricular outflow tract and complete relief of outflow obstruction in virtually all patients (16). Operative mortality is approximately 7 percent, and there is a small incidence of complete heart block and ventricular septal defect.

Almost all patients have experienced good or excellent symptomatic improvement after the Morrow operation. This is paralleled by hemodynamic improvement, and the resting gradient in virtually all patients is found to be absent or greatly reduced. Long-term followup reveals that a small number of patients, though improved early after operation, later develop symptoms again. About 6 percent of operative survivors have died in the late postoperative period, either suddenly or after prolonged congestive failure. Of all patients operated on, however, approximately 70 percent have maintained good symptomatic improvement during followup periods of up to 20 years (17).

Studies relating to IHSS have been the subject of nearly 100 publications from the Cardiology and Surgery Branches.

Valvular Heart Disease

Surgical treatment of valvular heart disease prior to the advent of the heart-lung machine was limited to commissurotomy for stenotic mitral and aortic valves and annulus reduction (narrowing of the orifice) for aortic regurgitation.

Charles Bailey performed the first successful closed mitral commissurotomy in the United States in 1943. Since the 1960s the operation has been largely replaced in this country by open-heart procedures. A large number of patients in our clinic, having undergone a closed mitral commissurotomy for treatment of rheumatic mitral stenosis, have been followed to determine whether and when to repeat a commissurotomy or mitral valve replacement. Long-term evaluation reveals good hemodynamic results in most patients if selected properly (18,19). Recently a review of 303 patients who had undergone a closed operation showed a 2 percent operative mortality and actuarial survival ranging from 95 percent at 5 years to 70 percent at 15 years after operation. Fifty-four patients (18 percent) required mitral valve replacement at a mean of 9.6 years after commissurotomy (range 1-26 years) (20). Advantages of the closed operation are that it does not require the heart-lung machine, normally takes less time to perform than the open operation, and allows relief of stenosis in the beating heart and immediate assessment of regurgitation. We still use the closed operation in selected patients, based on our clinical and hemodynamic data.

The introduction of the heart-lung machine in the late 1950s opened the door to the correction or palliation of almost all cardiac lesions. The first successful mitral valve replacement was performed in this clinic on March 11, 1960, using a flexible polyurethane prosthesis resembling the normal valve (21). Since that time the clinic has been involved in evaluating the results of mitral valve replacement with various prostheses (22-26). Of the first 100 patients who underwent replacement during 1961-1965 in this clinic, 83 survived the operation. Of those, 76 percent were alive at five years, and 64 percent at eight years. Sixteen of the late deaths were definitely attributed to the presence of the prosthesis: systemic arterial emboli in 8 patients, valve thrombosis in 2, perivalvular leak in 1, ball variance in 2, endocarditis in 2, and intracerebral hemorrhage due to anticoagulants in 1 (27,28). The major complications of the early ball valves were clot formation producing emboli, valve dysfunction secondary to thrombosis, and bleeding problems from the anticoagulants.

Systematic Evaluation of Prosthetic Heart Valves

The Clinic of Surgery made a major commitment to the development and evaluation of various prosthetic devices, both mechanical and tissue, used in the treatment of valvular heart disease. The program has been unique in the acquisition of pre- and postoperative hemodynamic data, and approximately 90 percent of patients who receive valve replacements continue to be followed, some up to 20 years. Serial catheterizations and studies have revealed various strengths and weaknesses of commonly used prosthetic devices, indicating either continued clinical use or abandonment. Usually valves are removed from clinical use because of various inherent problems, the solutions to which often produce others. Problems include unacceptable hydraulic function, emboli to cerebral or peripheral arteries, anticoagulation complications, valve failure from varying causes, anemia secondary to hemolysis, and prosthetic infection.

The evolution of the Starr-Edwards cage-ball valve is reviewed to illustrate the importance of systematic evaluation (see Figure 3). This valve type is not singled out as more problematic than others; it has simply been one of the major valves used in the Clinic of Surgery.

The Starr-Edwards 1000 series aortic valve was first implanted at NIH in 1961, and by 1966 reports of fatal degener-

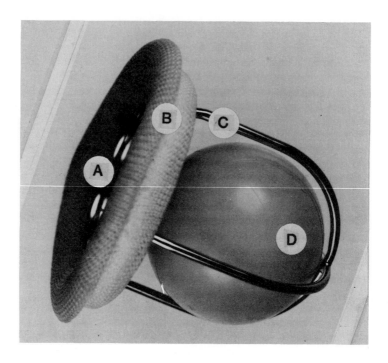

FIGURE 3. Starr-Edwards mechanical valve 6120. A. Valve orifice with metal studs to support ball. B. Dacron-covered
stent. C. Strut of valve cage. D. Ball, or "poppet."

ation of the silicone rubber ball (ball variance) appeared.
WILLIAM C. ROBERTS, Chief of Cardiac Pathology, has worked
in collaboration with the Clinic in the evaluation of heart
valves recovered at a repeat operation or at necropsy. Ball
variance was found in 12 patients who died within 24 months
after implantation of the Starr-Edwards 1000. Of these cases
11 showed that severe degeneration of the poppet, or ball, had
contributed to the patient's death (29).
    A diagnosis of potentially fatal ball variance could often
not be made by routine clinical examination or cardiac catheterization. Morrow suggested that the balls be made radio-
graphically visible or opaque, and therefore barium-containing
silicone rubber was used in the earliest ball valves. A noninvasive examination developed in this clinic utilized the
radiopaque ball to determine its percent excursion relative
to the cage length. This allowed detection of changes in ball
size (30). The examination provided information resulting in
elective change of the ball before a fatal complication occurred in six patients for whom other diagnostic criteria were

lacking. The 1000 series valve was implanted in a total of 121
patients, most of whom have had the valve or poppet changed or
have died.

The problem of ball variance was solved by changing the
cure process of the silicone rubber. The new valve was designated the 1200 and later the 1260 series. It has proved to
be virtually indestructible, and the Starr-Edwards 1260 aortic
and 6120 mitral continue in clinical use today.

Mechanical valves require lifelong anticoagulation to reduce embolization and, in some cases, to ensure continued
mechanical function. High thromboembolic incidence and the
inherent risk of prolonged anticoagulation stimulated collaborative research between this clinic and the Edwards Laboratory. A new valve covered with Dacron fabric allowed autogenous tissue ingrowth with subsequent inhibition of valvular
thrombosis (31-33). The cloth covering of the rigid prosthesis
did decrease the rate of embolization, obviating the need for
long-term warfarin in some instances and thus averting anticoagulation complications and death. These cloth-covered
valves were the 2300 series aortic and the 6300 series mitral
and tricuspid. Serial catheterizations of our patients implanted with 2300/6300 valves showed that some had developed
progressive prosthetic stenosis, requiring repeat valve replacement. Valves removed at operation revealed that stenosis
had resulted from a ring of scar tissue in the primary valve
orifice, thought to be due to direct seating of the ball on
autogenous tissue.

The solution to stenosis-producing tissue ingrowth was
the development of a composite seat providing a bed of metal
studs to support the ball. These valves were the 2310 and
6310 series. Their fate was to be cloth-wear of the struts,
producing severe hemolytic anemia secondary to increased shear
on the red blood cells. An attempt to correct this yielded
the "close clearance" 2310/6310 valve. Several early deaths
resulted when the ball stuck open in the cage, producing massive regurgitation, and the valve was promptly removed from
clinical use.

In the 2320/6320 series to follow, the distance between
the struts and the ball was increased to prevent sticking, but
unfortunately emboli and anemia due to cloth-wear required replacement of the valve in many patients. The 2400/6400 series
valves temporarily solved the anemia problem by having a metal
tract on the inside of the struts, but the exposed metal again
necessitated lifelong use of anticoagulants. Six patients have
required late replacement of the 2320 and 2400 series valves,
which have revealed wear of the metal studs of the valve seat
with resultant severe cloth-wear of the primary valve orifice.

Only valves of the 1260 and 6120 series are still manufactured.

Tissue valves, either fresh or fixed, appeared to offer a reasonable alternative to mechanical valves. Expected to be less thrombogenic, they would not require anticoagulants, and durability was the major concern for their clinical use. However, early formaldehyde-fixed porcine valves mounted on a rigid stent showed severe deterioration as early as six months after implantation in patients. A glutaraldehyde-fixed porcine valve mounted on a flexible stent was developed cooperatively by the Clinic and the Hancock Laboratory (34). It was first implanted in the mitral position in July 1970 (see Figure 4).

The five-year clinical experience with this valve in 85 patients who survived long-term with no postoperative anticoagulation showed that only one had an embolus. There was good hydraulic function in 54 patients studied pre- and postoperatively, and only one valve failure, at 56 months. Hemolysis or anemia of clinical significance had not been observed, and no valve had become infected (25). Use of the porcine bioprosthesis became standard for our mitral and tricuspid valve replacements and for aortic valve replacement in selected patients.

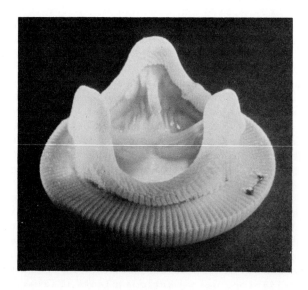

FIGURE 4. Hancock porcine bioprosthesis. This glutaraldehyde-fixed porcine valve mounted on a flexible dacron stent is now standard in the Clinic of Surgery for mitral, tricuspid, and some aortic valve replacements.

Continued long-term followup of approximately 111 patients who are 5-13 years postoperative shows a failure rate of 10 percent at an average of 78 months after implant (range 56 to 122 months) (26). Failure of the porcine valve tends to be gradual, and reoperations were performed on 9 of 10 failed patients, with 8 surviving the procedure. Prolonged clinical followup and serial catheterizations continue to be important in learning more about the natural history of the tissue valves, particularly in respect to when they fail and whether a repeat operation is needed. The embolic rate for tissue valves is similar to that for mechanical valves with anticoagulants, but avoidance of complications secondary to anticoagulants makes use of the tissue valve a lesser risk.

The mode of failure of a tissue valve is usually calcification, collagen degeneration, or thrombosis. Calcification is particularly troublesome in children and adults under 30 years of age. Lower calcification rates are claimed for third- and fourth-generation tissue valves now being manufactured, but our experience in adults indicates that at least six to eight years of implant time will be needed to gain the clinical knowledge for evaluation. Currently, an animal model used in our experimental laboratory provides accelerated testing of these valves to determine the relative effectiveness of various anticalcification processes (35).

The Clinic of Surgery continues to accumulate clinical and hemodynamic information for various prostheses, a unique function that will be vital until heart valves are perfected.

Other Collaborative Studies

Timing of heart surgery is critical. An operation too soon may result in an unnecessary death; too late, in less than an optimal result. In the 1970s operation was deferred for many patients with aortic regurgitation until either symptoms or marked cardiomegaly developed, in the hope of avoiding complications of prosthetic valves or cardiopulmonary bypass. Close analysis of a group of these symptomatic patients whose operation had followed long medical therapy revealed that a significant number either died or had persistent congestive heart failure in spite of a successful valve replacement (36).

Analysis of various risk factors revealed that a group of high-risk patients could be identified on the basis of left ventricular dimensions and of calculations of heart function from a noninvasive echo. On the basis of these findings, asymptomatic patients with aortic regurgitation were followed annually until certain dimensions were reached, then every six months until criteria were fulfilled for operative intervention. Long-term followup revealed improved survival and fewer patients with congestive failure in the postoperative period (37). Thus, timely intervention may produce a better long-term prognosis in certain individuals.

A second collaborative study is cited to demonstrate the need for a "second look" at patients previously studied. The role of aortic valve replacement without myocardial revascularization in patients with combined aortic valvular disease and coronary artery disease (CAD) was examined. We felt that the combined valve replacement with revascularization practiced in the early 1970s in several institutions might result in a higher operative mortality than valve replacement alone. Aortic valve replacement (AVR) alone was performed in 55 of our consecutive symptomatic patients with combined CAD and aortic valve disease and in 142 patients with aortic valve disease and no CAD. Results were compared with those published from other centers performing combined procedures. Operative mortality, operative infarction, recurrent angina, and survival at three-year followup in our patients with CAD having AVR alone were similar to those of patients having AVR and revascularization at other centers. The data at three years suggested that preoperative detection of CAD did not necessitate simultaneous revascularization in all patients at the time of AVR (38).

The same cohort of patients, reexamined after three additional years of followup, revealed a lower long-term survival after four years in patients with CAD who had not had simultaneous revascularization. Similar analysis from the other centers is not available, but in light of our second-look data, a combined operation is now performed.

Other collaborative protocols include evaluation of long-term coronary artery bypass graft patency (39) and radionuclide angiogram (RNA) evaluation following revascularization (40). RNAs involve injection of a radioactive material and scanning of the heart with a gamma camera to reveal elevated end-diastolic and end-systolic left ventricular volumes as well as a reduced ejection fraction. The technique is useful in assessing ventricular function and evaluating response to therapy.

Summary

The role of the Clinic of Surgery in the evolution of cardiovascular surgery spans the development of diagnostic tests, characterization of congenital abnormalities of the left ventricular outflow tract and its operative treatment, development of operative techniques, and evaluation of prosthetic devices, operative intervention timing, and efficacy of combined operations. Numerous new mechanical and bioprosthetic heart valves currently being manufactured should be subjected to studies conducted in this Clinic on earlier devices until a near-perfect valve is available. Continued development of noninvasive studies that provide predictors for the timing of operative intervention in congenital and acquired heart disease will continue to be an important goal for the Heart Institute.

References

1. Sanders, R.J., and A.G. Morrow. A new diagnostic method in the study of congenital heart disease: The krypton-85 test for circulatory shunts. Proceedings of the Second United Nations International Conference on the Peaceful Uses of Atomic Energy 26:99. Geneva: United Nations, 1958.

2. Braunwald, E., et al. A simplified indicator-dilution technic for the localization of left-to-right circulatory shunts: An experimental and clinical study of intravenous injection with right heart sampling. Circulation 20:875-880, 1959.

3. Morrow, A.G., et al. The assessment of operative results in congenital heart disease by intraoperative indicator-dilution curves. Circulation 33:263-269, 1966.

4. Morrow, A.G., et al. Left atrial pressure pulse in mitral valve disease. A correlation of pressures obtained by transbronchial puncture with the valvular lesion. Circulation 16:399-405, 1957.

5. Ross, J., Jr., E. Braunwald, and A.G. Morrow. Transseptal left atrial puncture: New technique for the measurement of left atrial pressure in man. Am J Cardiol 3:653-655, 1959.

6. Ross, J., Jr., E. Braunwald, and A.G. Morrow. Left heart catheterization by the transseptal route: A description of the technique and its application. Circulation 22:927-934, 1960.

7. Brochenbrough, E.C., et al. Percutaneous puncture of the left ventricle. Br Heart J 23:643-648, 1961.

8. Tanenbaum, H.L., E. Braunwald, and A.G. Morrow. Determination of cardiac output and pressure gradients at operation: A technic for the immediate assessment of the results of operation for stenotic valvular disease. N Engl J Med 258:527-530, 1958.

9. Roberts, W.C., and A.G. Morrow. Congenital aortic steno-
    sis produced by a unicommissural valve. Br Heart J 27:
    505-510, 1965.
10. Fisher, R.D., D.T. Mason, and A.G. Morrow. Results of
    operative treatment in congenital aortic stenosis. J
    Thorac Cardiovasc Surg 59:218-224, 1970.
11. Conkle, D.M., M. Jones, and A.G. Morrow. Treatment of
    congenital aortic stenosis. An evaluation of the late
    results of aortic valvotomy. Arch Surg 107:649-651,
    1973.
12. Morrow, A.G., et al. Discrete subaortic stenosis compli-
    cated by aortic valvular regurgitation. Clinical, hemo-
    dynamic, and pathologic studies and the results of opera-
    tive treatment. Circulation 31:163-171, 1965.
13. Braunwald, N.S., and A.G. Morrow. Incomplete persistent
    atrioventricular canal. J Thorac Cardiovasc Surg 51:71-
    80, 1966.
14. Goldfaden, D.M., M. Jones, and A.G. Morrow. Long-term
    results of repair of incomplete persistent atrioventric-
    ular canal. J Thorac Cardiovasc Surg 82:669-673, 1981.
15. Braunwald, E., A.G. Morrow, and W.P. Cornell. Idiopathic
    hypertrophic subaortic stenosis: Anatomic, hemodynamic,
    clinical and angiocardiographic factors. Trans Assoc Am
    Physicians 73:297, 1960.
16. Morrow, A.G., and E.C. Brochenbrough. Surgical treatment
    of idiopathic hypertrophic subaortic stenosis: Technic
    and hemodynamic results of subaortic ventriculotomy. Ann
    Surg 154:181-189, 1961.
17. Maron, B.J., et al. Long-term clinical course and symp-
    tomatic status of patients after operation for hyper-
    trophic subaortic stenosis. Circulation 57:1205-1213,
    1978.
18. Morrow, A.G., and N.S. Braunwald. Transventricular mitral
    commissurotomy: Surgical technique and a hemodynamic
    evaluation of the method. J Thorac Cardiovasc Surg 41:
    225-235, 1961.
19. Morrow, A.G., L.A. duPlessis, and B.R. Wilcox. Hemo-
    dynamic studies after mitral commissurotomy. Surgery
    54:463-470, 1963.
20. Rutledge, R., et al. Mitral valve replacement after
    closed mitral commissurotomy. Circulation 66:I,162-166,
    1982.
21. Braunwald, N.S., T. Cooper, and A.G. Morrow. Complete
    replacement of the mitral valve. Successful clinical
    application of a flexible polyurethane prosthesis. J
    Thorac Cardiovasc Surg 40:1-11, 1960.
22. Morrow, A.G., et al. Prosthetic replacement of the mitral
    valve. Operative methods and the results of preoperative

and postoperative hemodynamic assessments. Circulation 29:2-13, 1964.

23. Glancy, D.L., et al. Hemodynamic studies in patients with 2M and 3M Starr-Edwards prostheses: Evidence of obstruction to left atrial emptying. Circulation, Supplement 1-39:113-118, 1969.

24. Brown, J.W., et al. Clinical and hemodynamic comparisons of Kay-Shiley, Starr-Edwards No. 6520, and Reis-Hancock porcine xenograft mitral valves. Surgery 76:983-991, 1974.

25. McIntosh, C.L., et al. Atrioventricular valve replacement with the Hancock porcine xenograft: A five year clinical experience. Surgery 78:768-775, 1975.

26. Borkon, A.M., et al. Mitral valve replacement with the Hancock bioprosthesis: Five-to-ten year follow-up. Ann Thorac Surg 32:127-137, 1981.

27. Morrow, A.G., et al. Prosthetic replacement of the mitral valve. Preoperative and postoperative clinical and hemodynamic assessments in 100 patients. Circulation 35:962-979, 1967.

28. Levine, F.H., J.C. Copeland, and A.G. Morrow. Prosthetic replacement of the mitral valve. Continuing assessments of the 100 patients operated upon during 1961-1965. Circulation 47:518-526, 1973.

29. Roberts, W.C., and A.G. Morrow. Fatal degeneration of the silicone rubber ball of the Starr-Edwards prosthetic aortic valve. Am J Cardiol 22:614-620, 1968.

30. McIntosh, C.L., and W.H. Schuette. A noninvasive technique for determining aortic and mitral ball variance. Circulation, Supplement IV:117, 1973.

31. Braunwald, N.S., and A.G. Morrow. Tissue ingrowth and the rigid heart valve. J Thorac Cardiovasc Surg 56:307-319, 1968.

32. Bull, B., J.C.A. Fuchs, and N.S. Braunwald. Mechanism of formation of tissue layers on the fabric lattice covering intravascular prosthetic devices. Surgery 65:640-648, 1969.

33. Hannah, H. III, B. Bull, and N.S. Braunwald. The development of an autogenous tissue covering on prosthetic heart valves: Effect of warfarin and dextran. Ann Surg 168:1075-1078, 1968.

34. Reis, R.L., et al. The flexible stent. J Thorac Cardiovasc Surg 62:683-689, 1971.

35. Jones, M., et al. Experimental evaluation of bioprosthetic valves implanted in sheep. In Cardiac Bioprostheses, Proceedings of the Second International Symposium, pp. 275-292, L.H. Cohen and V. Gallucci (eds.). New York: Yorke Medical Books, 1982.

36. Henry, W.L., et al. Observations on the optimum time for operative intervention for aortic regurgitation. I. Evaluation of the results of aortic valve replacement in symptomatic patients. Circulation 61:471-483, 1980.

37. Bonow, R.O., et al. The natural history of asymptomatic patients with aortic regurgitation and normal left ventricular function. Circulation 68:509-517, 1983.

38. Bonow, R.O., et al. Aortic valve replacement without myocardial revascularization in patients with combined aortic valvular and coronary artery disease. Circulation 63:243-251, 1981.

39. Seides, S.F., et al. Long-term anatomic fate of coronary artery bypass grafts and functional status of patients five years after operation. N Engl J Med 298:1213-1217, 1978.

40. Kent, K.M., et al. Effects of coronary artery bypass on global and regional left ventricular function during exercise. N Engl J Med 298:1434-1439, 1978.

Introduction

THERAPEUTIC RESEARCH IN THE
NATIONAL CANCER INSTITUTE

Several chapters in this volume deal with aspects of cancer causation. In this one we consider treatment. The treatment of cancer divides into three modes: surgery, radiotherapy, and chemotherapy. By employing skillful blends of these, clinical oncologists are achieving significant progress against the group of diseases known as cancer, producing remissions in many patients not presently being cured. There are still tumors that are refractory to treatment, but because of advances in our ability to treat these in the past two decades, the keynote of the cancer therapist is optimism. Indeed, this field of medicine retains only scientists and physicians who are optimists.

The greatest achievements recorded in this chapter are in chemotherapy. A significant number of drugs are available that have proved efficacious, first in the experimental animal and then in humans. It has been established that these agents are more likely to achieve a beneficial effect when administered in combination with others. For each type of tumor, many combinations of drugs and many dosage schedules must be tested; the permutations are essentially limitless.

The quest for new drugs proceeds in several ways. Analogs of various metabolites, normal intermediaries of metabolism, have been found to interfere with essential cellular processes and thereby to inhibit tumor growth. In other instances new agents have been found through a broadly based search of many compounds known to damage cells—a hunting expedition. Clearly, as our understanding of tumors advances, as we learn more about their pathogenesis and the mechanism of metastasis, we may expect to discover new and even more effective anticancer drugs. Meanwhile, with increasing skill in the design of drugs, the uses of ionizing radiation, and the techniques of surgery, more tumors may be expected to yield to this three-pronged attack.

D. S.

25

THERAPEUTIC RESEARCH IN THE NATIONAL CANCER INSTITUTE

Vincent T. DeVita, Jr.

Abraham Goldin

Introduction

This chapter relates the contribution of the intramural
clinical research program of the National Cancer Institute to
the notable advances in cancer therapy up to the late 1970s.
Emphasis is on developments in cancer chemotherapy, which was
paramount in the program prior to the era of combined modality therapy. The opening of the NIH Clinical Center in 1953
offered an unparalleled opportunity for the exercise of tal-
ent and drive on the part of investigators, particularly in
clinical cancer research; and the clinical program benefited
greatly during the early years from its colocation with the
extramural cancer drug development program. Given these ideal
conditions, it is understandable that 10 of the 15 prestigious
Albert Lasker Medical Research Awards for cancer chemotherapy
have gone to scientists who worked in the clinical program of
the Cancer Institute.

In 1975 an NCI reorganization combined all of the treatment modalities into one organizational unit, the Clinical
Oncology Program, which in turn brought NCI's clinical research into the era of combined modality therapy.

A few words of background are in order. Ehrlich's discovery in 1898 of the first alkylating agent foreshadowed the
successes of chemotherapy, but it was some 50 years before
this observation found application in the chemotherapy of

---

*VINCENT T. DeVITA, Jr., M.D., Director, National Cancer Insti-
tute. ABRAHAM GOLDIN, Ph.D., Scientist Emeritus and former
Associate Director for International Treatment Research, Division of Cancer Treatment, NCI. Prepared with the editorial
assistance of ELEANOR M. RICE, Editorial Assistant, Office of
the Director, NCI.*

neoplasia. In 1900 very few cancer patients were being cured. But in the early part of this century, the widespread application of the radical mastectomy introduced by William Halsted, exemplifying the principle of en bloc resection, and of X-rays, discovered in 1895 by Wilhelm Roentgen, provided an alternative to surgery for certain tumors and contributed to a climate of cautious optimism that cancer could be cured. Meanwhile, the development of transplantable animal tumors offered a means for testing candidate antitumor drugs prior to their administration to humans. These three early achievements in place by 1915 must be acknowledged as crucial to later developments in cancer medicine.

By about 1930 an overall cancer cure rate of 20 percent had been achieved with improved surgical technique, anesthesia, and blood transfusions. Radiotherapy played a minor role in the overall cure of cancers at that time. Low-voltage radiotherapy equipment was so crude that, according to much of the literature, this treatment was too toxic to be useful, foreshadowing the criticism of anticancer drugs to come later. By 1955, the routine use of antibiotics, further improvement in surgery, cobalt radiotherapy, and then linear accelerators had combined to bring the overall relative survival rate for cancer patients to about 33 percent, but at that point progress plateaued. This impasse was correctly attributed to the progressive growth of micrometastases outside the surgical or radiation field, often before the disease was detectable clinically or at the time of initial treatment. It was clear to many that success would require systemic treatment to complement surgery and radiotherapy in those cancers for which local treatment did not produce cures.

The discovery in 1943 that systemic treatment with nitrogen mustard could exert antitumor effects in animal systems and then in patients with Hodgkin's disease and other lymphomas created a furor among physicians concerned with the treatment of cancer. In the late 1940s it became apparent that chemicals could elicit at least partial regression of tumor in some human cancers. Farber, in 1947, demonstrated that the folic acid antagonist aminopterin was effective in inducing impressive remissions in acute leukemia of childhood. Advances in the field of systemic treatment required additional anticancer drugs, but where were they to be found?

The Early Years, 1937–1953

The beginnings of cancer research in America were modest. When President Franklin D. Roosevelt signed the Bone-Magnuson

Bill in 1937, creating the Cancer Institute, he placed the battle against this dread disease in the public domain. As part of this effort, Government support for research in cancer treatment was initiated on a large scale. The new Institute, headed by CARL VOEGTLIN, pursued drug screening and evaluation under MURRAY SHEAR. One of Shear's first efforts was to isolate an active ingredient of Coley's mixed toxins. The screening program, however, remained loosely organized until much later. Studies begun by Shear's group during the 1930s were continued following World War II by JONATHAN HARTWELL, who isolated podophyllin derivatives which, though highly toxic, were effective against animal neoplasia. The group screened a series of colchicine analogs, and MORRIS BELKIN started screening plant extracts for antitumor activity. The extreme toxicity of all these drugs greatly limited their usefulness in patients.

At the Clinical Research Unit in Baltimore, ABRAHAM GOLDIN's group began a series of studies in which it was demonstrated that the tumor-bearing animal could be utilized in a quantitative manner to determine comparative drug effectiveness and dose-response effects. Applying the principles of the dose-response relationship with randomization of treatments using mice, the influence of the schedule of drug administration was investigated empirically. Metabolite-antimetabolite relationships were studied with a view toward controlling toxicity to the host while optimizing therapeutic effect. These data were later to become major components of the design of clinical trials of anticancer drugs at the Clinical Center.

In 1946 LLOYD LAW, who remains one of NCI's preeminent cell biologists, introduced the L1210 murine leukemia cell line, a tumor that became a mainstay in the cancer drug screening program and a tool for preclinical investigation of anticancer drugs. He conducted many fundamental studies with this rapidly growing neoplasm. His experiments in the 1950s were the earliest demonstrations of the now exceedingly important observation that resistance to antifols and other drugs can develop spontaneously in mammalian tissue.* With this in mind, clinicians can design protocols to circumvent resistance to drugs which, though initially active against a given tumor in some cancer patients, lose their effectiveness. The leukemia L1210 cell line was also used widely in comparative kinetic modeling studies designed to compare the relative growth characteristics of rodent tumors used for

---

*This observation followed on the heels of and confirmed the seminal work on bacterial resistance to phage by Luria and Delbruck.

identifying candidate drugs against human tumors, their ultimate target.

Before the Clinical Center was built, clinical research facilities in other institutions fulfilled its functions, but this was discontinued shortly after the new research hospital was completed on the Bethesda campus. When the Clinical Center was opened in July 1953, a highly successful effort in cancer therapeutic research was begun. Three separate branches, Medicine, Surgery, and Radiology, were established for the conduct of clinical cancer studies.

Development of a Full-Scale
Clinical Research Program, 1953-1972

Demonstrating Curative Chemotherapy

In 1954 GORDON ZUBROD became NCI's first Clinical Director as well as Chief of the new General Medicine Branch. The Branch has since played a central role in the development of cancer chemotherapy and has been led successively by EMIL FREI, SEYMOUR PERRY, PAUL CARBONE, VINCENT DeVITA, and ROBERT C. YOUNG. Zubrod brought a solid scientific background and excellent administrative skills. Moreover, he maintained a firm belief, based largely on the success of the malaria drug development program in World War II, that quantitative chemotherapy and pharmacology combined with the appropriate expertise would make progress in cancer chemotherapy inevitable. Zubrod's crucial contributions to clinical research in cancer were recognized in 1972 by the Albert Lasker Special Medical Research Award.

This early NCI effort was indeed the first truly successful, tightly focused program of clinical cancer research and, of equal importance, training in oncology. It attracted young, dynamic clinical investigators eager for opportunities in academic research in a controversial new field of medicine. Initially the major mission of the program was to attract and train physicians interested in cancer chemotherapy, to establish pharmacology laboratories, and to launch quantitatively based clinical trials. To these ends, Gordon Zubrod recruited Emil Frei, EMIL J. FREIREICH, and DAVID RALL. With this nucleus it became possible to attract a significant number of talented Clinical Associates to the field of drug research.

At the beginning, Frei, Freireich, and JAMES HOLLAND provided the clinical leadership. They were joined and succeeded by other investigators: Paul Carbone, Vincent DeVita, GEORGE

CANELLOS, JOHN ZIEGLER, EDWARD HENDERSON, the late MYRON
KARON, BRUCE CHABNER, PHILIP SCHEIN, Robert Young, and others.
All of these investigators, who first served as Clinical Associates in the Commissioned Corps of the U.S. Public Health
Service, assumed important leadership roles in cancer therapy
and therapeutic research both within NIH and in the wider community of academic medicine. An additional number of Clinical
Associates too numerous to mention here were trained in the
Medicine Branch and have since formed the nucleus for the new
subspecialty of internal medicine, medical oncology, which
was established in 1973.

The initial dramatic demonstration that therapy with drugs
such as nitrogen mustard and the folic acid antagonists would
have a significant effect against cancer provided a powerful stimulus to search for new and more effective antitumor
agents. In 1955 the Congress authorized $5 million for a can-
cer drug development program at NCI. Accordingly, the Cancer
Chemotherapy National Service Center was established within
the Institute to coordinate the first nationwide cooperative
cancer chemotherapy program. The CCNSC was first directed
by KENNETH ENDICOTT, who would later serve as Director, NCI.
This was the first large "special initiative" program within
the NIH structure.

In 1966 NCI was reorganized to coordinate related activities, and the CCNSC was integrated into a single chemotherapy
research program under Zubrod. The intramural clinical component of the program consisted of the General Medicine Branch
with two sections, one for clinical chemotherapy and the other
for pharmacology and experimental therapeutics. This Branch
was to give rise to the current NCI medical oncology branches
(one at the Clinical Center and the other at the National
Naval Medical Center) and the Pediatric Oncology, Dermatology,
Metabolism, Immunology, and Clinical Pharmacology Branches, as
well as the Laboratory of Chemical Pharmacology. The chemotherapy program, however, remained separate from the other
clinical specialties until 1975, when the surgery and radiation branches were combined in the current organization of
the Clinical Oncology Program.

There were additional features of the intramural clinical
research program that contributed to its success. A vacuum
existed in the field because most universities had no interest
in the medical aspects of cancer treatment and no cancer subspecialty in their departments of medicine. The climate in
academic medicine was generally hostile to the use of anticancer drugs and was pessimistic about cancer treatment in
general. This was due in part to the controversy over the
special congressional initiative establishing NCI's Drug Development Program, the empirical approach to drug develop-

ment, and the toxic nature of most anticancer drugs. The NIH Clinical Center was one of the few places where the field could evolve rapidly, driven by the imagination of young investigators unencumbered by more conservative academic constraints.

NCI intramural staff made substantive contributions to the drug development effort by participating in the initial choice of screening systems and the subsequent selection of new screening models. In 1956 Zubrod proposed dividing clinical trials involving new anticancer drugs into three phases (I, II, and III) to permit the focus of each trial on different criteria and problems pertaining at the successive stages unique to cancer drug development. David Rall and Gordon Zubrod drew up the initial preclinical toxicological guidelines to establish the accepted definition of "limiting toxicities" and the "safe starting dose" in man. These guidelines were adopted by the Food and Drug Administration and remained the standard for NCI and the pharmaceutical industry.

All of these factors fueled the movement to develop cures with drugs for significant fractions of patients with choriocarcinoma, acute leukemia of childhood, Hodgkin's disease, diffuse large cell lymphoma (the disease known then as reticulum cell sarcoma), Burkitt's lymphoma, and mycosis fungoides. Significant advances were also made in the identification of new treatments for islet cell cancer, adrenal carcinoma, ovarian and breast cancers, and chronic myelocytic leukemia. In addition, major contributions were made to the identification and treatment of infectious complications of cancer treatment. It was at the Clinical Center, in the main, that techniques to support intensive combination chemotherapy, such as platelet and white cell transfusions, and the appropriate protective environment were also developed. For this work the Lasker Award was given in 1972 to MIN CHIU LI, ROY HERTZ, EUGENE VAN SCOTT, Frei, Freireich, Carbone, DeVita, Ziegler, and Holland, as well as Zubrod. The principles of combination chemotherapy derived from these early studies have had a major and continuing impact on chemotherapy for other cancers, as well as the use of chemotherapy to complement surgery and radiotherapy in early stages of the disease. They also furthered the specialties of medical and pediatric oncology. A brief description of the salient features of this work follows.

Choriocarcinoma. Prior to 1957 choriocarcinoma was incurable unless excised when still localized, as rarely occurred, and then only by resorting to total hysterectomy. When metastatic, it was fatal within six months. The initial suggestion that chemotherapy could cure metastatic cancer

is attributed to the late Min Chiu Li. In 1956 Li employed
methotrexate because he had observed that a patient with malignant melanoma secreting chorionic gonadotropin had responded to this folic acid antagonist with a fall in titer.
His first choriocarcinoma patient was treated with a dose and
schedule he had designed. He was scolded severely for his
unorthodox approach, but the patient's response was dramatic.
Indeed, Li's colleagues attributed this initial success to
"spontaneous regression." Then, using the intermittent schedule of administration, Li observed a progressive drop of gonadotropin in the urine of women whose pulmonary metastases
regressed in response to treatment. Ultimately Li left NCI
under a cloud of the controversy over the toxicity of his
unusual treatment.

By 1963 Hertz's endocrinology group, then including MOR-
TIMER LIPSETT and GRIFF ROSS, reported a cure of 28 out of 63
patients, or almost 45 percent, at five-year followup. In
later studies at NCI, a cure rate of 88 percent was reported.
The success in choriocarcinoma as an indication that drugs
could cure cancer has remained controversial because the tissue of origin is fetal and therefore in part foreign to the
host. These early clinical observations, however, demonstrated several important principles that remain fresh today:

- That metastatic cancer is curable in humans by means of
  drugs;

- That quantitative measurements of a tumor marker could
  be used to anticipate and affirm complete regression and
  cure in a patient following drug treatment; and

- That determination of the scheduling characteristics of
  drugs is of prime importance—specifically, intermittent scheduling as a means, potentially, of increasing
  tumor cell kill while limiting bone marrow toxicity.

Acute Lymphocytic Leukemia. As one of the major malignancies of childhood, acute lymphocytic leukemia presented a
particularly poignant plea from both the small patients and
their families. James Holland was at NCI between 1953 and
1954 and, following his departure, was associated with Frei
and Freireich through a cooperative group, the Acute Leukemia Group B (ALGB), established by Zubrod to expand clinical
trials. There was a close interaction between preclinical
experimentalists and clinicians at NCI. The results of preclinical studies of combination chemotherapy, like those of
Skipper, Law, and Goldin, all found expression in the treat-

ment of acute lymphocytic leukemia of childhood where tissue
was readily accessible to evaluate the clinical impact of
these new studies.

The quantitative data from L1210 leukemia and related
screens focused on the importance of killing *all* tumor cells.
These data led to the strategy for achieving total tumor cell
eradication in the clinics. Protocols were developed that,
for the first time, specified methods for patient selection,
objective criteria for dosage, and dose adjustment. Quantitative criteria for terms like "complete remission" and "remission maintenance" were formulated. It was within the context of these studies that the first clear distinctions between "remission induction," "remission maintenance," and
other terms were made. Employing drugs in combination, Frei,
Freireich, and Karon at NCI, Holland with ALGB, and Pinkel
at St. Jude's Hospital in Memphis, Tennessee, were able to
maintain effective doses and improve survival. The forerunner
of all combination chemotherapies for childhood leukemia was
the VAMP program (vincristine, amethopterin,* 6-mercaptopu-
rine, prednisone) designed by Freireich, Karon, and Frei—
the first of its kind to admit openly to the attempt to cure
acute lymphocytic leukemia of childhood. It achieved a high
rate of prolonged, complete remissions.

With success against the initial disease came recognition
of the problem of relapse in pharmacologic sanctuaries—body
sites inaccessible to chemotherapy. NCI pathologist LOUIS
THOMAS with Freireich and others identified meningeal leukemia
as a major cause of treatment failure. Rall and his associates
defined the pharmacokinetic problems of intrathecal** therapy
with antifols while RALPH JOHNSON explored the use of central
nervous system irradiation. Identification of the syndrome
of meningeal leukemia and its effective management have had
subsequent application to other kinds of malignancies where
subarachnoid spread provides potentially fatal foci of residual disease.

The effectiveness of folic acid antagonists against overt
meningeal leukemia was demonstrated by a comparative study in
1964. Prophylactic use of intrathecal methotrexate reduced
the incidence of meningeal leukemia and thereby improved the
cure rate significantly. Now a 50 percent cure rate has been
achieved for this previously incurable disease by remission
induction with vincristine and prednisone, prophylactic administration of intrathecal methotrexate, brain irradiation,
and intermittent treatment with methotrexate and 6-mercapto-

---

*Later named methotrexate.
**Injection via the theca of the spinal cord into the sub-
arachnoid space.

purine during remission. By the 1970s national mortality from this disease had begun to fall as use of the treatment spread nationwide. For this ground-breaking effort, Frei and Freireich shared the General Motors Prize for cancer treatment in 1983.

Hodgkin's Disease. This is a malignancy of the lymphatic system which affects principally young adults. Although curable by radiotherapy in its most localized forms, it was seldom detected at that stage and, unless treated by chemotherapy, was fatal in the majority of patients who presented with advanced disease. Today over 80 percent of all patients with Hodgkin's disease are curable, and the national mortality has fallen dramatically.

The development of a drug cure for this solid neoplasm of adults represents a singular triumph. In the early 1960s, pessimism surrounded chemotherapy of Hodgkin's disease because the response to drugs, namely alkylating agents, was temporary. In addition, progress at NCI in the development of new protocols for the disease was initially hampered somewhat by rivalries between the specialties of radiation therapy and chemotherapy. And finally, the major emphasis in 1963 was on the exciting clinical studies of the Acute Leukemia Service of the Medicine Branch, while the Solid Tumor Service was occupied with early-stage (Phases I and II) drug testing.

The initial intensive study with curative intent using a four-drug combination was conducted as a 14-patient pilot project in 1963 and 1964 by DeVita, JOHN MOXLEY, and Frei. They were strongly influenced by the work of Skipper, Schabel, and Wilcox. The first drugs utilized were cyclophosphamide, vincristine (Oncovin), methotrexate, and prednisone. Later nitrogen mustard replaced cyclophosphamide and the regimen gained the acronym MOMP. When methotrexate was replaced by procarbazine, a new, more effective agent tested singly both in France and at the Clinical Center, the regimen became known as MOPP.

The MOMP regimen was initiated in the fall of 1963. The plan was rational, albeit radical for that time: By employing drugs with differing toxicities in combination, at full dosages, single-drug toxicity could be avoided and additive and possibly synergistic antitumor responses would result. On the basis of the kinetic considerations that human tumors did not grow as uniformly as transplantable rodent tumor L1210, the short $2\frac{1}{2}$-month MOMP regimen (based on the 42-day induction cycle of protocols in use at that time) was changed to prolonged administration—a 6-month period—with MOPP. It was hypothesized that the combination of four drugs acting via different mechanisms could also circumvent the development of drug resistance.

The most radical departure, as in acute lymphocytic leukemia, seems trite now: the goal of cure, not palliation, even in persons with metastatic disease. Chemical cure of Hodgkin's disease, even in its advanced form, was first reported in 1967 by DeVita and co-workers and was confirmed by others in the 1970s. In a followup of 155 patients treated at NCI who had achieved complete remission with the MOPP chemotherapy program, 82 percent were alive at 5 years and 72 percent at 10 years. The MOPP program provided a model for the treatment of other forms of cancer in adults.

Non-Hodgkin's Lymphoma (NHL).
This awkward name is given to those lymphomas of adults which are not Hodgkin's disease. While localized forms of these lymphomas were curable with radiotherapy, the majority of cases (90 percent) are detected as disseminated disease. The most aggressive form, which killed patients within two years of diagnosis, was called reticulum cell sarcoma. This disease was later designated, according to Henry Rappaport's classification, as diffuse histiocytic lymphoma and is now called diffuse large-cell lymphoma. When MOPP was being used in Hodgkin's disease, it was also used with all lymphoma patients referred to the Medicine Branch. Initially MOPP was abandoned in the treatment of NHL because the majority of early patients who had a slower-growing variety, follicular lymphoma, did not achieve durable remissions with this chemotherapy regimen. In 1967, however, it was noted that several patients with diffuse hystiocytic lymphoma had been rendered free of disease by treatment with MOPP and had remained so since 1964. Accordingly, the treatment program was modified and the study extended.

The drug cure of NHL with C-MOPP, a version employing cyclophosphamide instead of nitrogen mustard, was reported in 1975 by DeVita and others. With newer drugs and scheduling concepts, the majority of adults in advanced stages of diffuse large-cell lymphoma can now be cured. Disease-free survival at two years from the termination of treatment is tantamount to cure for this aggressive tumor. A current Medicine Branch protocol with alternating cycles of two combinations of drugs (ProMACE-MOPP) to circumvent the spontaneous development of drug resistance has increased the remission rate in patients with advanced disease to 74 percent, with 60 percent of all patients free of disease at three years. Again, on the heels of this achievement, national mortality for patients with diffuse lymphomas has begun to fall.

Burkitt's Lymphoma. This is a malignancy of the lymphatic system found principally among children in Africa. Denis Burkitt, a British surgeon, had described the disease in 1958, noting its sensitivity to chemotherapy. When Burkitt left Uganda, he asked that NCI lend partial support to the clinical unit at Makerere University to study this disease. Encouraged by the report of impressive results achieved with chemotherapy in a small percentage of patients, NCI staff members Carbone, Ziegler, and CHARLES VOGEL went to Uganda to establish a lymphoma unit at Makerere Hospital. In 1970 Ziegler's group reported that 60 percent of patients in favorable stages of Burkitt's lymphoma could be cured with cyclophosphamide and began to define prognostic groups. In 1979, at 10-year followup, cures were reported for 38 percent of 192 patients in all stages for whom followup had been feasible. The NCI staff convincingly described an American counterpart of Burkitt's lymphoma also responsive to chemotherapy, and a new combination chemotherapy regimen has resulted in an increase of the cure rate to 70 percent.

Mycosis Fungoides. In the early 1960s Van Scott and NCI radiotherapist J. ROBERT ANDREWS began studying and treating the lymphoma of the skin known as mycosis fungoides with electron beam radiation, using the giant Van de Graaff accelerator at the Clinical Center. The results in early disease were encouraging. These studies continue with more sophisticated sources of electron beams, under the direction of the Radiation Branch's present chief, ELI GLATSTEIN, and his medical oncologist colleague PAUL BUNN.

Van Scott and co-workers also began to experiment with the use of topical chemotherapy. They showed that complete remissions could be achieved by applying the alkylating agent nitrogen mustard to the skin of patients in early and superficial stages of mycosis fungoides. Many patients remained free of disease, and thus the more serious, resistant stages were avoided. This approach was similarly employed in epidermoid and basal cell carcinomas by Edmund Klein at Roswell Park Memorial Institute in Buffalo. He obtained excellent results in these common skin cancers with topical applications of 5-fluorouracil, a treatment in use today. For this work Van Scott and Klein shared in the 1972 Lasker prize.

Other Advances in the Medical Treatment of Cancer

Not all cancers studied in the NCI intramural clinical program proved curable by drugs, surgery, or radiotherapy.

Some, such as multiple myeloma, served as perplexing models and sources of tissue and serum that made possible some early important work in structure and function of immunoglobulins. For other cancers, significant advances in management continue to influence their treatment today.

Adrenal Cortical Cancer.   This malignancy of the adrenal cortex, or outer edge of the adrenal gland, is fatal unless detected at a stage where all of the malignant tissue can be removed surgically. Therefore, DELBERT BERGENSTAL and Hertz's demonstration that op'DDD, a derivative of the insecticide DDT, inhibited steroid synthesis and produced tumor regression in advanced adrenal cortical cancer was an important early achievement. Although not curative when the disease is metastatic, complete clinical remissions occur, and this is still the treatment of choice for metastatic adrenal cancer. It has also stimulated interest in the search for drugs with selective organ toxicity. Because of the rarity of adrenal cortical cancer, op'DDD has not been tested as an adjuvant to surgery, where it might actually prove to be curative.

Islet Cell Tumors of the Pancreas.   The story of the treatment of islet cell tumors of the pancreas is analogous to that of adrenal cancer. The NCI intramural program led by Philip Schein played a major role in the development of streptozotocin, the first drug effective against this rare tumor. Streptozotocin is an antibiotic isolated from a strain of *Streptomyces achromogenes* by investigators at Upjohn. It turned out to be a naturally occurring nitrosourea, 1-methyl-1-nitrosourea, with a glucose molecule attached. This compound was shown, quite incidentally, to be diabetogenic in rats, probably because the glucose moiety afforded entry into the islet cells. It also had the property, unusual among anticancer drugs, of sparing the bone marrow. These observations led to its development and use in treatment of the rare islet cell carcinoma. As a primary treatment of metastatic islet cell tumor, the compound proved capable of producing durable complete remissions. These studies demonstrated how specific a cancer drug could be for a particular tumor type.

This critical observation later resulted in modification of the extramural clinical trials program. New anticancer drugs are now tested on specific tumors in cases where the preclinical toxicologic effects indicate organ specificity. The practice had a marked effect on the development of the now widely used anticancer drug diamminedichloroplatinum (cisplatin). This very useful anticancer agent was at first thought to be inactive, since tests showed little effect against common tumors. Careful study of the drug in rarer tumors identified its dramatic effect in testicular cancer. Because data from controlled clinical trials were limited for such a rare tumor, the Food and Drug Administration approved the new drug application for cisplatin only after much debate. Marketed specifically for the treatment of testicular cancer, it has had a dramatic effect on national mortality from this disease. Subsequent tests of the use of cisplatin in combination with other drugs have shown that its spectrum is indeed much wider than originally anticipated.

Chronic Myelogenous Leukemia (CML). CML is a malignancy of bone-marrow stem cell proliferation and the first shown to have a characteristic chromosome marker, the so-called Philadelphia chromosome. Freireich became interested in this disease as part of his pioneer investigations into leukocyte procurement for experimental transfusion in patients rendered aplastic by chemotherapy. Incidental allogeneic grafts of CML cells were observed in some patients given transfusions of peripheral cells from CML patients as supportive care. This was one of the early demonstrations that the peripheral leukocytes of such patients are capable of surviving as stem cells for subsequent engraftment, a feature which has been explored subsequently in autologous engrafting of cryopreserved peripheral leukocytes with intensive chemotherapy of the blastic phase.

NCI staff conducted important studies on the efficacy of hydroxyurea, an agent which has become a standard drug for the treatment of the chronic phase of the disease. These investigations demonstrated it to be free of the undesirable delayed myelosuppressive effects of busulfan. The extreme heterogeneity of the blastic phase of the disease was first described at NCI by Canellos and other members of the Medicine Branch. Investigations of the evolution of CML to its blastic phase undertaken by Carbone, Canellos, and DeVita defined the extent of myelofibrosis as a complication and the detection of aneuploidy* to herald the onset of the blastic phase and influence the outcome of treatment.

In 1967 NCI staff demonstrated that the blast cells of approximately 30 percent of patients in blastic crises had morphologic characteristics of lymphoblasts. This observation, coupled with the demonstration that vincristine/prednisone (an antilymphoblastic treatment program) produced complete remissions for about two-thirds of such patients, stimulated subsequent investigations leading to the conclusion that CML can be viewed clinically as a disease of the totipotential stem cell. Subsequent work in other laboratories confirmed

---

*Deviation from the normal number of chromosomes.

the presence of lymphoid enzymes (terminal transferase) and immunologic surface markers characteristic of acute lympho-blastic leukemia.

Adult Acute Leukemia. During the early 1960s, acute leu-kemia in adults was a rapidly fatal malignancy with a re-mission rate of only 20 percent. Unlike the remissions of childhood leukemia, these were not durable and few patients lived longer than six months. In parallel with their studies in children, Frei, Freireich, and Edward Henderson showed that a four-drug combination, POMP—prednisone, vincristine (On-covin), methotrexate, and 6-mercaptopurine (Purinethol)—produced a higher rate of complete remission and some durable remissions. Further studies by others in the intramural pro-gram defined the role of arabinoside cytosine and daunorubicin in this disease. Using newer combinations of these drugs, more recent investigations throughout the United States, particu-larly by Freireich after moving to the M.D. Anderson Hospital in Houston, have seen a doubling of the complete remission rate and median survival, with a population of long-term disease-free survivors, very likely cured.

Ovarian Cancer. Because it is "silent," ovarian cancer, curable by surgery when truly localized, is particularly dif-ficult to diagnose early. Often tumors appear to be localized when they have already spread. In the late 1960s the role of medical oncologists in managing this disease was as limited as were the drugs effective in its treatment. At that time only L-phenylalanine mustard (L-PAM) was adequately tested for the treatment of patients with disseminated ovarian cancer. A seminal observation made in the Medicine Branch changed the staging of this disease dramatically (see Peritoneoscopy be-low). NCI's clinical trials program, under the guidance of Robert Young and Vincent DeVita, has since identified several other agents effective against advanced ovarian carcinoma: 5-fluorouracil, methotrexate, hexamethylmelamine, adriamycin, and cisplatin.

In the early 1970s a Medicine Branch controlled clinical trial indicated that the addition of hexamethylmelamine to a three-drug combination of cyclophosphamide, methotrexate (amethopterin), and 5-fluorouracil (Hexa-CAF) yielded results superior to those achieved with L-PAM alone in Stages III and IV ovarian cancer. There was a higher percentage of complete remissions, and one-third of the patients had complete dis-appearance of tumor. Sixty-five percent of those treated with this new drug combination are alive at five years. The re-sults appear to indicate long-term disease-free survival of at least 10 percent of patients in the trials, and others have now confirmed these results.

Ovarian cancer is also unusual among malignancies in that it kills by local invasion within the abdominal cavity rather than by distant metastases. Failure to control the local disease is related to failure to destroy every malignant cell within the nooks and crannies of the abdominal cavity, even with radiotherapy. Utilizing the extraordinary pharmacologic expertise in the intramural program, NCI achieved another first by employing the technique of peritoneal dialysis to exploit the different pharmacokinetics of renal clearance and peritoneal diffusion capacity of large volumes (2-4 liters) of intraperitoneally administered drugs. This intraperitoneal chemotherapy, the so-called "bellybath" approach, has proved feasible with several agents and produced a 25- to 300-fold excess of the drug within the peritoneal space as compared with plasma concentrations. The bellybath approach is now under investigation as a postoperative adjuvant treatment at several other institutions.

Small Cell Lung Cancer. This is the malignancy of the lung which had the poorest prognosis in the 1960s. Prior to 1972, there was no effective treatment for small cell lung cancer, but it is now yielding to a combination of intensive chemotherapy and radiotherapy. Such treatment has rendered about 20 percent of patients whose cancer is limited to the chest free of disease long enough to be considered cured. To minimize chances of relapse, prophylactic irradiation of the central nervous system is also being employed. The laboratory work conducted by JOHN MINNA and his colleagues, paralleling the clinical trials, has identified a specific karyotypic (chromosomal) abnormality in this disease and the expression of the *myc* oncogene* in a specific subset. They discovered that bombesin, a neuropeptide, is produced by this tumor and may provide a mechanism for autoregulation of growth.

Brain Tumors. Brain tumors were previously treatable only with surgery and radiotherapy. David Rall opened up the field of drug treatment of brain tumors by bringing a series of neurosurgeons into the Laboratory of Experimental Therapeutics and Chemical Pharmacology to collaborate in pioneering studies of the blood-brain barrier. Rall and his colleagues encouraged the design of lipid-soluble anticancer drugs that might be effective in brain tumor patients. John Montgomery at Southern Research Institute in Birmingham, Alabama, synthesized a whole

---

*See chapters by Paul and Waldmann (Section V), Rauscher and Shimkin, and Scolnick.

series of nitrosourea compounds, some of which are marketed today.

In 1971 Rall organized the Brain Tumor Study Group, composed of neurosurgeons interested in using chemotherapy to supplement methods of local control. They observed that treatment with radiation and nitrosourea chemotherapy following surgery elicited modest but definite improvement among patients with highly malignant glioblastoma multiforme. Since then, a search has been under way for drugs that specifically exert effects against tumors of the central nervous system. One such drug is the aziridine benzoquinone derivative AZQ synthesized by JOHN DRISCOLL and his group in the intramural Pharmacology Program of the Laboratory of Medicinal Chemistry. It has been shown to be effective against murine brain tumors and is undergoing preliminary clinical investigations with encouraging results.

Breast Cancer. The principles of combination chemotherapy in lymphoma and leukemia were first applied to the treatment of metastatic breast cancer by EZRA GREENSPAN in New York City and by RICHARD COOPER in Buffalo. Cooper reported a very high complete remission rate with a continuously administered five-drug regimen. NCI staff led by George Canellos, seeing potential benefit in the use of cyclical drug combination chemotherapy as an adjuvant to surgery, developed the CMF program: cyclophosphamide, methotrexate, and 5-fluorouracil. This combination, tested by Bonadonna and others in Milan, Italy, under contract with NCI, is still standard for the adjuvant drug treatment of breast cancer.

Peritoneoscopy. Used by gastroenterologists and gynecologists for many years, peritoneoscopy was introduced at the Clinical Center by DeVita as a tool for medical oncologists. An instrument inserted through a small incision permits visualization of internal organs and determination of the spread of tumor. It has proved effective as a substitute for surgical staging* of lymphoma patients in studies first reported by members of the Medicine Branch and for staging and following results of treatment in patients with ovarian cancer.

Through use of peritoneoscopy, some ovarian cancer patients assumed to have only localized disease were found by C. M. BAGLEY and DeVita to have "hidden" metastases on the undersurface of the diaphragm. The possibility of recurrence in these patients was high, since they would otherwise have received no further therapy or would have been given limited

---

*The determination of distinct phases or periods in a particular disease.

radiation up to the lower edge of the liver. This crucial
observation led to the wider use of adjuvant chemotherapy,
including the "bellybath" technique, and the proper extension
of radiotherapy to cover the dome of the diaphragm. The observation of hidden metastases is credited with a large share
of the decline in national mortality from ovarian cancer in
this country during the past decade.

Advances in Supportive Care

Platelet and Granulocyte Transfusion. Platelet transfusions, pioneered by Freireich's group at NCI and Isaac
Djerassi at Children's Hospital in Boston, have made a significant contribution to supportive therapy of cancer patients throughout the world. In the early years, the use of
platelet transfusions at the Clinical Center created much
controversy because it was unproven and placed a strain
on the blood bank. To compensate, the Cancer Institute
provided its own platelet procurement program for most of
the 1970s. Freireich and his colleagues were the first to
demonstrate the correlation between platelet level and increased risk of hemorrhage and the use of platelet transfusion to prevent hemorrhagic death. This program first implemented regular platelet replacement in the treatment of acute
leukemia and thereby drastically reduced mortality due to
hemorrhage.

The utility of histocompatible platelets was demonstrated
by RONALD YANKEE and others in the NCI intramural program.
They were able to show that HLA*-matched platelet transfusions can be given for long periods without risk of isosen-
sitization. Their routine use has been a significant advance
in the care of patients requiring repeated transfusions.

Freireich's group, using granulocytes from donors with
chronic granulocytic leukemia, was the first to perform therapeutically effective granulocyte transfusions. This treatment
proved modestly effective in some patients with established
infections. Then a contract was initiated which resulted in
the development of the IBM 2990 blood cell separator, still
the most effective means for collecting adequate numbers of
leukocytes from normal donors for both research and treatment.

The Life Island. The first clinically usable germ-free
environment was introduced by Freireich at NCI in the 1960s.

---

*Human leukocyte antigen, important in cross-matching
procedures and partially responsible for tissue rejection.

This plastic bubble provided means of preventing infection in patients who had received myelosuppressive* chemotherapy. The modern laminar air rooms currently in wide use stem from these early pioneering studies.

Diagnosis and Treatment of Infectious Disease

As hemorrhage declined as a cause of death, infection killed most cancer patients who either did not respond to treatment or were temporarily vulnerable to infection while undergoing the new, more aggressive treatment in use at the Clinical Center in the 1950s and 1960s. It proved to be more complicated to collect and administer white cells for transfusion than platelets. Antibiotics were still the first line of defense. Effective management of these problems in cancer patients began with the recognition that a different spectrum of infectious diseases was occurring in the immunocompromised host.

Staphylococcal infections troubled most of the academic medical world in the 1960s, but cancer patients were dying from pseudomonas septicemia. Studies pioneered in the early 1960s by Freireich, GERALD BODEY, CLAUDE FORKNER, and others in the Medicine Branch placed gram-negative sepsis, particularly from pseudomonas, in perspective, and identified heretofore uncommon forms of this disease such as diffuse pneumonitis with vasculitis and perirectal abscesses. Clinical Associates in the Medicine Branch were taught to assume that this infection was present in all cancer patients with fever and leukopenia and, contrary to the generally accepted practice, to administer combinations of antibiotics in advance of culture results. These combinations always included the drug colimycin, the only antipseudomonas agent available at that time. Because adequate serum levels were difficult to obtain with the recommended intramuscular use, colimycin was administered intravenously (though prohibited on the label). Nonetheless, prompt empirical treatment of presumed pseudomonas septicemia saved the lives of patients who were on their way into remission and changed the approach to the management of the febrile leukopenic cancer patient.

As bacterial infections were recognized and treated, even more unusual infections began to appear. It turned out that one-quarter of all patients who died from their cancer in the Clinical Center were shown by autopsy to have disseminated candidiasis. Amphotericin B, the antifungal antibiotic hereto-

---

*Inhibiting bone marrow activity, which results in decreased production of blood cells and platelets.

fore reserved for the treatment of cryptococcal meningitis, was pressed into use to treat patients who were febrile without identified bacterial or viral causes. This treatment too was controversial, but is known today to prevent candidiasis deaths.

Another fungus, *Aspergillus fumigatus,* appeared in peculiar forms in the immunosuppressed cancer patient. DeVita recounts an illustrative experience that occurred after he left the NCI Clinical Associate program to complete his residency training. A leukemic patient with lobar pneumonia was diagnosed by house staff and consulting faculty as having klebsiella pneumonia despite the fact that aspergillus was growing freely in the sputum. Aspergillus lobar pneumonia, having been seen in Bethesda, was the proper diagnosis, but was dismissed as not a known manifestation of aspergillosis. The patient succumbed to both his illnesses, and autopsy revealed invasive aspergillosis lobar pneumonia. On returning to Bethesda, DeVita and Young, then a new Clinical Associate, collected seven similar cases and offered them for publication. The report was rejected by one of the leading experts on lobar pneumonia as presenting an impossible association but was finally accepted for publication in another journal. A paper reporting 98 cases was later published and remains the definitive work on infection by aspergillus in cancer patients.

Another then-unusual but now topical infection, *Pneumocystis carinii* pneumonia, was first described and successfully treated in adult cancer patients on the Medicine Branch wards. A woman whose Hodgkin's disease was progressing in spite of combination chemotherapy (MOMP) died of an undefined pneumonitis. The Cancer Institute's astute pathologists searching for a cause did the proper silver stains and made the diagnosis of *Pneumocystis carinii* pneumonia, but a visiting pathologist from Africa about to attend the regular Wednesday rounds where the case was to be presented said that this diagnosis was impossible since *Pneumocystis* pneumonia afflicted only premature infants. The diagnosis, however, proved correct. As a result, needle aspiration biopsy of the lung was applied in the diagnosis of other patients with diffuse pneumonias of unknown etiology, and the first two successfully treated cases were reported in the *New England Journal of Medicine*.

Shortly thereafter, Hughes and his associates at St. Jude's Hospital recognized the epidemic nature of this disease in leukemic children, a circumstance reminiscent of the later discovery of Legionnaire's disease. The treatment of choice for *Pneumocystis carinii* pneumonia was the drug pentamidine isethionate, then available only from the Centers for Disease Control in Atlanta. Experience with the drug

was limited to infants in Hungary and patients with sleeping
sickness in Africa. With access to frequent cases of *Pneumocystis carinii* pneumonia and with the help of PHILIP WAALKES,
who had joined the Medicine Branch for a time, an assay was
developed for pentamidine isethionate and was used to describe
its pharmacokinetics. The compound remained the mainstay of
treatment until it was replaced by the much-easier-to-use commercial combination of sulfanilamides and antifols.

The ironic aspect of this is that *Pneumocystis carinii*
pneumonia was soon shown to occur more often in patients who
had attained remission with aggressive chemotherapy than in
those who were dying of their cancer. The infection occurred
while they were being withdrawn from treatment, suggesting
that the pulmonary manifestations were a result of a returning
immune and inflammatory response. Thus the identification
and successful treatment of this disease with pentamidine
isethionate saved the very patients who had the best response
to more aggressive drug treatment. Today *Pneumocystis carinii*
pneumonia has reemerged as an important infectious complication of patients with acquired immune deficiency syndrome
(AIDS), and pentamidine isethionate has reemerged as a very
useful backup treatment.

Surgery and Radiotherapy at NCI:
Selection of Primary Treatment Based on the
Availability and Effectiveness of Other Modalities

The Surgery Program was established in 1953 and headed by
ROBERT SMITH, who conducted studies on the significance of
circulating tumor cells to the process of metastasis. This
early approach investigated possible causes of surgical failure unrelated to the technical details of the surgical procedures. Fragmentation of tumor was studied microscopically,
both in the wound area and in the blood. It was frequently
observed that, following surgery, drainage of tumor cells
from the wound area occurred for several days. NCI pathologists and surgeons demonstrated that cancer cells could be
found in the blood of patients whose cancer had been localized, even those who remained tumor-free.

Later, NCI surgeons led by ALFRED KETCHAM concerned themselves principally with radical surgery of uterine tumors,
cancers of the head and neck, soft-tissue and bone sarcomas,
and melanomas. These investigators were also involved very
early with studying the effects of laser radiation on normal
and neoplastic cells. Ketcham developed a craniofacial surgi-

cal approach, an important contribution to en bloc removal of
cancer of the ethmoid sinus. Still in use, the procedure has
resulted in improved survival for that tumor. In addition,
there was considerable experimental reconstructive surgery of
the head and neck using extended shoulder and deltopectoral
full-thickness skin flaps, and early successful work in total
mandibular replacement.

In the experimental treatment of melanomas, surgeons grap-
pled with the problem of distant metastases, the primary cause
of the overall mortality of 51 percent at five years. There
were preliminary efforts by DONALD L. MORTON and others, in
collaboration with the Immunology and Medicine Branches, to
assess the effectiveness of various combinations of treatment
in melanoma and to evaluate the effectiveness of immunotherapy
or chemotherapy in patients with minimal residual disease.

In 1974 STEVE ROSENBERG, appointed chief of the Surgery
Branch, brought with him a background in laboratory science
unique amongst cancer surgeons. His ability to engage the
skills of persons from a variety of disciplines has since
served as a model for cancer surgery programs around the world
and has resulted in innovative clinical research efforts already impacting on previously refractory cancers. Rosenberg
placed emphasis on combining treatments by tailoring the surgical procedure to the availability and effectiveness of both
radiotherapy and chemotherapy. The ultimate outcome has been
less radical surgery and more live, intact patients.

The intramural surgical program at NCI continues to pioneer work on soft tissue sarcoma, moving away from the radical
surgical approach used in the early years of the program. With
soft tissue sarcomas of the extremities, survival had been 40
percent at three to five years, with a local recurrence rate
between 20 and 40 percent. In 1977, in collaboration with the
Radiation and Medicine Branches, Rosenberg's group began a
prospective randomized trial to evaluate the efficacy of adjuvant radiotherapy and of chemotherapy with adriamycin, cyclophosphamide, and high-dose methotrexate. Those patients who
received chemotherapy have been shown to have a continuous
disease-free survival of 91 percent at three years by actuarial analysis and an overall survival of 93 percent. This
improvement in disease-free survival is significant when the
experimental patients are compared with the randomized control
group that had not receive chemotherapy.

The addition of chemotherapy to surgical treatment has
resulted in a definite decrease in the rate of recurrence
and an enhanced prospect for disease-free survival. Employing
a strategy in which surgery to achieve negative resection mar-
gins is followed by radiotherapy and chemotherapy, NCI surgeons and radiotherapists have reported data showing that

there have been no local recurrences since 1975 in patients who meet these criteria. It can be inferred, therefore, that this treatment is effective for control of micrometastases as well as for local control without sacrificing the affected limb.

After a fitful start elsewhere, beginning with the resection of pulmonary metastases of renal cancer, surgical treatment of metastatic cancer has been established as standard therapy by Rosenberg's group. In patients with osteosarcoma, removal of pulmonary metastases with staged thoracotomy has demonstrated that long-term disease-free survival is possible, even with numerous metastases and regardless of growth rate. This is a radical departure from past concepts of the ultimate outcome of patients with any evidence of metastases. These studies are changing our conceptions of the biology of metastases and altering surgical treatment of metastatic cancer at other sites.

The early years of the Radiotherapy Program saw PHIL RUBIN, HERMAN SUIT, and other prominent radiotherapists begin their careers at NCI. Studies by MORT ELKIND on the shoulder of the dose-response survival curve were a major milestone in radiation biology. That the cells' repair mechanism can repair sublethal damage from radiation within 4 to 6 hours is undoubtedly one of the major findings in the area of cellular response to radiation.

Ralph Johnson followed J. Robert Andrews as chief of NCI's Radiation Branch in 1963. His early demonstration that the combination of chemotherapy and central nervous system irradiation was more effective than either modality alone in increasing the survival time of mice with leukemia L1210 constituted a significant contribution to the central nervous system treatment of leukemias of childhood. It is also a major reason why central nervous system irradiation was incorporated into the "total treatment" protocols for acute leukemia of childhood both at NCI and St. Jude's Hospital. Johnson's early studies in the radiotherapy of Hodgkin's disease made an additional important contribution by demonstrating, in one of the first controlled trials in this disease, that lesser amounts of radiation would suffice in patients with Stages I and II cancers who had the nodular sclerosing variety of the disease.

The clinical program in radiation oncology at NCI entered a new era in 1977 with the arrival of Eli Glatstein from Stanford. Glatstein is conducting a direct comparison of radiotherapy with chemotherapy in early-stage lymphomas. Studies by the Radiation Oncology Branch now center on innovative ways to integrate radiotherapy with other forms of treatment. These studies include the use of intraoperative radiotherapy and radiosensitizing compounds such as misonidazole. In collaborative studies, radiation therapy with preservation of the breast for Stages I and II mammary cancer patients and of the limbs of sarcoma patients is compared with surgery. Other unique combined modality programs are the study of small cell carcinoma of the lung (with the NCI-Navy Medical Oncology Branch), the continuing study of electron beam therapy for mycosis fungoides, and collaboration with the Pediatric Oncology Branch on combined modality treatment of rhabdomyosarcoma and Ewing's sarcoma.

Conclusion

The remarkable flexibility of NCI's intramural therapeutic research program during the past two decades—its ability to respond to changing demands, pressures, and opportunities—has produced a milieu conducive to and supportive of scientific enterprise. This has been a major factor in the development of cures for over a dozen cancers with chemotherapy alone. Between 1955 and 1970, a single question occupied most of NCI's clinical investigators: Could drugs, as the sole treatment modality, cure cancer? The answer is Yes. The implications of this answer in the affirmative are important to our understanding of the biology of the cancer cell itself.

In the telling, it seems easier than it was in the doing. There was major resistance to these experiments both within and outside the NIH community. All of the investigators who fulfilled their aspirations at NIH owe a debt of gratitude to those who provided the protected environment for the then-radical concepts taking shape. Those provider-protectors include Kenneth Endicott, Director of NCI from 1960 until 1969, and C. Gordon Zubrod, both of whom possess the wisdom, judgment, and clarity of vision to see over the horizon something invisible to others—and the courage to act on that vision.

Suggested Readings

General History and Background

Law, L. Resistance in leukemic cells to an adenine antagonist 6-mercaptopurine. Proc Soc Exp Biol Med 84:409-412, 1953.
Goldin, A., J.M. Venditti, S.R. Humphreys. Modification of treatment schedule in the management of advanced mouse leukemia with amethopterin. J of NCI 17:203-212, 1956.

Rieselbach, R.E., et al. Subarachnoid distribution of drugs after lumbar puncture. N Engl J Med 267:127, 1962.

Skipper, H.E., et al. Experimental evaluation of potential antitumor agents. On the criteria and kinetics associated with curability of experimental leukemia. Cancer Chemother Rep 35:1, 1964.

Zubrod, C.G., et al. The chemotherapy program of the National Cancer Institute: History, analysis and plans. Cancer Chemother Rep 50:349-540, 1966.

Freirich, E.J., et al. Quantitative comparison of toxicity of anticancer agents in mouse, rat, hamster, dog, monkey and man. Cancer Chemother Rep 50:219-244, 1966.

Malmgren, R.A. Studies of circulating cancer cells in cancer patients. In Mechanism of Invasion in Cancer, International Union Against Cancer Monographs, Volume 6, P. Dennoix (ed.), pp. 108-117. Berlin: Springer-Verlag, 1967.

Yankee, R.A., et al. The cell cycle of leukemia L1210 cells in vivo. Cancer Res 27(1):2381-2385, 1967.

Schein, P.S., et al. The evaluation of anticancer drugs in dogs and monkeys for the prediction of qualitative toxicities in man. Clin Pharmacol Ther 11:3-40, 1970.

DeVita, V.T. Cell kinetics and the chemotherapy of cancer. Cancer Chemother Rep, Part 3(2)(1):23-33, 1971.

DeVita, V.T., and P.S. Schein. The use of drugs in combination for the treatment of cancer: Rationale and results. N Engl J Med 288(19):998-1006, 1973.

DeVita, V.T. The evolution of therapeutic research in cancer. N Engl J Med 298:907-910, 1978.

DeVita, V.T., et al. The drug development and clinical trials programs of the Division of Cancer Treatment, National Cancer Institute. Cancer Clin Trials 2:195-216, 1979.

Goldin, A., et al. Historical development and current strategy of the NCI Drug Development Program. In Methods in Cancer Research, H. Busch and V.T. DeVita (eds.), vol. 16, pp. 165-245. New York: Academic Press, 1979.

DeVita, V.T., J.E. Henney, and S.M. Hubbard. Estimation of the numerical and economic impact of chemotherapy in the treatment of cancer. Proceedings of the 1980 International Symposium on Cancer. In Cancer Achievements and Prospects for the 1980's, J.H. Burchenal and H.S. Oettgen (eds.), pp. 859-880. New York: Grune and Stratton, 1981.

Choriocarcinoma

Hertz, R. Interference with estrogen induced tissue growth in the chick genital tract by a folic acid antagonist. Science 107:300, 1948.

Li, M.C., R. Hertz, and D.B. Spencer. Effect of methotrexate upon choriocarcinoma and chorioadenoma. Proc Soc Exp Biol Med 93:361-366, 1956.

Hertz, R., J. Lewis, and M.B. Lipsett. Five years experience with chemotherapy of metastatic trophoblastic diseases in women. Am J Obstet Gynecol 86:808-814, 1963.

Li, M.C. Trophoblastic disease: Natural history, diagnosis and treatment. Ann Intern Med 74:102-113, 1971.

Leukemias of Childhood

Freireich, E.J., M. Karon, and E. Frei III. VAMP combination chemotherapy in the treatment of childhood acute leukemia. Proc Am Assoc Cancer Res 5:50, 1964.

Frei, E. III, and E.J. Freireich. Progress and perspectives in the chemotherapy of acute leukemia. Adv in Chemother 2:269-298, 1965.

Frei, E. III, et al. The effectiveness of combinations of antileukemic agents in inducing and maintaining remission in children with acute leukemia. Blood 26:642-656, 1965.

Pinkel, D. The ninth annual David Karnofsky lecture: Treatment of acute lymphocytic leukemia. Cancer 48:1128, 1979.

Lymphomas: Hodgkin's Disease

DeVita, V., et al. Intensive combination chemotherapy and x-irradiation in the treatment of Hodgkin's disease (abstract), Proc Amer Assoc Cancer Res 6:15, 1965.

Moxley, J.H. III, et al. Intensive combination chemotherapy and x-irradiation in Hodgkin's disease. Cancer Res 27:1258-1263, 1967.

DeVita, V.T., A. Serpik, and P.P. Carbone. Combination chemotherapy in the treatment of advanced Hodgkin's disease. Ann Intern Med 73:881, 1970.

DeVita, V.T., et al. Peritoneoscopy in the staging of Hodgkin's disease. Cancer Res 31:1746-1750, 1971.

DeVita, V.T. Science citation index classic: Combination chemotherapy in the treatment of Hodgkin's disease. Curr Contents 12:10, March 19, 1979.

DeVita, V.T., et al. Curability of advanced Hodgkin's disease with chemotherapy. Ann Intern Med 92:5, May 1980.

DeVita, V.T. The consequences of the chemotherapy of Hodgkin's disease. The tenth David A. Karnofsky memorial lecture. Cancer 47(1):1-13, 1981.

Non-Hodgkin's Lymphomas

Lowenbraun, S., V.T. DeVita, and A.A. Serpick. Combination chemotherapy with nitrogen mustard, vincristine, procarbazine, and prednisone in lymphosarcoma and reticulum cell sarcoma. Cancer 25(5):1018-1025, 1970.

Carbone, P.P., et al. Burkitt's tumor: A comparative study in Africa and the United States. Recent Results Cancer Res 36:126-136, 1971.

DeVita, V.T., et al. Advanced diffuse histiocytic lymphoma, a potentially curable disease. Results with combination chemotherapy. Lancet 1(7901): 248-250, 1975.

Fisher, R.I., et al. Diffuse aggressive lymphomas: Increased survival after alternating flexible sequence of ProMACE and MOPP chemotherapy. Ann Intern Med 98:304-309, 1983.

Ovarian Cancer

Bagley, C.M., et al. Ovarian carcinoma metastatic to the diaphragm—frequently undiagnosed at laparotomy. Am J Obstet Gynecol 116(3):397-400, 1973.

Rosenoff, S.H., et al. Peritoneoscopy: A valuable tool in ovarian carcinoma. Ann Inter Med 83(1):37-41, 1975.

Dedrick, R.L., et al. Pharmacokinetic rationale for peritoneal drug administration in the treatment of ovarian cancer. Cancer Treat Rep 62(1):1-11, 1978.

Young, R.C., et al. Advanced ovarian adenocarcinoma. A prospective clinical trial of melphalan (L-Pam) versus combination chemotherapy. N Engl J Med 299(23):1261-1266, 1978.

Miscellaneous Malignancies

Hutter, A.M., Jr., and D.E. Kayhoe. Adrenal cortical carcinoma. Results of treatment with o,p'DDD in 138 patients. Am J Med 41(4):581-92, 1966.

Ketcham, A.S., et al. Treatment of advanced cancer of the ethmoid sinuses. Nobel Symposium No. 10, Disorders of the Skull Base Region (monograph). Almqvist and Wiksell (eds.), pp. 320-334. New York: Wiley, 1969.

Canellos, G.P., et al. Hematologic and cytogenetic remission in blastic transformation in chronic granulocytic leukemia. Blood 38(6):671-679, 1971.

Schein, P., et al. Streptozotocin for malignant insulinomas and carcinoid tumor. Arch Intern Med 132:555-561, 1973.

V. T. DeVITA, JR., AND A. GOLDIN

Canellos, G.P., et al. Cyclical combination chemotherapy for
advanced breast carcinoma. Br Med J (England) 1(901):
218-220, 1974.

Vonderheid, E.C., et al. A 10-year experience with topical
mechlorethamine for mycosis fungoides: Comparison with
patients treated by total skin electron beam radiation
therapy. Cancer Treat Rep 63(4):681-689, 1979.

Moody, T.W., et al. High levels of intracellular bombesin
characterize human small-cell lung carcinoma. Science
214:1246-1248, 1981.

Whang-Peng, J., et al. Specific chromosome defect associated
with human small-cell lung cancer: Deletion 3p(14-23).
Science 215:181-182, 1982.

Rosenberg, S.A., et al. Prospective randomized evaluation of
adjuvant chemotherapy in adults with soft tissue sarcomas
of the extremities. Cancer 52(3):424-434, 1983.

Little, C.D., et al. Amplification and expression of the
c-myc oncogene in human lung cancer cell lines. Nature
306(10):194-196, 1983.

Infectious Complications of Malignancy
and Supportive Care

Gaydos, L.A., E.J. Freireich, and N. Mantel. The quantitative relation between platelet count and hemorrhage in
patients with acute leukemia. N Engl J Med 266:905-909,
1962.

Freireich, E.J., et al. The function and rate of transfused
leukocytes from donors with CLM in leukopenic recipients.
Ann NY Acad Sci 113:1081-1090, 1964.

Hersh, E.M., et al. Cause of death in acute leukemia: A 10-
year study of 414 patients. J Am Med Assoc 194:105-109,
1965.

Levin, R.H., et al. Erythroid homografts following leukocyte
transfusion in a patient with acute leukemia. Blood 26:
587-609, 1965.

Freireich, E.J. Continuous flow in vivo blood cell separator.
Lab Management 6:20-23, 43-48, 1968.

DeVita, V.T., et al. Pneumocystis carinii pneumonia: Successful diagnosis and treatment of two patients with associated malignant processes. N Engl J Med 280:287-291, 1969.

Waalkes, T.P., C. Denham, and V.T. DeVita. Pentamidine: Clinical pharmacologic correlations in man and mice. Clin
Pharmacol Ther 11(4): 505-512, 1970.

Young, R.C., et al. Aspergillosis: The spectrum of the disease in 98 patients. Medicine 49(2):147-173, 1970.

26

EPILOGUE

J. E. Rall

I arrived at the National Institutes of Health in 1955 and experienced what was common for most physicians coming from an academic medical center. At NIH, instead of the pressures of a large clinic—urgent consultations, teaching responsibilities, patients to be seen in the general wards— one was concerned only with patients referred for research. Another early impression: the awesome immensity of the place and diversity of research interests. One was quickly swept, however, into the particular ambience that characterized NIH during the halcyon days of the 1950s and 1960s. If the pace today is more measured and rather less hectic, the ambience is no less stimulating.

A very early and important aspect of life at NIH is the journal club. Perhaps the most influential was the one in biochemistry and enzymology started by ARTHUR KORNBERG with HERBERT TABOR, EARL STADTMAN, BERNIE HORECKER, and LEON HEPPEL. A story about it, probably apocryphal, concerns JAY SEEGMILLER, as dedicated and hard-working a scientist as ever there was. The club's meeting date is said to have fallen on December 25, and Jay, with a wife and young children, felt obliged to have Christmas dinner at home. Afterward Arthur Kornberg is said to have remarked, "Jay is really a good scientist, but I'm not sure he's serious."

The journal clubs took many forms. For any given laboratory, there might be one that would meet three or four times a week. There were inter-Institute journal clubs centered, for instance, around immunology, endocrinology, physical or organic chemistry. I remember one devoted to studying journals on organic chemistry in Japanese. Sometimes these clubs were quite informal, as when HERMAN KALCKAR came by and said to GORDON TOMKINS and me, "You know, I don't think we really know any statistical mechanics." I couldn't think of a truer statement, so we organized then and there a journal club on

---

J. E. RALL, M.D.; Ph.D., Deputy Director for Intramural Research, National Institutes of Health.

ISBN 0-12-667980-0

statistical mechanics to meet every Monday. The clubs that
originated at NIH were widely exported, since a modest number
of NIH scientists in the 1950s and 1960s had sabbaticals in
laboratories throughout the world and almost invariably took
journal clubs with them.

An interesting aspect of early NIH was the fifth-floor
library in the Clinical Center. It was open 24 hours a day,
every day, and frequently one saw people working there in the
small hours of the morning. As a residue of the great influence of chemistry at the early NIH, a section of the library
was devoted exclusively to chemical literature. For anyone
with a fondness for chemistry, this was a great convenience;
but it was, alas, lost when the library moved to more spacious
quarters on the first and basement floors. Unfortunately, its
greater accessibility and the growth of NIH necessitated restrictions such as limited hours. The latter change, as one
might suppose, brought an outcry from the scientists.

The staff has often expressed concern that we are not
fully utilizing the wide range of available talents in our
midst. Various devices have been introduced to promote constructive interaction. In the Arthritis Institute, for ex-
example, teas were held in various laboratories for a number of years. It was at those that I first saw the NMR and
the electron spin resonance apparatus and all the instrumentation and talents of the Laboratory of Chemical Physics, set up
by TED BECKER and now ably run by rotating section chiefs.

An important feature of NIH for more than three decades
has been the NIH Lecture series, which consists of four or
five evening lectures a year by outstanding scientists. While
rich in scientific content, the presentations usually include
a sufficiently broad introduction to render them meaningful to
an intelligent laity. So, from early times, scientists have
brought nonscientist spouses and friends.

There was some concern in the late 1950s about the
decision-making process at NIH. Since all the scientists had
come from universities, we expected to find more or less demo-
cratic control by the senior staff through something like a
faculty senate. The institution, however, was structured in a
hierarchical manner, and there was little opportunity for
decision-making, or even input, from the average tenured professional investigator. This was felt by senior people, such
as HANS STETTEN, as well as by the more junior. As a result,
each Institute gradually formed what were called Assemblies of
Scientists, coordinated by an Inter-Assembly Council. Open to
everyone with a professional degree, the Assemblies met with
varying frequency to discuss and comment on certain aspects
of NIH policy.

A notable action of the Assemblies occurred when ED KORN

was the Council's President. A rather grandiose and poorly thought-out scheme had been proposed to deal with purchasing at NIH. The scheme as outlined would have computerized everything and abolished the telephone charge order. It was the Assembly of Scientists that analyzed the scheme in a professional, managerial way and succeeded in averting this ill-advised venture. On the other hand, I am glad to report that NIH's own Division of Computer Research and Technology subsequently generated the necessary software to allow purchasing to be automated. The system is now operative and has vastly improved acquisition at NIH.

The Assemblies have been interested in diverse things. In the 1950s a matter causing considerable concern was the difficulty of minorities, particularly blacks, in obtaining housing convenient to NIH. Numerous petitions, protests, and resolutions were passed. While perhaps unrelated to these, fair housing was adopted in Montgomery County and the situation has vastly improved.

The Clinical Center was opened in 1953, and the unsubstantiated rumor at the time was that the NIH Director, addressing the rather small clinical staff, said, "I hope you'll be able to admit patients who won't die." Arrangements were casual for the first few years with respect to who was to take care of patients. There were a few senior M.D.'s, but no consistent provision for recruiting residents. Rather haphazardly, one would call friends at Massachusetts General, or New York Hospital, or Columbia Presbyterian and say, "Do you have some good intern or resident who would like to come to NIH?" In those glorious days, the quid pro quo was a commission in the Public Health Service that would satisfy the draft requirements.

In the mid 1950s the patient population increased and the medical staff had to be expanded. A more formal program for training young graduates was instituted. In the 1960s and early 1970s, some four or five hundred of the best and brightest medical students would descend on NIH every spring for a hectic week of interviews. The chosen few would arrive at NIH approximately two years later to start their training as Clinical Associates. Over the two-year training period, about half their time was spent in the laboratory and half on the wards. This program played an important role in setting the standards for clinical and clinically oriented basic research in medical schools throughout the country.

The research training process was greatly facilitated by the design of the Clinical Center, where about 40 percent of a large building housed the 500-odd patients and 60 percent was devoted to laboratories. The latter included not only the facilities of M.D.'s doing clinical investigation, but

also highly professional laboratories in basic science—those
of BERNARD (STEVE) BRODIE, JULIE AXELROD, BOB BERLINER, MAR-
SHALL NIRENBERG, CHRIS ANFINSEN, LIZ NEUFELD, GILBERT ASH-
WELL, Bernie Horecker, Herman Kalckar, etc. Often the taste
of sophisticated laboratory research became addictive, and
the Clinical Associates decided to stay a third or fourth
year or, indeed, to make a career of research at NIH.

In the early 1960s a new category of associates was devised, the so-called Research Associates. These were physicians whose sole obligation was to do research. In those
days a substantial proportion of physicians received relatively minor training in chemistry, biochemistry, and biology
in undergraduate school; and in medical school, the training
was, perforce, not as intensive as that of a Ph.D. in any of
these fields. Hence, various seminars and courses were suggested. When Chris Anfinsen returned to NIH in 1963, he became particularly interested in this program and set up a
dynamic series of evening seminars limited to 10 or 12 students and run by several dozen NIH scientists. In one of
them, Chris, DAVID DAVIES, and the class constructed models
of ribonuclease and several other proteins. Seminars were
given in any field that was highly active at the time, as well
as in areas not particularly exciting but of fundamental importance, such as organic chemistry, differential equations,
matrix analysis. Attendance at the seminars was hotly con-
tested, and numerous associates felt that they were unfairly
denied the advantage of participation.

An important part of NIH's efforts to pull itself up by
its academic bootstraps was the establishment of the Foundation for Advanced Education in the Sciences (FAES). This was
a private, nonprofit educational organization that Stetten,
Berliner, and a few other far-sighted people set up in the
late fifties to run a night school. It was a graduate school
in which innumerable courses but no degrees were given. At
present the Foundation offers on the order of 120 courses,
in subjects ranging from nuclear magnetic resonance methodology to advanced Russian to techniques in molecular biology.
The registration is usually in excess of 2000 students.

These represent a potpourri of the NIH community and can
often contribute to the teaching process. I well remember a
course given by ARTHUR PATCHETT many years ago. After some
five minutes of moving electrons around on the blackboard,
Patchett declared, "And now you see why this reaction is base-
catalyzed." However, an older organic chemist said, "I've run
the reaction and it goes much better in acid." Thus, a mixture of young M.D.'s who need further courses, older Ph.D.'s
who want exposure to the latest concepts in chemistry, biol-

ogy, physics, or what-have-you, and some bright technicians band together once or twice a week to learn.

Another aspect of the Foundation that has been important in giving the scientists at NIH a feeling of community has been the Sunday afternoon concert series begun by GIULIO CANTONI in 1968. These concerts, generally by chamber music groups or soloists, are open to subscription by the public. With Giulio's and Paola Saffiotti's persuasive efforts, outstanding performers have been seen and heard in the Masur Auditorium—among them, Isaac Stern and Rudolf Serkin.

One of the problems recognized at NIH early in the 1950s was that the U.S. Civil Service system was ill adapted to the kind of academic life that scientists entering NIH had been used to and considered more or less optimal for doing productive research. Most vigorous scientific enterprises require that a large proportion of scientists be graduate students or postdoctoral fellows available without long-term commitment. NIH is not a university and, lacking graduate students, has an even greater need for postdoctoral fellows. The problem was that the system granted tenure within a year, precluding continual replacement. Fortunately, it was discovered that NIH had the statutory authority to award fellowships, and so the Staff Fellowship Program was devised. This is basically a postdoctoral program that has been extended and now permits younger scientists to work at NIH for as long as seven years without tenure. It has been very useful in maintaining a flow of young scientists to and from NIH. This has been largely a program for Ph.D.'s because for many years the Clinical and Research Associate programs, restricted to M.D.'s, used the Commissioned Corps mechanism as an employment device.

In the turbulent 1960s, scientists in Federal institutions were affected by the great civil rights movement and the prolonged conflict in Vietnam, very much as were their counterparts in universities throughout the country. Hence, there was a Vietnam Moratorium Committee at NIH and picketing of the Clinical Center. The Committee had invited Benjamin Spock to speak on a balmy spring afternoon, and his speech drew a thousand or more people. This was during the Nixon era, when BOB MARSTON was NIH Director. With consummate skill Bob was able to satisfy the activists at NIH and simultaneously comply with most Administration policies. This happy state, however, was abruptly terminated when, shortly after the reelection of President Nixon, Marston was suddenly discharged. This gave rise to enormous concern by NIH scientists. In the past the directorship of NIH had been a totally nonpolitical job, and though I think almost no one knew Marston's party affiliation (certainly, I didn't), it was strongly suspected that he had been fired for political reasons. There was an emotional meeting in the Masur Auditorium, where Bob Berliner, Deputy Director for Science and a close associate of Marston's throughout the latter's regime, decried this unfortunate, ill-advised, and certainly unjust move.

Change has always been a part of life at NIH. One need for change, more and more evident in the seventies, was in the mode of caring for patients, since the Clinical Center as a hospital had been designed in the late 1940s. The surgical suites were grossly inadequate by modern standards. No provision had been made for intensive-care facilities, though the Cancer Institute, by removing three or four walls, was able to improvise a postsurgical intensive-care unit. The X-ray department was overcrowded; the clinical pathology laboratory also, and beginning to usurp research space. Little provision had been made for outpatients in the design of the Clinical Center, and more and more were being seen in improvised outpatient departments, which were so crowded that no new clinics could be set up. When Charlie Edwards was Assistant Secretary for Health and TED COOPER was his assistant, we drew their attention to some of these problems and took Edwards, who had practiced surgery, through the operating room to see the conditions first hand. Finally, authorization was obtained and the Ambulatory Care Research Facility designed. Surprisingly, the ACRF was constructed almost on time and within budget.

What of the future of the NIH intramural program? Clearly, one can note several trends in the United States as a whole that will have an impact on how the intramural NIH does its work. One of the major trends is the decreasing interest of medical students in entering biomedical research. The reason is surely economic. The cost of medical education is so tremendous these days that the average medical student is reported to graduate with a debt of $30,000. Extrapolating, one sees that in a very few years the average graduate will receive a bill for some $50,000 along with the M.D. degree. Given the considerable income advantage to be expected from private practice over research, it is only reasonable to assume that many students will be deflected from a research career.

Another trend, probably related, is that the proportion of research grants going to principal investigators who are M.D.'s has been declining for some years. And perhaps even more significant, the American Federation for Clinical Research—which requires for membership the publication of a single paper, seeks to enroll all physicians interested in medical research, and retires members at age 40—has shown a drop in active membership in the last two years. While NIH

has quite a few services that provide splendid clinical training, it is heavily research-oriented. Accordingly, the intramural program at NIH, particularly the clinical program, will
have a difficult time attracting first-rate physicians who de-
sire training for careers in research or in academic medicine.
So far, we have been fortunate. The pool, though diminishing,
has been adequate to meet NIH's needs.

Another concern for research institutions such as NIH,
which does not have a graduate school and depends heavily on
postdoctoral fellows as components of its research teams, is
the prospect for scientific staffing in the long run. In a
steady-state universe of biomedical science, the average Ph.D.
will spend 3 to 5 years as a postdoctoral fellow and about 35
years as a senior investigator. Senior investigators are
interested in employing their own postdoctoral fellows. If one
assumes that as many Ph.D.'s are produced as drop out of the
research pool, it follows that the average Ph.D. staying in
research would be entitled to only about a tenth of a postdoctoral fellow per year. But the average senior investigator
at NIH sponsors two to four postdoctoral fellows at any given
time. There clearly looms a problem.

Obviously, these figures have to be corrected for a number
of factors. Many Ph.D.'s, for example, go into industry, administration, or teaching at a nonresearch school and therefore do not hire postdoctoral fellows. Furthermore, NIH can
continue to employ foreign scientists. Yet it does appear
that within the next decade or so, NIH and most research institutions will face a paucity of postdoctoral fellows available for work in their laboratories.

There are, of course, university graduate students working at NIH—perhaps 50 to 100 at any given time. Most are
getting their Ph.D. either at The Johns Hopkins University
through a cooperative arrangement with the FAES, which provides for stipends, or at one of the local universities.
Nonetheless, it is apparent that NIH cannot count on the
number of graduate students that a major university would
expect to have. The problem of professional staffing is one
that NIH must cope with intramurally in the ensuing decades.

A perennial issue at NIH, as in many university medical
schools, is the balance between clinical and basic research.
This surfaced when the Clinical Center was opened in the early
1950s, because it was clear that an organization previously
concerned almost exclusively with basic research was venturing
boldly into large-scale clinical research. The future, however, seems relatively stable with respect to this potential
conflict, as there are no plans to expand the clinical areas
of NIH, with the possible exception of the outpatient department. Given, therefore, steady-state funding (which may be

optimistic), the ratio between clinical and basic research should probably not change much in the 1980s and 1990s.

Related to the balance between basic and clinical research is the organizational structure of NIH. At least 25 laboratories are involved in what one might call biochemistry, and probably a dozen in cell biology. From time to time, there are proposals that all the biochemistry at NIH be gathered into a single Department of Biochemistry, all the cell biology into a Department of Cell Biology, etc. This is clearly at odds with the organizational structure, which tends to be disease oriented. And because of public and congressional interest in disease-oriented medical research, it is doubtful that this structure will be changed. We will continue to pursue investigations along the lines of scientific opportunities and disciplines (as represented generally by the chapters in this book) within a mission-oriented structure dedicated to the conquest of cancer, heart disease, arthritis, and other major health problems.

Perhaps a dozen new Institutes have been proposed for NIH and, as of this writing (fall 1983), it seems likely that at least one will be added to the present 11. It is not clear that Institutes are usually formed in response to scientific opportunities, and one suspects that the more venal aspects of the political process are often involved. A current Institute of Medicine study of the organizational structure of NIH is addressing this issue.

As with most great institutions, NIH has been in process of change since the creation of its antecedents on Staten Island in 1887. At times it has followed the political winds, at times generated its own changes. Economic and social trends have sometimes forced NIH into different courses. Nonetheless, the underlying theme and mission of NIH has been constant: to investigate life processes so as to improve the health of mankind.

INDEX OF NAMES